Biodentine™

Imad About
Editor

Biodentine™

Properties and Clinical Applications

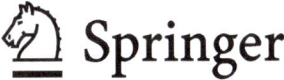 Springer

Editor
Imad About
Aix Marseille University
CNRS, ISM, Institute of Movement Science
Marseille
France

ISBN 978-3-030-80934-8   ISBN 978-3-030-80932-4   (eBook)
https://doi.org/10.1007/978-3-030-80932-4

This Springer imprint is published by the registered company Springer Nature Switzerland AG
The registered company address is: Gewerbestrasse 11, 6330 Cham, Switzerland

Acknowledgments

I wish to thank Springer for the fruitful collaboration on the project and for giving the opportunity to make it happen. My sincere thanks to the contributing authors for their thoughtful input, excellent contribution, and reactivity. I would also like to address my special thanks to the reviewers. Thanks to their expert evaluation, the peer-review process ran smoothly and allowed to further improve the content organization and presentation.

Contents

1   Biodentine™ Microstructure and Composition   1
    Josette Camilleri

2   Biodentine™ Physico-Chemical Properties: From
    Interactions with Dental Tissues to Ageing 11
    Amre R. Atmeh and Timothy F. Watson

3   Biocompatibility and Bioactive Properties of Biodentine™ 31
    Matthias Widbiller, Charlotte Jeanneau, Kerstin M. Galler, Patrick
    Laurent, and Imad About

4   Biodentine™ in Inflammation and Pain Control 51
    Fionnuala T. Lundy, Thomas Giraud, Ikhlas A. El-Karim,
    and Imad About

5   Biodentine™ Clinical Applications in Vital Pulp Therapy
    in Permanent Teeth 67
    Avijit Banerjee and Montse Mercadé

6   Biodentine™: Applications in Pulpotomy of Deciduous Teeth 87
    Sivaprakash Rajasekharan

7   Biodentine™ Applications in Traumatology and Fractures 103
    Luc Martens and Rita Cauwels

8   Biodentine™ Applications in Irreversible Pulpitis
    Management in Children and Adults 121
    Nessrin Taha and Papimon Chompu-inwai

9   Calcium Silicate-Based Cement (Biodentine™) as a Bioactive
    Material for the Long-Term Preservation of Pulp Vitality
    in Restorative Dentistry and Prosthodontics 147
    Athina Bakopoulou, Anna Koutrouli, and Imad About

10 **Biodentine™ Applications in Furcation Perforation
    and Root Resorption** 177
    Till Dammaschke and Mariusz Lipski

11 **Clinical Application of Biodentine™ in Regenerative
    Endodontics/Revitalization** 207
    Kerstin M. Galler and Tatiana M. Botero

Contributors

Imad About Aix Marseille University, CNRS, ISM, Institute of Movement Science, Marseille, France

Amre R. Atmeh Department of Restorative Dentsitry, Hamdan Bin Mohammed College of Dental Medicine, Mohammed Bin Rashid University of Medicine and Health Sciences (MBRU), Dubai, United Arab Emirates

Athina Bakopoulou Department of Prosthodontics, School of Dentistry, Faculty of Health Sciences, Aristotle University of Thessaloniki (AUTh), Thessaloniki, Greece

Avijit Banerjee Cariology and Operative Dentistry, Centre for Oral Clinical Translational Sciences, Faculty of Dentistry, Oral and Craniofacial Sciences, King's College London/Guy's and St. Thomas' Hospitals Trust, London, UK

Tatiana M. Botero Cariology, Restorative Sciences and Endodontics, University of Michigan, School of Dentistry, Ann Arbor, MI, USA

Josette Camilleri School of Dentistry, Institute of Clinical Sciences, College of Medical and Dental Sciences, University of Birmingham, Birmingham, UK

Rita Cauwels Department of Paediatric Dentistry, Ghent University, Ghent, Belgium

Papimon Chompu-inwai Division of Pediatric Dentistry, Department of Orthodontics and Pediatric Dentistry, Faculty of Dentistry, Chiang Mai University, Chiang Mai, Thailand

Till Dammaschke Department of Periodontology and Operative Dentistry, Westphalian Wilhelms-University, Münster, Germany

Ikhlas A. El-Karim The Wellcome-Wolfson Institute for Experimental Medicine, School of Medicine, Dentistry and Biomedical Sciences, Queen's University Belfast, Belfast, UK

Kerstin M. Galler Department of Conservative Dentistry and Periodontology, University Hospital Regensburg, Regensburg, Germany

Thomas Giraud Aix Marseille University, CNRS, ISM, Institute of Movement Science, Marseille, France

Assistance Publique-Hôpitaux de Marseille, Pôle Odontologie, Hôpital Timone, Marseille, France

Charlotte Jeanneau Aix Marseille University, CNRS, ISM, Institute of Movement Science, Marseille, France

Anna Koutrouli Department of Paediatric Dentistry, School of Dentistry, Faculty of Health Sciences, Aristotle University of Thessaloniki, Thessaloniki, Greece

Patrick Laurent Aix Marseille University, CNRS, ISM, Institute of Movement Science, Marseille, France

Assistance Publique-Hôpitaux de Marseille, Pôle d'Odontologie, Hôpital Timone, Marseille, France

Mariusz Lipski Department of Preclinical Conservative Dentistry and Preclinical Endodontics, Pomeranian Medical University, Szczecin, Poland

Fionnuala T. Lundy The Wellcome-Wolfson Institute for Experimental Medicine, School of Medicine, Dentistry and Biomedical Sciences, Queen's University Belfast, Belfast, UK

Luc Martens Department of Paediatric Dentistry, Ghent University, Ghent, Belgium

Montse Mercadé Department of Dentistry, Universitat de Barcelona, Barcelona, Spain

Researcher at IDIBELL Institute, Barcelona, Spain

Private Practice Limited to Endodontics and Dental Traumatology in Barcelona, Barcelona, Spain

Sivaprakash Rajasekharan Department of Paediatric Dentistry and Special Care, PAECOMEDIS Research Cluster, Ghent University, Ghent University Hospital, Ghent, Belgium

Nessrin Taha Department of Conservative Dentistry, Jordan University of Science and Technology, Irbid, Jordan

Timothy F. Watson Centre for Oral, Clinical and Translational Sciences, Faculty of Dentistry, Oral and Craniofacial Sciences, King's College London, London, UK

Matthias Widbiller Department of Conservative Dentistry and Periodontology, University Hospital Regensburg, Regensburg, Germany

About the Editor

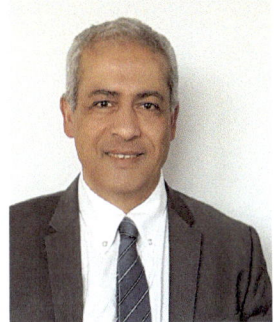

Imad About is Head of the Research Laboratory and of Basic Sciences at the Faculty of Dentistry, Aix-Marseille University, France. Professor About gained his PhD in Biochemistry from Aix-Marseille University in 1992 and subsequently joined the university as an assistant professor, later becoming Professor of Oral Biology in 2002. He was President of the Pulp Biology and Regeneration Group of the International Association of Dental Research and is currently President of the Continental European Division. He is Associate Editor of Clinical Oral Investigations and was guest editor of a special issue published in Stem Cells International in 2017 and a special issue of the Journal of Endodontics published in 2020. Professor About's research group is involved in investigating the role of progenitor and non-progenitor cells in dentin-pulp regeneration and the effects of biomaterials on these events.

He was the winner of the European Society of Endodontology annual research grant in 2012 and received the "Distinguished Scientist Award 2018" from the Pulp Biology and Regeneration Group. Professor About is actively involved in developing dental materials and is one of the leading academics involved in Biodentine development. He is also a well-recognized expert in pulp stem cells and tissue regeneration. He has published more than 220 peer-reviewed papers, abstracts, and book chapters and is a renowned speaker who has frequently been invited to major international conferences.

Introduction

Taking advantage of tricalcium silicate's biological effects, Biodentine™ has been designed as a bioactive bulk dentin substitute and as a temporary enamel replacement material. While the material has a short history being released in 2010, it raised a big interest in the dental and scientific communities. A testimony of this interest is the increasing number of publications in the scientific as well as the clinical fields, which appears to be ascribed to the material unique properties. Unlike other dentin substitutes, Biodentine application does not require any conditioning of the dentin surface, and the subsequent sealing is provided by micromechanical retention as Biodentine penetrates the dentin tubules forming tag-like structures.

Due to the technology used for its development, Biodentine is the only resin-free tricalcium silicate-based material which has high mechanical properties after a short setting time. Indeed, Biodentine mechanical properties after setting are close to those of the dentin, so that it can be cut and reshaped like the natural dentin. Additionally, Biodentine can be bonded with different types of adhesives before finishing the final restoration with a composite resin.

It is also important to highlight that the material sets upon hydration, a process which leads to ion/molecule release. These so-called by-products inhibit bacterial growth and interact with the underlying soft and hard tissues, leading to dampening of the inflammatory reaction and inducing tissue healing/regeneration.

Thus, given the number of published original manuscripts on Biodentine, the editor felt that it was time to put together the current knowledge on the material in this book in a synthetic manner by bringing together a combined knowledge from scientific and clinical research.

The content of this book reminds us of several facts: (1) that restorative materials are applied on injured/inflamed/infected tissues which do not behave in a similar way to that of healthy ones; (2) that the material is not inert but interacts with the underlying tissue modulating its inflammatory reaction and healing potential; (3) that the host tissue response needs to be taken into consideration. Indeed, dental tissues have a well-demonstrated healing potential thanks to the presence of stem cells, and recent data highlighted that pulp cells can even kill cariogenic bacteria and subsequently regulate the pulp inflammation. These facts constitute the scientific basis for understanding the recent paradigm shift in the way irreversible pulpitis is defined and treated. So, this book is unique in demonstrating how our scientific knowledge from the advanced material science and cell biology research combined with the material interaction with the underlying tissue can bring a significant change to the clinical practice.

The first part of the book (Chaps. 1–4) aims at presenting this material highlighting its specific characteristics and the subsequent host responses to its application. These chapters are written by scientists known for their extensive scientific investigations of tricalcium silicate's chemistry, biocompatibility, and interactions with biological soft and hard tissues. All chapters are signed by authors having a significant track record and high-level publications in this field. Chapter 1 provides an overview on the material technology, classification, microstructure/composition, and essential characteristics. The second chapter reports on the material properties describing its interactions with hard tissues and how it penetrates the dentin tubules to provide a marginal sealing. The third chapter is devoted to the material biocompatible properties. It reports on the material-specific interactions with the underlying tissues and how it induces the target tissue healing. Chapter 4 provides insights on Biodentine effects on the inflammation control and on pain receptors' expression and functional activity in vitro. This chapter also provides a link between the experimental data in vitro and an overview of clinical reports summarizing the current evidence on pain reduction in clinic with Biodentine.

The second part of the book (Chaps. 5–11) is written and illustrated by well-recognized clinicians having a significant experience in Biodentine applications in primary and permanent dentitions as well as in material applications in vital pulp therapy and endodontics. All clinical chapters contain clinical protocols based on the authors' experience, which represent an additional added value to the readers of this book. Biodentine applications in vital pup therapy are reported in Chaps. 5–9. Chapter 5 reports on its application in permanent teeth while Chap. 6 focuses on its use in pulpotomy of deciduous teeth. Chapter 7 illustrates Biodentine applications in dental traumatology and fractures. Chapter 8 updates the rapidly advancing knowledge on treating irreversible pulpitis. This chapter provides evidence that treating irreversible pulpitis is not a taboo anymore. A critical analysis of irreversible pulpitis diagnosis is provided, and the current evidence on the clinical effectiveness of irreversible pulpitis treatment in primary and permanent teeth is detailed. Chapter 9 focuses on the clinical applications of Biodentine in prosthetic dentistry. The endodontic applications of Biodentine are reported in the last two chapters. While Chap. 10 describes its applications in furcation perforation and root resorption treatment, the last chapter reports on its application in regenerative endodontics/revitalization procedures.

The book is intended to be used as a guide for the scientific and clinical communities and to represent a solid backbone of knowledge on the material itself and on its clinical applications to all dental students, clinicians, and academics.

Imad About

Biodentine™ Microstructure and Composition

Josette Camilleri

1.1 Introduction

Biodentine (Septodont, Saint-Maur-des-Fossés, France) is a hydraulic cement developed as a dentine replacement material and specifically targeted for vital pulp therapy. This procedure has been classically managed by using liner materials with calcium hydroxide being the material of choice. In the latest guidelines issued by the European Society of Endodontology for the management of the vital pulp [1], calcium hydroxide has not been indicated as the material of choice for vital pulp therapy. Water-based hydraulic calcium silicate cements have been specifically suggested as the most appropriate materials by the guidelines [1] based on the superior histological [2, 3] and clinical outcomes compared with calcium hydroxide in the treatment of the exposed pulp [4–7].

There are a number of hydraulic cements available clinically. Their use in dentistry dates back to the nineteenth century [8, 9] with Witte, a German dentist, describing the filling of a root canal with Portland cement [8]. This method was also described in detail by Schlenker in 1880, indicating the use of a mixture of Portland cement, added to water, creosote and carbolic acid to make a dark brown paste [9]. Even in these early communications, it was reported that the material consistency was crumbly and this made its clinical use challenging. The invention was no longer mentioned until Mahmoud Torabinejad investigated the use of Portland cement for repair of root perforations [10] and also as a root-end filling material [11]. The invention was patented [12, 13] and the material was called mineral trioxide aggregate (MTA). The main scope of using Portland cement was its hydraulic nature; it is mixed with water and undergoes a hydration reaction and can be used in a wet environment without deteriorating. Since then a number of materials have been

J. Camilleri (✉)
School of Dentistry, Institute of Clinical Sciences, College of Medical and Dental Sciences, University of Birmingham, Birmingham, UK
e-mail: J.Camilleri@bham.ac.uk

© Springer Nature Switzerland AG 2022
I. About (ed.), *Biodentine*™, https://doi.org/10.1007/978-3-030-80932-4_1

introduced and researched. A classification of hydraulic cements used in dentistry has been proposed [14]. These are classified either based on their clinical application (intra-coronal, intra-radicular, extra-radicular) or according to their chemistry as indicated in Fig. 1.1a.

Biodentine used as a dentine replacement material is an intra-coronal hydraulic calcium silicate material [14] and this defines its interaction with the substrate and the clinical environment. Furthermore, in the chemical classification outlined in Fig. 1.1a [14], Biodentine is tricalcium silicate based, is aqueous and includes reaction modifiers making it a Type 4 cement (Fig. 1.1b). All hydraulic calcium silicates used in dentistry have to be radiopacified to enable postoperative radiographic follow-up. MTA (ProRoot, Dentsply) is a Type 1 cement (Fig. 1.1b). It is made up of Portland cement (tricalcium silicate, dicalcium silicate, tricalcium aluminate, calcium sulphate) and bismuth oxide radiopacifier and is water based [15].

Biodentine's microstructure and chemistry will be discussed and compared to MTA to enable the understanding of how the materials differ regardless of both being hydraulic cements.

1.2   Presentation and Mixing

Biodentine is composed of a powder and liquid which are presented in a capsule and vial format as shown in Fig. 1.2. The powder is composed of 80% tricalcium silicate, 15% calcium carbonate and 5% zirconium oxide [16]. The liquid is composed of water, calcium, chlorine, sodium and magnesium [17]; a hydro-soluble polymer is also included in the liquid, but this is organic and thus it cannot be detected with X-ray fluorescence method used in the published research [17]. The specific surface area of Biodentine powder is higher than that of other commercial hydraulic cements as the particles are smaller sized [16].

Five drops of liquid from the vial are added to the powder in the capsule. The capsule is agitated mechanically using a Septodont mechanical mixer vibrated at 4500 rpm (Fig. 1.3) for 30 s to achieve a homogenous mixture.

1.3   Chemical Composition

The main features of Biodentine as a Type 4 cement are its cement base (tricalcium silicate), the use of an alternative radiopacifier to bismuth oxide used in MTA, the use of reaction modifiers and mixing with water for hydration.

1.3.1   Cement Base

Biodentine is based on tricalcium silicate which makes up 80% of the powder. Tricalcium silicate is the main constituent of Portland cement which is the cement base of MTA [18]. The use of industrial Portland cement in MTA has raised some

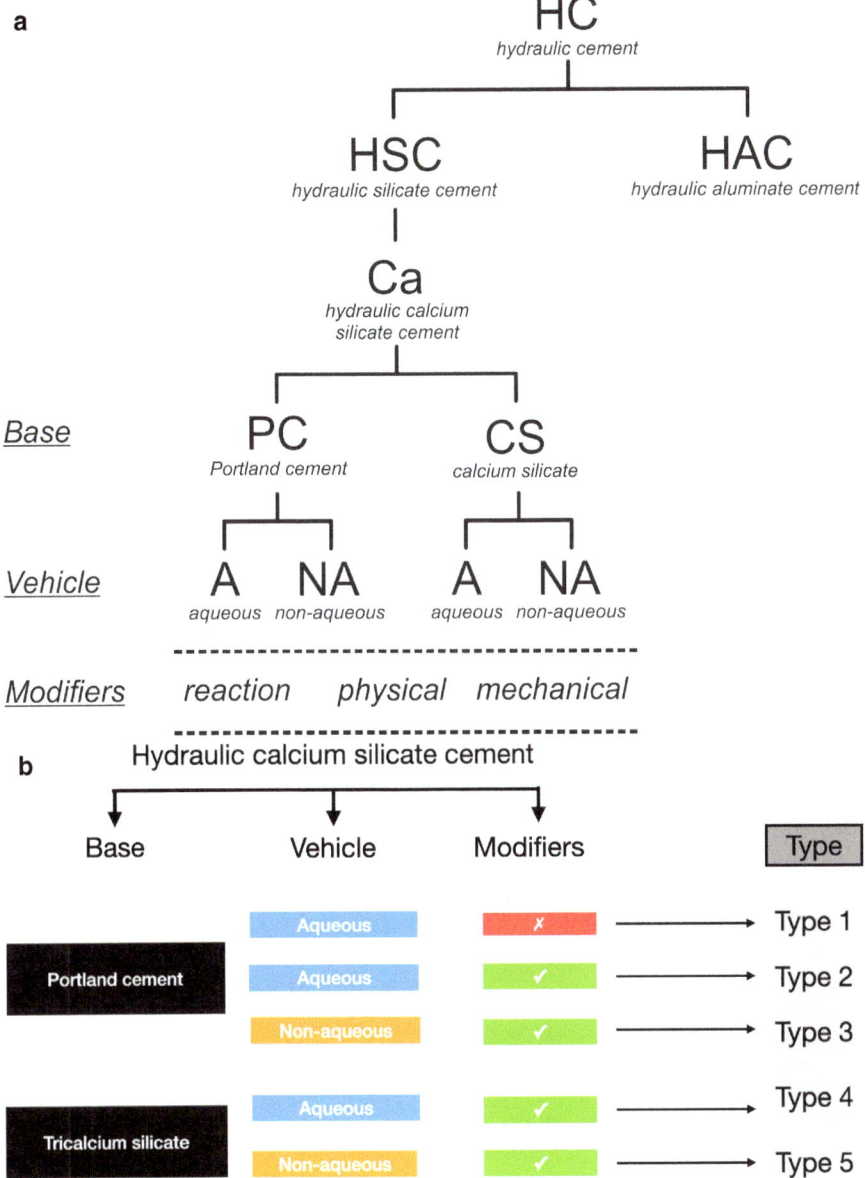

Fig. 1.1 (**a**) Schematic showing the chemical classification of hydraulic cements used in dentistry (Reproduced from Camilleri J. Classification of hydraulic cements used in dentistry. Front. Dent. Med. 2020;1:9. doi: https://doi.org/10.3389/fdmed.2020.00009 [14]); (**b**) schematic showing the subdivisions of the hydraulic calcium silicate cements in clinical use based on the base, vehicle and modifiers leading to five subtypes of material

Fig. 1.2 Biodentine presentation showing the capsules with the powder and vials of liquid. (Courtesy of Septodont)

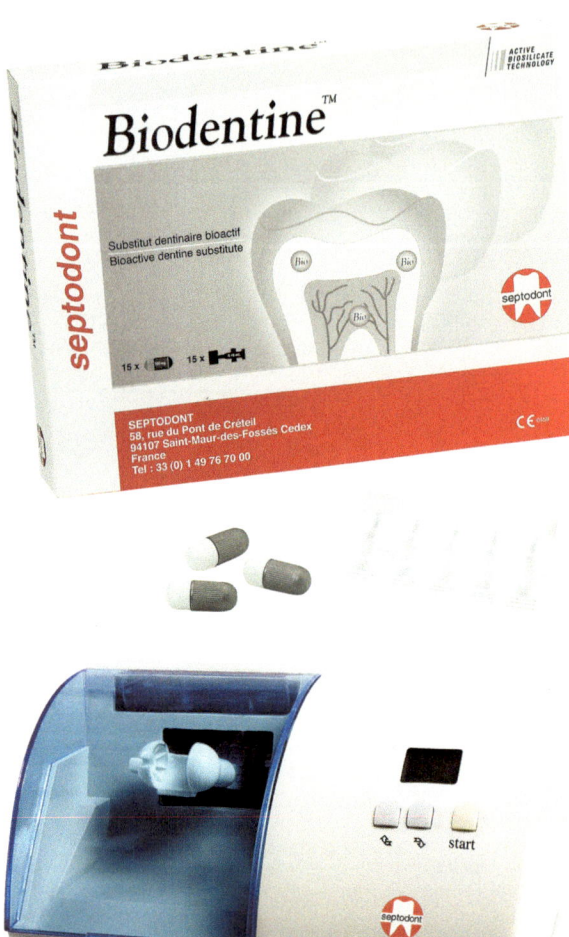

Fig. 1.3 Septodont Biodentine automatic mixer. (Courtesy of Septodont)

concerns due to the trace heavy metals found in industrial cements which are due to the use of natural minerals used in the cement manufacture and the use of wastes as fuels to fire the kilns where the cements are manufactured. Arsenic, lead and chromium have been detected in dental cements based on Portland cement [19, 20] but negligible amounts were leached in physiological solution [17, 19–24]. The other concern with Portland cement is the presence of an aluminium phase which results in leaching of aluminium in solution and has been traced in serum and main organs in animal models [25–28]. In Biodentine, laboratory-grade tricalcium silicate without trace elements and aluminium-based phase is used.

The hydration reaction of Biodentine is different from that of MTA as only the tricalcium silicate hydration occurs in the former [18]. Industrial Portland cement

[29–31] and MTA [32, 33] have other phases and thus other reactions occur. The hydration reaction of the tricalcium silicate in Biodentine is shown in Eq. (1.1):

$$2\left(3CaO\cdot SiO_2\right)+6H_2O \rightarrow \underset{\text{calcium silicate hydrate}}{3CaO\cdot 2SiO_2\cdot 3H_2O}+\underset{\text{calcium hydroxide}}{3Ca\left(OH\right)_2} \tag{1.1}$$

The end product of hydration of tricalcium silicate in Biodentine is calcium silicate hydrate and calcium hydroxide while that of MTA includes also ettringite and monosulphate.

1.3.2 Modifiers

Biodentine includes 5% zirconium oxide as radiopacifier [16] resulting in a radiopacity of 5 mm aluminium thickness. The zirconium oxide does not seem to participate in the hydration reaction [16] unlike the bismuth oxide in MTA [33]. The zirconium oxide particle does not interact with the reaction by-product present in the cement matrix (Fig. 1.4) and does not leach in solution [34]. Thus, zirconium oxide can be considered as an inert filler and imparts the necessary radiopacity to Biodentine.

The reaction modifiers in Biodentine include the calcium carbonate which is present in 15% proportion [16] in the powder, and the hydro-soluble polymer and the calcium chloride present in the liquid. The calcium carbonate enables the early release of calcium ions in solution in higher amounts than the unmodified tricalcium

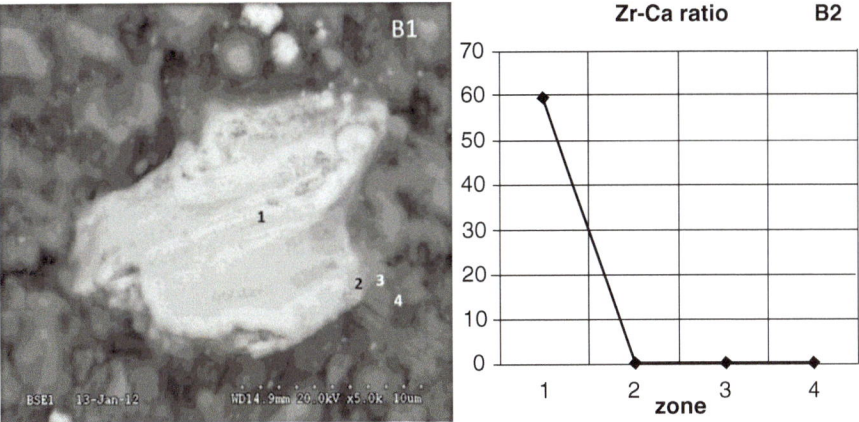

Fig. 1.4 Back scatter scanning electron micrograph of zirconium particle in Biodentine cement matrix indicating the zones that were analysed by energy-dispersive spectroscopy to generate data on calcium and zirconium levels to enable the working out of Ca-Zr ratios indicating any interaction of the zirconia particles with the reaction by-product in Biodentine matrix. (Reproduced with permission from Camilleri J, Sorrentino F, Damidot D. Investigation of the hydration and bioactivity of radiopacified tricalcium silicate cement, Biodentine and MTA Angelus. Dent Mater. 2013 May;29(5):580–93 [16])

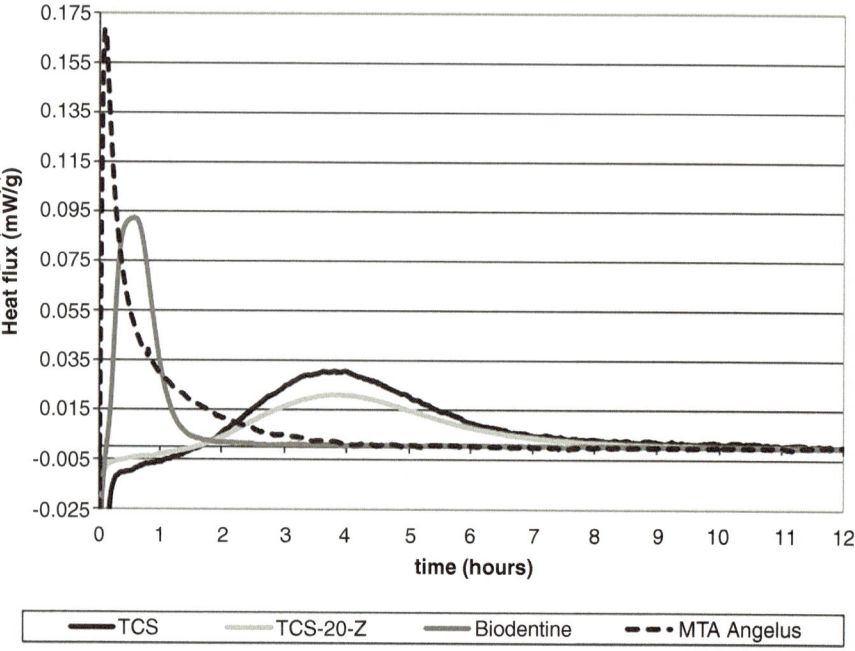

Fig. 1.5 Graphical representation of heat flux generated with time for Biodentine and unmodified tricalcium silicate to show the effect of the calcium carbonate on Biodentine hydration. (Reproduced with permission from Camilleri J, Sorrentino F, Damidot D. Investigation of the hydration and bioactivity of radiopacified tricalcium silicate cement, Biodentine and MTA Angelus. Dent Mater. 2013 May;29(5):580–93 [16])

silicate [35] and this affects the reaction kinetics of Biodentine [16]. Compared to an unmodified tricalcium silicate, Biodentine shows a rise in heat flux in the early stages of the hydration reaction (Fig. 1.5).

The calcium chloride reduces the setting time [36, 37]. The hydro-soluble polymer in the liquid has a dual role. It allows a reduced water-powder ratio and this results in enhanced material strength as has been evidenced [37]. Furthermore, the hydro-soluble polymer increases material flow and improves material handling.

1.4   Biodentine Microstructure

The phase composition of Biodentine gives it a very specific microstructure [38]. The calcium carbonate in Biodentine has a dual role. It is responsible for the early high calcium ion release [35], and also serves as a nucleating agent. This is very clear in Fig. 1.6 where the reaction by-product composed of calcium silicate hydrate and calcium hydroxide is deposited around the calcium carbonate particle. Further

Fig. 1.6 Back scatter scanning electron micrograph of Biodentine after 28 days of hydration showing the main phases. The microstructure and particle arrangement are very ordered and also exhibit very low porosity. Specific microstructural components are shown: (A) calcium carbonate particle; (B) zirconium oxide; (C) reaction by-product

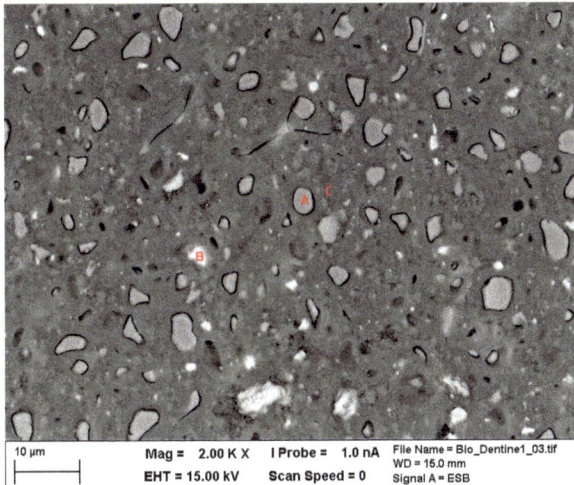

reaction by-product is present in the material matrix together with the zirconium oxide and the calcium hydroxide is precipitated on the material surface and in solution [34]. This specific composition results in a material with a very ordered microstructure (Fig. 1.6) and low porosity [39].

Since Biodentine is recommended for use as a dentine replacement material, it may not have the optimal amount of environmental fluids and this may impair its hydration as hydraulic cements require a moist environment for optimal hydration. This was investigated using a whole tooth model and Biodentine hydration was not impaired by the environmental moisture [35]. Figure 1.7a shows the experimental set-up where Biodentine was used as a pulp capping material in a tooth kept in culture media, thus maintaining the pulp vital. The teeth were sectioned after 15 days and the material microstructure is assessed by scanning electron microscopy and compared to the microstructure of Biodentine stored fully immersed in Hanks' balanced salt solution (Fig. 1.7b). Biodentine used as a pulp capping material in a vital tooth assessed using a whole-tooth model was shown to hydrate and its hydration was more advanced than the material stored fully immersed [35].

1.5   Conclusions

Biodentine is a hydraulic calcium silicate cement that has been optimized to exhibit an ordered microstructure and aims at improved physical, chemical and biological properties.

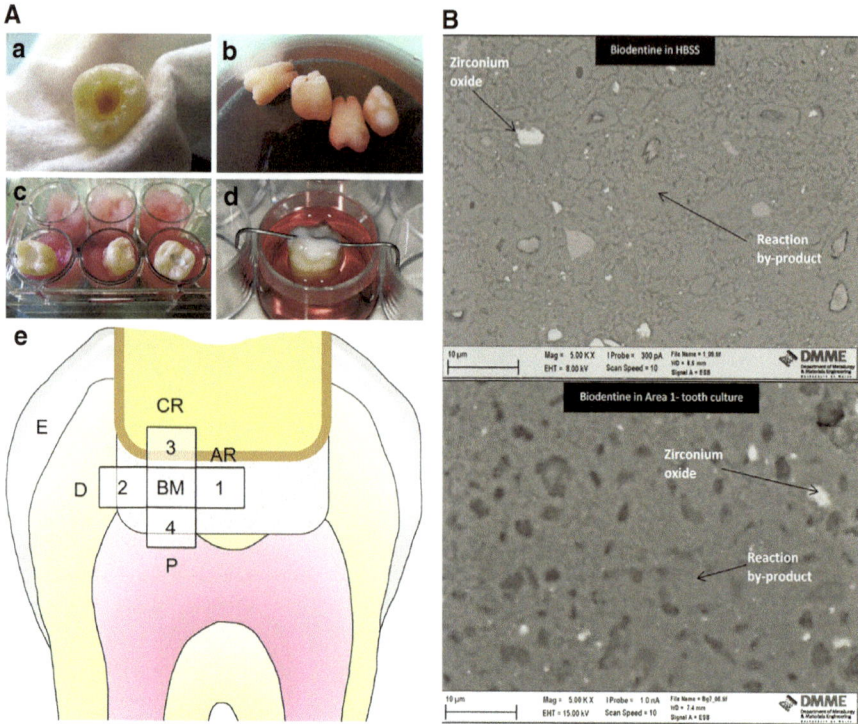

Fig. 1.7 (**A**) Pulp capping and entire tooth culture (a–e). Immature teeth were collected and cleaned, and pulp cavities were prepared (a). Teeth with pulp cavities were placed in culture medium (b). Pulp capping was performed, and teeth were placed onto sterile absorbent cotton soaked with culture medium for setting (c). After bonding and placing the composite resin, teeth were then suspended in 12-well culture plates and cultured for 14 days (d). (e) Schematic representation of the capped tooth indicating the examined areas. Four representative areas indicated by numbers were examined: (1) within the biomaterial, (2) at the biomaterial/dentin interface, (3) at the biomaterial/composite resin interface, and (4) at the biomaterial/pulp interface. (**B**) Back scatter scanning electron micrographs of Biodentine extracted from the whole-tooth culture model and compared to material stored in simulated body fluid for 14 days. *AR* adhesive resin, *BM* pulp-capping biomaterial, *CR* composite resin, *D* dentin, *E* enamel, *P* pulp. (Reproduced with permission from Camilleri J, Laurent P, About I. Hydration of Biodentine, Theracal LC, and a prototype tricalcium silicate-based dentin replacement material after pulp capping in entire tooth cultures. J Endod. 2014 Nov;40(11):1846–54 [35])

References

1. Duncan HF, Galler KM, Tomson PL, Simon S, El-Karim I, et al. European Society of Endodontology position statement: management of deep caries and the exposed pulp. Int Endod J. 2019;52:923–34.
2. Aeinehchi M, Eslami B, Ghanbariha M, Saffar AS. Mineral trioxide aggregate (MTA) and calcium hydroxide as pulp-capping agents in human teeth: a preliminary report. Int Endod J. 2003;36:225–31.

3. Nair PNR, Duncan HF, Pitt Ford TR, Luder HU. Histological, ultrastructural and quantitative investigations on the response of healthy human pulps to experimental capping with mineral trioxide aggregate: a randomized controlled trial. Int Endod J. 2008;41:128–50.
4. Cho SY, Seo DG, Lee SJ, Lee J, Lee SJ, Jung IY. Prognostic factors for clinical outcomes according to time after direct pulp capping. J Endod. 2013;39:327–31.
5. Hilton TJ, Ferracane JL, Mancl L, Northwest Practice-Based Research Collaborative in Evidence-Based Dentistry (NWP). Comparison of CaOH with MTA for direct pulp capping: a PBRN randomized clinical trial. J Dent Res. 2013;92:16S–22S.
6. Mente J, Hufnagel S, Leo M, et al. Treatment outcome of mineral trioxide aggregate or calcium hydroxide direct pulp capping: long-term results. J Endod. 2014;40:1746–51.
7. Kundzina R, Stangvaltaite L, Eriksen HM, Kerosuo E. Capping carious exposures in adults: a randomized controlled trial investigating mineral trioxide aggregate versus calcium hydroxide. Int Endod J. 2017;50:924–32.
8. Witte DR. The filling of a root canal with Portland cement. German quarterly for dentistry. J Cent Assoc German Dent. 1878;18:153–4.
9. Schlenker M. Fuellen der Wurzelkanaele mit Portland-Cement nach Dr Witte [Classification of clinically available hydraulic calcium silicate cements]. Deutsche Vrtljschr F Zahnh. 1880;20:277–83.
10. Lee SJ, Monsef M, Torabinejad M. Sealing ability of a mineral trioxide aggregate for repair of lateral root perforations. J Endod. 1993;19(11):541–4.
11. Torabinejad M, Watson TF, Pitt Ford TR. Sealing ability of a mineral trioxide aggregate when used as a root end filling material. J Endod. 1993;19(12):591–5.
12. Torabinejad M, White JD. Tooth filling material and method of use. Patent number: 5415547, 1993.
13. Torabinejad M, White JD. Tooth filling material and method of use. Patent number: 5769638, 1995.
14. Camilleri J. Classification of hydraulic cements used in dentistry. Front Dent Med. 2020;1:9. https://doi.org/10.3389/fdmed.2020.00009.
15. Camilleri J, Montesin FE, Brady K, Sweeney R, Curtis RV, Pitt Ford TR. The constitution of mineral trioxide aggregate. Dent Mater. 2005;21:297–303.
16. Camilleri J, Sorrentino F, Damidot D. Investigation of the hydration and bioactivity of radiopacified tricalcium silicate cement, Biodentine and MTA Angelus. Dent Mater. 2013;29(5):580–93.
17. Camilleri J, Kralj P, Veber M, Sinagra E. Characterization and analyses of acid-extractable and leached trace elements in dental cements. Int Endod J. 2012;45(8):737–43.
18. Camilleri J. Characterization and hydration kinetics of tricalcium silicate cement for use as a dental biomaterial. Dent Mater. 2011;27(8):836–44.
19. Chang SW, Shon WJ, Lee W, Kum KY, Baek SH, Bae KS. Analysis of heavy metal contents in gray and white MTA and 2 kinds of Portland cement: a preliminary study. Oral Surg Oral Med Oral Pathol Oral Radiol Endod. 2010;109(4):642–6.
20. Schembri M, Peplow G, Camilleri J. Analyses of heavy metals in mineral trioxide aggregate and Portland cement. J Endod. 2010;36(7):1210–5.
21. Monteiro Bramante C, Demarchi AC, de Moraes IG, Bernadineli N, Garcia RB, Spångberg LS, Duarte MA. Presence of arsenic in different types of MTA and white and gray Portland cement. Oral Surg Oral Med Oral Pathol Oral Radiol Endod. 2008;106(6):909–13.
22. De-Deus G, de Souza MC, Sergio Fidel RA, Fidel SR, de Campos RC, Luna AS. Negligible expression of arsenic in some commercially available brands of Portland cement and mineral trioxide aggregate. J Endod. 2009;35(6):887–90.
23. Kum KY, Zhu Q, Safavi K, Gu Y, Bae KS, Chang SW. Analysis of six heavy metals in Ortho mineral trioxide aggregate and ProRoot mineral trioxide aggregate by inductively coupled plasma-optical emission spectrometry. Aust Endod J. 2013;39(3):126–30.
24. Duarte MA, De Oliveira Demarchi AC, Yamashita JC, Kuga MC, De Campos Fraga S. Arsenic release provided by MTA and Portland cement. Oral Surg Oral Med Oral Pathol Oral Radiol Endod. 2005;99(5):648–50.

25. Demirkaya K, Can Demirdöğen B, Öncel Torun Z, Erdem O, Çetinkaya S, Akay C. In vivo evaluation of the effects of hydraulic calcium silicate dental cements on plasma and liver aluminium levels in rats. Eur J Oral Sci. 2016;124(1):75–81.
26. Demirkaya K, Demirdöğen BC, Torun ZÖ, Erdem O, Çırak E, Tunca YM. Brain aluminium accumulation and oxidative stress in the presence of calcium silicate dental cements. Hum Exp Toxicol. 2017;36(10):1071–80. https://doi.org/10.1177/0960327116679713. Epub 2016 Nov 27.
27. Simsek N, Bulut ET, Ahmetoğlu F, Alan H. Determination of trace elements in rat organs implanted with endodontic repair materials by ICP-MS. J Mater Sci Mater Med. 2016;27(3):46.
28. Garcia LDFR, Huck C, Magalhães FAC, Souza PPC, Souza Costa CA. Systemic effect of mineral aggregate-based cements: histopathological analysis in rats. J Appl Oral Sci. 2017;25(6):620–30. https://doi.org/10.1590/1678-7757-2016-0634.
29. Taylor HFW. Cement chemistry. London: Thomas Telford; 1997. p. 113–225.
30. Odler I. Hydration, setting and hardening of Portland cement. In: Hewlett PC, editor. Lea's chemistry of cement and concrete. London: Arnold; 1998. p. 241–84.
31. Moir GK. Cements. In: Newman J, Choo BS, editors. Advanced concrete technology; constituent materials. Elsevier Butterworth Heinemann: Oxford; 2003. p. 3–45.
32. Camilleri J. Hydration mechanisms of mineral trioxide aggregate. Int Endod J. 2007;40(6):462–70.
33. Camilleri J. Characterization of hydration products of mineral trioxide aggregate. Int Endod J. 2008;41(5):408–17.
34. Arias-Moliz MT, Farrugia C, Lung CYK, Schembri Wismayer P, Camilleri J. Antimicrobial and biological activity of leachate from light curable pulp capping materials. J Dent. 2017;64:45–51.
35. Camilleri J, Laurent P, About I. Hydration of Biodentine, Theracal LC, and a prototype tricalcium silicate-based dentin replacement material after pulp capping in entire tooth cultures. J Endod. 2014;40(11):1846–54.
36. Kaup M, Schäfer E, Dammaschke T. An in vitro study of different material properties of Biodentine™ compared to ProRoot MTA. Head Face Med. 2015;11:16.
37. Grech L, Mallia B, Camilleri J. Investigation of the physical properties of tricalcium silicate cement-based root-end filling materials. Dent Mater. 2013;29(2):e20–8.
38. Grech L, Mallia B, Camilleri J. Characterization of set intermediate restorative material, Biodentine, bioaggregate and a prototype calcium silicate cement for use as root-end filling materials. Int Endod J. 2013;46(7):632–41.
39. Camilleri J, Grech L, Galea K, Keir D, Fenech M, Formosa L, Damidot D, Mallia B. Porosity and root dentine to material interface assessment of calcium silicate-based root-end filling materials. Clin Oral Investig. 2014;18(5):1437–46.

Biodentine™ Physico-Chemical Properties: From Interactions with Dental Tissues to Ageing

2

Amre R. Atmeh and Timothy F. Watson

Abbreviations

C2S   Di-calcium silicate
C3S   Tri-calcium silicate
CH   Calcium hydroxide
CSC   Calcium silicate cement
CSH   Calcium silicate hydrate
GIC   Glass ionomer cements

2.1   Introduction

With the introduction of Biodentine, another type of restorative material was added to the clinician's armamentarium, to be used as a provisional coronal restorative and permanent dentine replacement material. The arrival of a new material with such scope of applications inevitably triggers the exploration of its interface with the dental tissues as well as its interaction with the surrounding environment. Although Biodentine, as with other calcium silicate-based dental cements, shares some of its basic constituents with the original grey MTA developed by Mahmoud Torabinejad in the early 1990s (ProRoot MTA) [1], they vary in the composition, manufacturing,

A. R. Atmeh (✉)
Department of Restorative Dentsitry, Hamdan Bin Mohammed College of Dental Medicine, Mohammed Bin Rashid University of Medicine and Health Sciences (MBRU), Dubai, United Arab Emirates
e-mail: amre.atmeh@mbru.ac.ae

T. F. Watson
Centre for Oral, Clinical and Translational Sciences, Faculty of Dentistry, Oral and Craniofacial Sciences, King's College London, London, UK
e-mail: timothy.f.watson@kcl.ac.uk

behaviour, and even their properties [2]. Hence the use of the term "hydraulic calcium silicate cements" could be more descriptive and inclusive for this family of cements that share being calcium silicate based rather than just imitations of MTA.

Before understanding the interaction with the tooth as well as the surrounding environment, it is essential to understand certain aspects and properties that are closely related to the cement's behaviour inside the mouth.

2.2   Properties of the Cement

Similar to other calcium silicate-based cements (CSCs), Biodentine undergoes a hydration reaction upon mixing with water. The resultant mixture is principally composed of a calcium silicate hydrate (CSH) gel that binds unreacted silicate phases and other solid components [3, 4]. This mixture contains another important component, which is the ion-rich water that fills the spaces and pores within the paste [5]. This composition and structure are essential to bear in mind when trying to appreciate the relation between this type of cement and the dental tissues. It is also essential to take note of the reactivity of this mixture with the surrounding environment, which is determined by the ions leaching out of the cement and the ions present in the curing environment. In fact, this structure is what makes calcium silicate-based cements unique among other restorative materials such as resin composites and glass ionomer cements (GICs). Although CSCs are comparable to GIC in their water-based nature, that is where the resemblance stops, and hence some have preferred to use the term "bio-interactivity" to distinguish the ions released by GICs from the ion release that is associated with apatite formation in CSCs [6].

The physico-chemical properties of Biodentine have been thoroughly investigated involving the different components or "phases" of the paste. Hence, for the sake of simplicity, we are discussing the main properties of Biodentine related to the "gel phase" that forms the CSH matrix and the "liquid phase" composed of the ion-rich water in the paste.

2.2.1   The CSH Gel

The CSH gel forms the matrix that holds other solid constituents in the Biodentine paste together after mixing [7]. It forms on the surface of the solid calcium silicate particles (tri-calcium silicate) upon hydration [8]. The hydration (setting) reaction is basically a dissolution-precipitation process that begins with the gradual dissolution of un-hydrated calcium silicate particles (C3S) to release calcium, hydroxyl, and silica ions into the liquid phase. It occurs through the hydrolysis of silicate and oxygen ions on the particles' surface, and as a result CSH gel precipitates on that surface after the liquid phase is oversaturated [9]. Meanwhile, calcium hydroxide (CH) is produced and precipitates in proximity to the CSH gel or within the water-filled spaces of the cements [5, 10].

Microstructurally, CSH is believed to be a semi-crystalline nonstoichiometric solid composed of layered molecular structures with poorly aligned and poorly

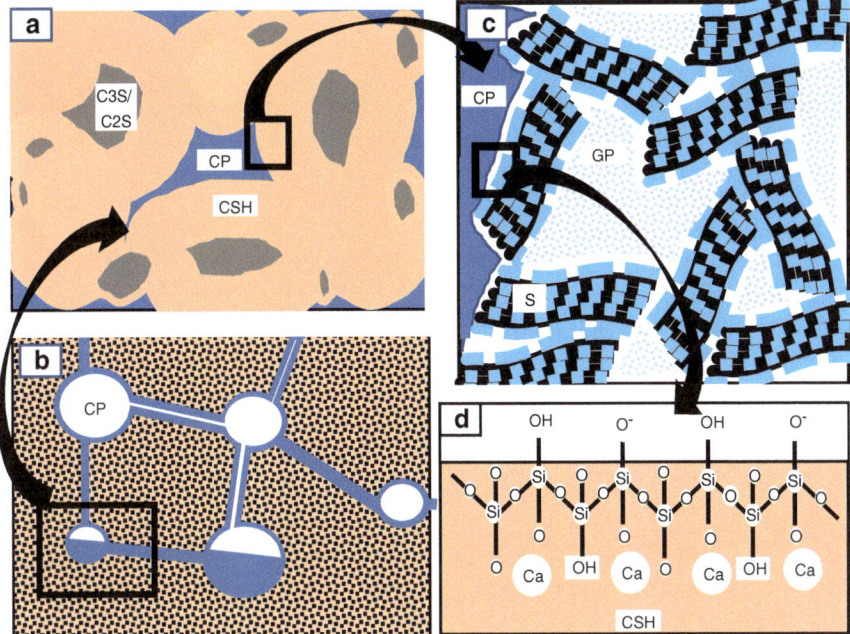

Fig. 2.1 The structure of hydrated Biodentine. (**a**) Hydrated Biodentine is composed of CSH gel surrounding non-hydrated C3S and C2S particles. The CSH gel allows aggregating these particles together during the setting and hardening process forming spaces (capillary pores—CP) interconnected with small channels. (**b**) This system of interconnected pores and channels forms a network within the hydrating cement that connects it with the outer environment. The pore solution that fills these spaces is the mobile phase of the cement that can exchange its content through this network with the outer environment. (**c**) The CSH gel is composed of layered molecular structures with poorly crystallised sheets (S) that are separated by narrow interlayer spaces. Water in these spaces is chemically bound, while spaces between the aggregated sheets are called gel pores (GP) that contain free water, as the bigger capillary pores. (**d**) The molecular structure of the CSH showing silanol groups on the CSH gel

crystallised sheets that are separated by 0.3 nm wide spaces [9, 11] (Fig. 2.1). Within this structure, relatively larger spaces or pores may exist (Fig. 2.1). As a gel, CSH is associated with hydrophilic surfaces provided mainly by the non-bridging oxygen atoms that can create hydrogen bonds. Additionally, the CSH surface is rich with hydroxyl groups from silanols (Si–OH) or calcium hydroxide, which can both be susceptible to hydrogen bond formation [12]. Such a hydrophilic structure will maintain some water chemically bound as part of the gel. The CSH phase of Biodentine, therefore, may act as a bonding medium with the tooth structure that is principally composed of hydroxyapatite, as will be discussed later.

2.2.1.1 Setting Time

The setting of mixed Biodentine is initiated by the hydration of calcium silicate particles and initial formation of CSH. This transforms the mixture into a plastic workable paste that hardens over time. The setting time is strongly related to the rate of calcium silicate dissolution and CSH precipitation [9].

Biodentine's setting time has been reported to be in the range of 6.5–86 min. These values, however, may represent two different setting times that describe different degrees of setting: the "initial" and "final" setting time [13]. The initial setting time ranges between 6.5 and 16 min, which is close to what is stated by the manufacturer (12 min) [14–16]. For the final setting time, it takes mixed Biodentine 45–86 min to become rigid solid [15, 17, 18]. However a shorter final setting time of 13–15 min has been reported [19, 20]. Using electrical impedance spectroscopy for the setting time measurement, Villat et al. [21] reported that the electrical resistivity of Biodentine was increasing over 2 weeks. This was attributed to the continuous maturation of the cement, which could be described as the hardening stage of the cement that involves continuous reduction of pore size and change in ionic composition of the pore solution [22, 23].

From a clinical point of view, both setting times matter. The "initial setting time" describes the duration at which the mixed cement remains plastic and adaptable. Practically, this could be considered as the working time. Hence, once Biodentine is mixed it should be applied while it is initially setting with adequate flowability; beyond that, the paste should not be manipulated until it is fully set and hardened.

The relatively shorter setting time of Biodentine in comparison with other CSCs indicates that CSH forms much quicker. This is due to different factors related to the nature and formulation of Biodentine that makes it set faster [24]. The purity of its phases, the high percentage of C3S that has a faster hydration than C2S, the presence of calcium carbonate, and, most importantly, the presence of $CaCl_2$ in the liquid along with solubilising polymers that reduce the water needed for hydration are all responsible for the shorter setting time of Biodentine [10, 25, 26].

It should be pointed out that all the reported values of setting time are based on lab testing under controlled conditions, which may vary from the clinical situation. Intra-orally, the setting time may be extended due to different factors such as inappropriate moisture control and contamination with blood. When Biodentine is applied as a coronal therapeutic material, a clean excavated dental cavity should be maintained with a proper rubber dam isolation. Blood contamination is another concern that may also occur during the placement of Biodentine as a root repair or root-end filling material, or even as a direct pulp capping material. Blood contamination was found to extend the setting time from 16 min up to 6 h [27, 28].

2.2.1.2 Viscosity and Flowability

As a freshly mixed paste, Biodentine maintains a plastic consistency to be manipulated within the limits of the initial setting time. Beyond that, the paste gradually transforms into a rigid and harder state composed of hydrating solids with reduced deformability. The hydration reaction causes more contacts between the hydrating solid components and less water-filled spaces and porosity, during which the paste gradually obtains increasing modulus of elasticity [9]. These changes are associated with changes in the rheological properties of the cement. In their study, Ha et al. [13] found that within the initial setting time of Biodentine, the paste develops 90%

of its plateau elastic modulus, which reflects the change in the cement's rheological properties at this stage.

As rheological properties of CSC depend primarily on its water/cement ratio [29], Biodentine has the advantage of the pre-proportioned powder and liquid that are mechanically mixed; this should maintain a consistent ratio [18]. Additionally, the hydro-soluble polymer in the liquid reduces the water/cement ratio to provide a reasonably thick paste with favourable handling properties [30].

Clinically, the viscosity of Biodentine and dental cements, in general, may strongly affect their clinical performance when applied and packed in contact with the dental tissues. Thicker mixes, associated with a lower water/cement ratio, have higher porosity and include more voids, while a more flowable consistency may adapt better to the dentine surface and may permeate through the dentinal tubules. Hence, the success of the treatment is strongly affected by the consistency of the cement, whether as a root-end filling material, direct pulp capping material, or dentine replacement material. Also, the time of application after mixing is critical, especially when using Biodentine during endodontic surgical repairs, where placing the root-end filling may take a longer time, potentially making the cement less adaptable: mixing should therefore be carefully timed in this clinical application.

2.2.1.3 Porosity

With the ongoing hydration of Biodentine after mixing, CSH forms on the unhydrated calcium silicate particles that aggregate together to form a porous mass with water-filled spaces. The porous structure of the paste is composed of a pore system of different sizes interconnected through channels and spaces. Pores are distributed in the cement in three forms [31, 32] (Fig. 2.1):

1. Gel pores (<10 nm), which are the smallest and form part of the CSH structure as intermolecular spaces between the gel sheets.
2. Capillary pores (up to 10 μm), which are water-filled spaces that exist in the cement as interconnected channels. They change with continuous deposition of CSH and ageing.
3. Air voids (>10 μm), which are usually created during the mixing or application of the cement.

Using mercury intrusion porosimetry (MIP), Camilleri et al. [33] reported 13.4% total porosity of Biodentine compared with 24.59% reported by Milutinović-Smiljanić et al. [34]. Total porosity was reported to be 6.2% [35] and 22.9% [36] using a water absorption method and ranged between 1.75% and 26.3% using microcomputed tomography (micro-CT) [34, 37–39].

This variation in reported porosity is due to the different methods that were used to assess the porosity of Biodentine. MIP is the most efficient for measuring the widest range of pore sizes ranging from 2.5 nm to 0.3 mm; hence it is expected to give the highest values of porosity in comparison with other techniques [40]. Water absorption, however, can only measure pores of 30 nm and above; hence it does not measure the "gel pores" and part of the capillary pores [31]. For micro-CT, pore detection is highly dependent on the spatial resolution reached by micro-CT, which is insufficient to detect gel pores and the majority of capillary pores; therefore the measured porosity is largely underestimated [41]. This was evident in the studies that compared between more than one methodology [34].

From a clinical point of view, the porous structure of Biodentine, and CSC in general, is important as it creates what looks like an internal transportation network connecting the internal cement's constituents with the external environment through the percolating water. Such movement can be described as "permeability", which allows the interaction and ion exchange between Biodentine and the surrounding tissues or saliva [23]. Hence porosity is tightly related to water absorption in wet conditions such as in the mouth. A higher porosity is associated with a larger surface area involved in the leaching process and more water absorption [42].

2.2.2   The Ion-Rich Water (Pore Solution)

Water in the pore spaces does not represent the only water content in the cement; rather it is distributed in the cement as [9, 11, 12] (Fig. 2.1):

1. Chemically bound interlayer water within the structure of the CSH gel, also described as non-evaporable water
2. Chemically bound water in the form of hydroxyl ions within the crystalline structure of CH
3. Surface-adsorbed water, lining the pores
4. Free water that fills the gel pores, capillary spaces, and voids in the hardened cement, which is also described as capillary water

Our discussion mainly concentrates on the free water that forms the ion-rich pore solution in Biodentine. The pore solution could be considered as the cement's active mobile phase that influences its chemical and biological properties. It mediates ion exchange between the cement and the surrounding environment (peri-radicular tissues, pulpal tissues, dentine, and saliva) during the setting process, or even afterward upon hardening [43].

The composition of Biodentine's pore solution depends on three factors: water availability from the surrounding environment that is described as sorption, ions released by the cement that depends on the solubility of the cement's constituents, and penetration of salts and ions from the outer environment. Solubility and sorption of Biodentine will be discussed here, while the penetration of outer ions will be discussed later as part of the effect of the cement curing environment.

2.2.2.1 Water Sorption
During the setting and hardening of Biodentine, water can still move into the cement through the pore system that connects it with the external environment (Fig. 2.1). This water movement, described as "sorption", takes place through capillary action that allows dynamic water movement with dentine and surrounding tissues [43].

Biodentine was reported to take up around 7–13% of its weight [35, 36, 44] and 0.007–0.014% of its volume [19, 39] through water sorption. These values, however, were reported to be lower in comparison with other CSCs, probably due to lower porosity [39]. Water uptake is higher during the first days of setting, during which the highest rate of ion exchange is expected to take place, subsequently dropping gradually with the continuing hydration and reduced porosity of the cement [19, 35].

2.2.2.2 Solubility

With the dynamic movement of water between Biodentine and the surrounding environment, soluble constituents of the cement could be washed out. Hence, it has been suggested that "elution of water-soluble material" rather than "solubility" is a preferred way to describe this process in CSCs [20]. Solubility of the set cement is highly dependent on the composition of the cement as well as the porosity and water dynamics, which eventually dictate the composition of the pore solution. Based on weight changes, Biodentine solubility was reported as 2.74% after 1 day [45], 6.7–5.4% after 1 week [22, 39], 4.6–7.3% after 1 month [20, 44], and 6.68% after 2 months [45]. While based on volumetric changes, Grech et al. [17] and Torres et al. [39] reported 4-week solubility of 0.002% and 0.012%, respectively. These values reflect the progressive change in the cement's mass upon soaking in a fluid with time, rather than the change in the solubility behaviour of the cement upon storage. This can explain the bioactive nature of these cements, which require ion and fluid exchange with the surrounding environment.

It has been argued that lab conditions in which solubility is tested, such as the use of distilled water, will give higher solubility values than what would be expected in the clinical situation [15]. Negative values of solubility (which indicate increase in the mass) were reported when physiological solutions were used [19, 20]. Additionally, the loss of mass may occur due to reasons other than dissolution [20]. Therefore, these values should be carefully interpreted, as they may reflect the highest solubility of the cement achieved in non-clinical conditions: in reality the cement's behaviour could be different and be less soluble intra-orally than in vitro.

2.2.2.3 Pore Solution pH

The main ionic composition of the pore solution is contributed by the dissolved calcium hydroxide, which exists in equilibrium with its precipitate distributed throughout the hydrating cement. Hence, the pH level of the pore solution is primarily dependent on its content of calcium hydroxide and reflects the progress of the hydration reaction [46]. With the progress of the hydration reaction, the production of calcium hydroxide will maintain a high pH and alkaline conditions for the cement and adjacent tissues. During the first few days, Biodentine exhibits the highest levels of pH (11.6–12.3), which drops gradually after 1 week to reach 8.9–10.7 within 4 weeks [17, 35, 36, 46, 47]. This is due to the hydration dynamics of CSCs that sees a gradual drop in calcium hydroxide formation [9], but some studies reported no change in pH during the first 2 weeks [19, 22].

Although the cement's pH is principally determined by the rate of calcium hydroxide formation, the solubility of other components of the cement and the levels of other ions can be affected by the pH levels. Alkaline pH is associated with higher levels of Si ions [48]. Biodentine was reported to release lower levels of calcium in weak acidic conditions [49] and exhibited lower pH levels in the presence of bicarbonate ions [46]. Therefore, the pH level of the pore solution might affect not only the pH of adjacent substrates, but also the nature of ion exchange over time.

2.2.2.4 Ca and Si Ions

Upon mixing the Biodentine powder with its liquid, calcium and silicon ions are rapidly released into the solution before precipitating in the form of CSH and CH [9]. While calcium hydroxide is the main source of calcium in the pore solutions, other sources such as calcium carbonate and CSH can also contribute.

Calcium ion release plays a pivotal role in the bioactive properties of Biodentine and CSCs. It is the primary source of calcium, besides the hydroxyl ion, that will tip the balance towards mineral precipitation and remineralisation [29]. This is in addition to other roles played by calcium in intercellular signalling and antimicrobial action [29]. The Ca ion level released by Biodentine was found to be the highest during the first 3 days [22, 35, 36, 46, 50], after which it drops profoundly to reach around 50% of its initial levels after 1-month storage. This change, as with the pH, reflects the drop in CH production associated with the slowing down of the hydration reaction with time [46]. Such changes are also associated with changes in the structure of the cement that includes reduced porosity and surface carbonation. Reduced porosity can limit the fluid movement and ion exchange with the outer environment, while surface carbonation can alter the surface structure affecting ion exchange and limiting pore solution movement [46]. The presence of $CaCl_2$ in the fluid of Biodentine could be one of the factors that are speculated to enhance the Ca ion release reported previously in comparison with MTA [51, 52].

Other ions, such as the Si ion, could also be released by Biodentine. Silicon ions play an important role in signalling as one of the cement's means of bioactivity and dentine remineralisation [29, 53]. Examining the level of leached Si ion of Biodentine stored in deionised water, we found that the cement maintained a constant level of Si (7.1 ppm) after 4-week storage, but it was significantly lower (<2 ppm) in samples stored in carbonation-encouraging conditions [46]. A study by Han and Okiji reported 0.7% atomic percentage of Si in dentine underneath Biodentine after 1-day storage in Ca- and Mg-free PBS, which increased gradually to reach 3.2% after 90 days [51].

2.3   Ageing and the Effect of Curing Environment on Biodentine

As discussed in the previous sections, the high pH and ion release by Biodentine drop gradually with time. In the first few days, the levels of calcium and hydroxyl ions are principally dependent on the rate of calcium hydroxide production that is related to the cement hydration rate. Calcium hydroxide production and release diminish profoundly after few days with the reduction in the hydration reaction rate [54]. At this stage, the calcium ion level may principally rely on the dissolution of solid constituents of the hydrated cement such as CSH, calcium carbonate, and precipitated calcium hydroxide. Furthermore, with the reducing porosity of the cement upon ageing, water availability will be affected. This reduction in the volume of water-filled pores means that water movement will decrease between the cement and surrounding environment. Hence, the first few days of the cement are the most critical for its function to induce tissue healing (as a pulp therapeutic material or root-end filling material), or dentine remineralisation (as a dentine replacement material). This period is critical for the body and immune system as well when the healing process is initiated [55].

Upon applying the freshly mixed Biodentine into the tooth, the cement is placed in direct contact with the surrounding physiological fluids, including saliva and blood. As a bioactive material, CSCs interact with these fluids through ion exchange [56], which reflects on the composition and structure of its pore system [43]. The nature and outcome of this interaction are dictated by the ions leaching out of the cement, on one side, and the ionic content of the surrounding fluids (saliva, plasma, or interstitial fluids) on the other side [57]. Hence, it is important for the clinician to understand the nature of such interactions as well as their impact on the cement. These aspects are particularly important for Biodentine as a root repair or root-end filling material where a reliable and durable seal is primarily dependent on the cement and its behaviour upon ageing in such conditions.

2.3.1 Phosphate-Rich Media

Phosphate is an important ion in physiological fluids such as saliva, plasma, and interstitial fluids. It plays an essential role as a buffering system, besides its other roles in maintaining homeostasis. Hence, phosphate ion is considered an essential component in the setting media of CSCs, especially when evaluating their bioactivity. In its simplest and most basic definition, bioactivity can be assessed based on the cements' ability to form apatite minerals when placed in a phosphate-rich medium [58]. Once the cement is stored in such an environment, which mimics the physiological conditions encountered by the cement in vivo, calcium ions leach out to precipitate as calcium phosphate minerals upon association with surrounding phosphate ions. Such precipitation takes place on the surface of the cement covered with silanol groups resulting from hydrolysis and ion exchange [56].

It is interesting that there is no consensus on the nature of the immersing media that have been used to store CSCs for assessing their bioactivity. The most commonly used phosphate-rich medium is phosphate-buffered saline (BPS), which contains 10 mmol/L PO_4^{3-}, compared to 0.7 mmol/L in Hanks' balanced salt solution (HBSS) [59]. The phosphate ion concentration in the latter is comparable to the concentration in the interstitial fluid and plasma (0.6–1.5 mmol/L) [60]; therefore it can mimic the actual situation when the cement is placed as a retro-filling material or pulp capping material. The phosphate ion level in saliva is higher (5.6 mmol/L) [61, 62]; hence it would be more suitable to use the PBS for immersing the cement when studying the Biodentine as a dentine replacement material. In addition to the formation of calcium phosphate minerals, the presence of phosphate may also lead to more calcium ion release from the Biodentine but may also reduce the porosity as a result of surface mineral deposition [63, 64].

The ability of Biodentine to induce the precipitation of calcium phosphate and hydroxyapatite minerals is the link between the cement's physico-chemical properties and its function inside the mouth. Mineral deposition can be responsible for the micromechanical retention of the cement through the formation of tag-like crystalline structures within the dentinal tubules [50]. It is also responsible for the mineralising potential of Biodentine on demineralised dentine [65], and the deposition of interfacial minerals that may improve the seal provided by the cement as a root repair or coronal dentine replacement material, or as a retrograde filling [59].

2.3.2   Carbonation and the Bicarbonate Ion

Carbonation is a widely investigated phenomenon in relation to Portland cement used in building construction, which occurs as a result of dissolution of atmospheric carbon dioxide into the pore water of hydrating CSC to form aqueous CO_2 [5]. The dissolved CO_2 reacts with calcium hydroxide and other hydration products of the cement to precipitate on its surface as calcium carbonate [46, 66]. In the oral cavity, conditions such as higher temperature and moisture can induce carbonation. In addition to that, carbonation increases in the presence of bicarbonate (HCO_3^{2-}) ions that are found in saliva, plasma, and interstitial fluid.

In the presence of bicarbonate ions, originally present in physiological fluids, calcium hydroxide leaching out of Biodentine will be consumed to precipitate in the form of calcium carbonate on the cement's surface [67]. This can reduce the surface porosity where larger crystals of calcium carbonate can occupy part of the pores. These crystals are also stronger than the replaced calcium hydroxide crystals; hence the compressive strength of the cement is improved [46] (Fig. 2.2).

As a result of surface carbonation and reduced porosity, ion exchange with the surrounding is affected leading to reduced release of Ca, Si, and OH ions. This effect can be either directly due to the consumption of calcium and hydroxyl ions or indirectly due to the reduced porosity that will limit ion leachability. Surface carbonation can also alter the surface chemical characteristics of the cement by the deposition of calcium carbonate. Such alterations may provide more favourable conditions for calcium phosphate deposition, acting as nucleation sites for apatite formation [68]. It may also improve cell adhesion to the cement's surface [69] or may enhance the osteogenic differentiation and proliferation of bone marrow-derived mesenchymal stem cells [70].

Fig. 2.2 Carbonation and calcium carbonate formation on Biodentine. SEM micrographs for Biodentine surface (white arrowheads) after ageing in a bicarbonate-rich medium showing calcium carbonate crystals (black arrowheads) covering the cement when imaging an intact surface (top) or fractured surface (bottom)

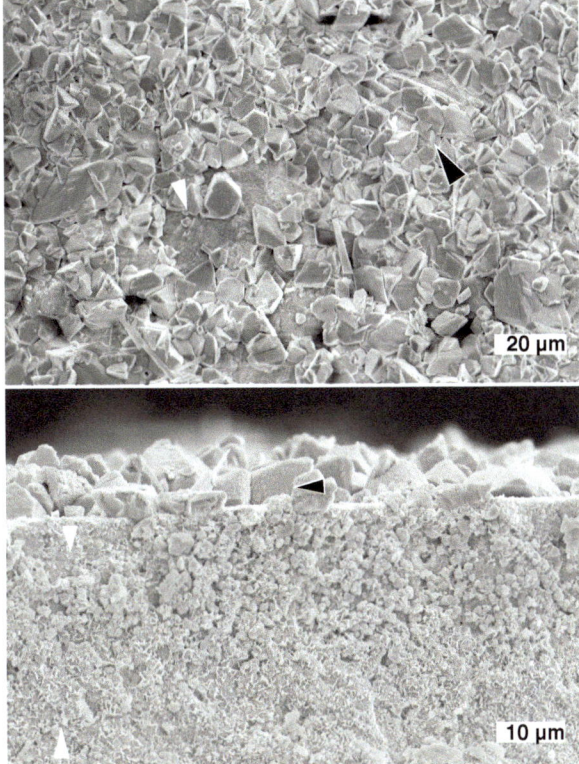

2.3.3 pH of the Surrounding Environment

In weak acidic conditions (pH = 5.5), Biodentine was found to have reduced surface hardness associated with surface erosion and altered porosity [71–73]. However, this was not found to affect the compressive strength of the cement [74]. Interestingly, it was reported that Ca ion release may drop in such conditions [49], while the sealing ability of the cement is enhanced [75].

2.4 Biodentine in Relation to Dentine

As a bio-interactive material, Biodentine is a rich source of highly alkaline calcium hydroxide (pH = 12.5) diffusing out of the cement into the surrounding environment and adjacent structures such as dentine, pulpal tissues, and bone. Besides the high pH, hydrating Biodentine is a rich source of ions, such as calcium, silicon, and carbonate. By diffusing into the surrounding environment, these ions can modify the equilibrium towards the formation and precipitation of minerals on the cement's surface or within the structure of adjacent tissues. This interaction with the surrounding environment is also associated with changes in the conditions that would affect or trigger different biological processes directly or indirectly and may even alter the structure of dentine underneath [76, 77]. These changes, collectively, mediate and potentiate the bioactive properties of the cement in physiological conditions, triggering cellular and metabolic pathways in favour of regeneration, mineralisation, and bone formation.

The most interesting aspect about the interface between dentine and Biodentine is the alkaline nature of the cement. Biodentine and calcium silicate-based cements are distinguished by their high alkalinity in comparison with other restorative materials. The widely used resin-bonded restorations rely on acid etching of dentine to expose the organic collagenous matrix and create a hybrid transitional layer between the composite and dentine. Glass ionomer cements are also acidic in nature in contrast to Biodentine, which implies different nature of interaction with dentine.

2.4.1 Interaction with Sound Dentine

As a dentine replacement and root repair material, Biodentine is applied in direct contact with dentine. Such physical proximity to dentine is essential for the cement to provide a good seal and achieve a successful outcome for treating a troubled pulp or repairing a perforated root. This anticipated seal will block the access of infecting bacteria and their products and prevent them from reaching the vital but vulnerable tissues inside the root canal system or adjacent peri-radicular tissues. Biodentine's adaptation to dentine, however, is not the sole factor in achieving this seal; rather it is the result of a combination of micromechanical as well as chemical interaction between the two substrates.

2.4.1.1 Tag-Like Structures

These structures can form within the dentinal tubules of interfacial dentine, which may reflect a micromechanical retentive mechanism to hold the cement in place [51, 67, 77]. The formation of tag-like structures results from the flow and penetration of freshly mixed paste into open dentinal tubules, which transform into crystalline clusters with time (Fig. 2.3). The formation of tag-like structures may play an important role in providing micromechanical retention for Biodentine, with a similar strength as the bonding of glass ionomer cement to dentine [20, 78]. This can explain the improved shear bond strength to dentine with time. The crystalline cluster formation may include apatite or carbonate salts as the paste encounters the phosphate- and bicarbonate-rich tubular fluid permeating from the pulp towards the interface, which may enhance the retention [50]. Such retention might also be potentiated by a chemical interaction with the adjacent dentine that involves its organic component. Clinically, these tag-like structures may also enhance the seal provided by the cement by extending the dentine-cement interface into the tubular lumen.

Fig. 2.3 Interfacial characteristics of the dentine-Biodentine interface. (**a**) SEM micrograph showing tag-like structures (*) forming inside the dentinal tubules in interfacial dentine. (**b**) A layer of structurally altered dentine (white arrowheads) that can be noticed underneath Biodentine (black arrowheads) in fractured dentine

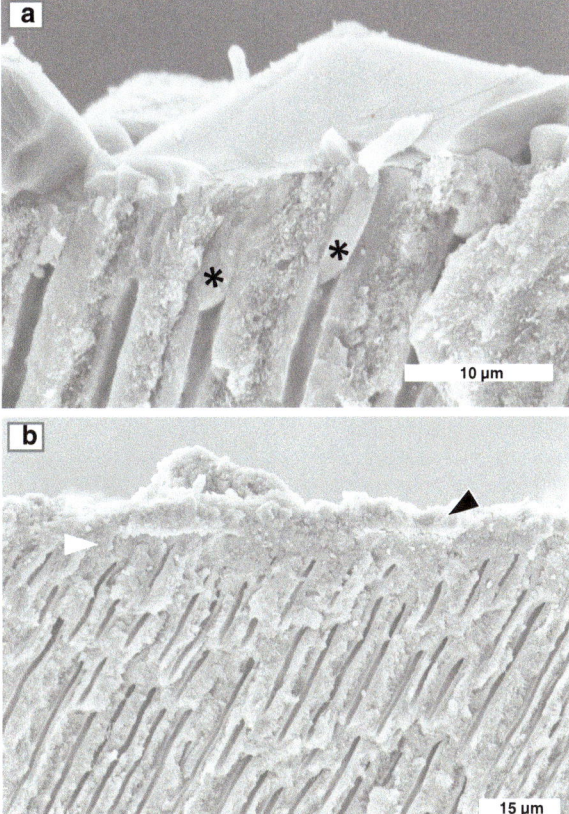

2.4.1.2 Structurally Altered Dentine Layer (Mineral Infiltration Zone)

The dentine-Biodentine interface is water permeable that allows fluids to permeate through the dentinal tubules from the pulp chamber to reach and infiltrate into the superficial layer of the cement close to the interface (Fig. 2.4) [77]. With the high water uptake of the freshly mixed cement, this will favour ion exchange between the two substrates, especially for the phosphate ion from the body fluids that can reach the interface to precipitate interfacial calcium phosphate minerals [79, 80].

Water movement can also take place in the opposite direction, as fluids from the cement may infiltrate into the dentine. Such fluid movement was confirmed by the formation of a richly dye-infiltrated dentine layer (of around 6.5 μm thickness) underneath fluorescein-labelled Biodentine using subsurface confocal laser scanning microscopy (CLSM) [77]. This layer of dentine appeared structurally altered on scanning electron microscope (SEM) images with altered collagen fibrils as detected by two-photon autofluorescence and second harmonic generation (SHG) imaging (Fig. 2.3) [67]. Such changes are the result of dual effect of the highly alkaline and ion-rich pore solution of Biodentine infiltrating the interfacial dentine.

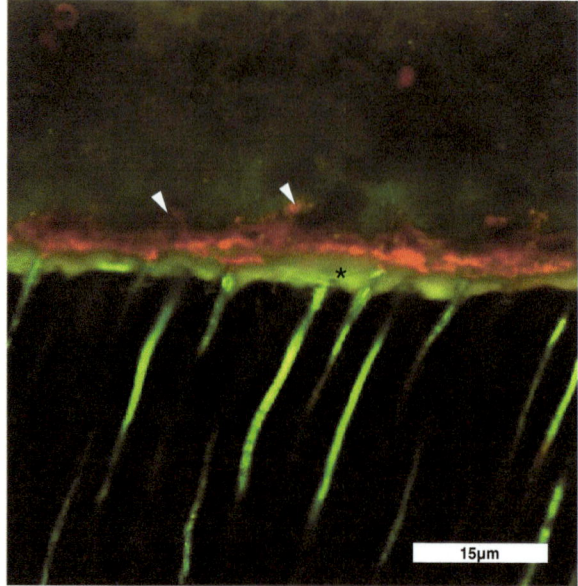

Fig. 2.4 Dentine-Biodentine interface. A fluorescence-mode CLSM image for the dentine-Biodentine interface showing the formation of the mineral infiltration zone within the structure of dentine (*). The fluorescein-labelled Biodentine (green) and its alkaline and ion-rich pore solution permeated through the dentinal tubules as well as the intratubular dentine. Rhodamine-labelled water (red) could also permeate from the pulp chamber to infiltrate into the superficial layer of the cement close to the interface (white arrowheads)

The fluid movement from Biodentine is associated with an alkaline caustic effect on the dentine leading to the degradation of collagen proximal to the cement. The alkaline pore solution infiltrating dentine may induce the breakdown of intermolecular bonds of collagen fibrils and distortion of the three-dimensional configuration of the protein, which increase their water absorption [81–83]. Structural changes in the interfacial dentine were also found to be associated with the release of matrix proteins such as transforming growth factor-β1 (TGF-β1) mediated by collagen degradation [76], which may trigger different reactionary processes to protect the pulp.

The "mineral infiltration zone" is the term used to describe the layer of structurally altered dentine formed underneath Biodentine. This term should not be confused or attributed to the bioactive potential of Biodentine, as it describes the cement's interaction with dentine regardless of the formation of calcium phosphate and apatite minerals [59]. As a result of the alkaline etching effect of Biodentine and accompanying structural changes of dentine, mineral uptake by interfacial dentine will be facilitated leading to ion infiltration into the intratubular dentine [77]. Interfacial dentine underneath Biodentine was found to take up Ca, Si, and CO_3 ions leaching out of the cement [50, 51, 75, 84]. After 1 week, Ca and Si ions may reach a penetration depth of around 74 and 46 µm, respectively [50], while the carbonate ion was detectable at a depth of around 48 µm over the same duration [77].

2.4.2 Interaction with Carious or Demineralised Dentine

Carious dentine is complex in its structure and remineralisation is challenging to study using in vitro models, with few of these representing all of the dynamic interactions occurring within the tooth [65, 85–87]. In particular, they rarely model the effect of the vital pulp response to the carious lesion and the tissue fluid dynamics/ remineralisation phenomena occurring within the dentine tubules over significant time periods, although there are models that get close to this [87]. In some respects, a simple demineralisation model may suffice for showing the remineralisation potential of materials [65], showing that the remineralisation capability of Biodentine is superior to that of GICs when a totally demineralised matrix is present. However, this is at the extreme of the various processes and there will be intermediate stages of remineralisation/demineralisation within the dentine.

The challenge of using real carious dentine as a substrate is therefore its inherent variability, so methods of characterising the extent of caries removal within the lesion and the relative position of the tooth restoration interface within the treated lesion are beneficial for introducing some degree of consistency to the results arising from a variable substrate. The use of biophotonics-based techniques such as Raman spectroscopy and fluorescence lifetime imaging may help to characterise the dentine caries substrate. Studies using natural carious lesions have shown that Biodentine is capable of remineralising caries-infected dentine when compared with GIC, with little difference between them when applied to caries-affected dentine [88]. At an ultrastructural level, the quality of remineralisation will be dependent upon whether it is "bottom up" or "top down" [87, 89]. However, in the management of an active carious lesion involving a pulp that can be managed to maintain vitality, the use of materials such as Biodentine that favour "top-down" mineralisation and its well-recognised therapeutic potential would be doubly beneficial.

2.5   Conclusion

While Biodentine shares comparable physico-chemical properties with calcium silicate-based cements, this material has significantly higher mechanical properties and has the advantage of a shorter setting time allowing its use as a therapeutic coronal restorative material besides its applications in endodontics. Biodentine is biointeractive with the surrounding environment and tissues through the ion-rich pore solution enriched with calcium and hydroxyl ions. This solution is responsible for the alkaline etching of dentine as we well as the production of apatite minerals and calcium carbonate in the presence of body fluids. Such interactivity may grant an improved seal for the cement-dentine interface combined with the biological and antimicrobial effects of released ions. Based on its physico-chemical properties, Biodentine can be an invaluable component of the practitioner's armamentarium bridging restorative and endodontic applications.

References

1. Torabinejad M, White DJ, Inventors, Loma Linda University, assignee. Tooth filling material and method of use. United States patent US 5,769,638, 23 Jun 1998.
2. Rajasekharan S, Martens LC, Cauwels RG, Verbeeck RM. Biodentine™ material characteristics and clinical applications: a review of the literature. Eur Arch Paediatr Dent. 2014;15(3):147–58.

3. Jennings HM, Parrott LJ. Microstructural analysis of hydrated alite paste. J Mater Sci. 1986;21(11):4053–9.
4. Taylor HF. Proposed structure for calcium silicate hydrate gel. J Am Ceram Soc. 1986;69(6):464–7.
5. Taylor H. Cement chemistry. London: Thomas Telford Publishing; 1997.
6. Gandolfi MG, Siboni F, Polimeni A, Bossù M, Riccitiello F, Rengo S, Prati C. In vitro screening of the apatite-forming ability, biointeractivity and physical properties of a tricalcium silicate material for endodontics and restorative dentistry. Dent J. 2013;1(4):41–60.
7. Camilleri J. Investigation of Biodentine as dentine replacement material. J Dent. 2013;41(7):600–10.
8. Camilleri J, Laurent P, About I. Hydration of Biodentine, Theracal LC, and a prototype tricalcium silicate-based dentin replacement material after pulp capping in entire tooth cultures. J Endod. 2014;40(11):1846–54.
9. Beaudoin O. Hydration, setting and hardening of Portland cement. In: Hewlett P, Liska M, editors. Lea's chemistry of cement and concrete. Oxford: Butterworth-Heinemann; 2019.
10. Kjellsen KO, Justnes H. Revisiting the microstructure of hydrated tricalcium silicate—a comparison to Portland cement. Cem Concr Compos. 2004;26(8):947–56.
11. Pinson MB, Masoero E, Bonnaud PA, Manzano H, Ji Q, Yip S, Thomas JJ, Bazant MZ, Van Vliet KJ, Jennings HM. Hysteresis from multiscale porosity: modeling water sorption and shrinkage in cement paste. Phys Rev Appl. 2015;3(6):064009.
12. Roosz C, Gaboreau S, Grangeon S, Prêt D, Montouillout V, Maubec N, Ory S, Blanc P, Vieillard P, Henocq P. Distribution of water in synthetic calcium silicate hydrates. Langmuir. 2016;32(27):6794–805.
13. Ha WN, Nicholson T, Kahler B, Walsh LJ. Mineral trioxide aggregate—a review of properties and testing methodologies. Materials. 2017;10(11):1261.
14. Butt N, Talwar S, Chaudhry S, Nawal RR, Yadav S, Bali A. Comparison of physical and mechanical properties of mineral trioxide aggregate and Biodentine. Indian J Dent Res. 2014;25(6):692.
15. Lucas CD, Viapiana R, Bosso-Martelo R, Guerreiro-Tanomaru JM, Camilleri J, Tanomaru-Filho M. Physicochemical properties and dentin bond strength of a tricalcium silicate-based retrograde material. Braz Dent J. 2017;28(1):51–6.
16. Ha WN, Nicholson TM, Kahler B, Walsh LJ. Rheological characterization as an alternative method to indentation for determining the setting time of restorative and endodontic cements. Materials. 2017;10(12):1451.
17. Grech L, Mallia B, Camilleri J. Investigation of the physical properties of tricalcium silicate cement-based root-end filling materials. Dent Mater. 2013;29(2):e20–8.
18. Kaup M, Schäfer E, Dammaschke T. An in vitro study of different material properties of Biodentine compared to ProRoot MTA. Head Face Med. 2015;11(1):1–8.
19. Jang YE, Lee BN, Koh JT, Park YJ, Joo NE, Chang HS, Hwang IN, Oh WM, Hwang YC. Cytotoxicity and physical properties of tricalcium silicate-based endodontic materials. Restor Dent Endod. 2014;39(2):89–94.
20. Dawood AE, Manton DJ, Parashos P, Wong RH, Palamara JE, Stanton DP, Reynolds EC. The physical properties and ion release of CPP-ACP-modified calcium silicate-based cements. Aust Dent J. 2015;60(4):434–44.
21. Villat C, Tran VX, Pradelle-Plasse N, Ponthiaux P, Wenger F, Grosgogeat B, Colon P. Impedance methodology: a new way to characterize the setting reaction of dental cements. Dent Mater. 2010;26(12):1127–32.
22. Soroka I. Portland cement paste and concrete. London: Macmillan International Higher Education; 1979.
23. Gopalan R, Venkappayya D, Nagarajan S. Textbook of engineering chemistry. New Delhi: Vikas Publishing House; 2010.
24. Camilleri J, Kralj P, Veber M, Sinagra E. Characterization and analyses of acid-extractable and leached trace elements in dental cements. Int Endod J. 2012;45(8):737–43.

25. El Elaouni B, Benkaddour M. Hydration of C3A in the presence of CaCO3. J Therm Anal Calorim. 1997;48(4):893–901.
26. Huan Z, Chang J. Novel bioactive composite bone cements based on the β-tricalcium phosphate–monocalcium phosphate monohydrate composite cement system. Acta Biomater. 2009;5(4):1253–64.
27. Alhodiry W, Lyons MF, Chadwick RG. Effect of saliva and blood contamination on the biaxial flexural strength and setting time of two calcium-silicate based cements: Portland cement and Biodentine. Eur J Prosthodont Restor Dent. 2014;22:20–3.
28. Moosani GKR, Manduri CS, Sampathi NR, et al. Evaluation of setting time of mineral trioxide aggregate and Biodentine in the presence of human blood and minimal essential media—an in vitro study. J Evid Based Med Healthc. 2017;4(94):5849–52. https://doi.org/10.18410/jebmh/2017/1177.
29. Koutroulis A, Batchelor H, Kuehne SA, Cooper PR, Camilleri J. Investigation of the effect of the water to powder ratio on hydraulic cement properties. Dent Mater. 2019;35(8):1146–54.
30. Camilleri J. Evaluation of selected properties of mineral trioxide aggregate sealer cement. J Endod. 2009;35(10):1412–7.
31. Aligizaki KK. Pore structure of cement-based materials: testing, interpretation and requirements. London: CRC Press; 2005.
32. Hearn N, Hooton D, Nokken M. Pore structure, permeability, and penetration resistance characteristics of concrete. In: Lamond JF, Pielert JH, editors. Significance of tests and properties of concrete and concrete-making materials. West Conshohocken, PA: ASTM; 2006. p. 238–53.
33. Camilleri J, Grech L, Galea K, Keir D, Fenech M, Formosa L, Damidot D, Mallia B. Porosity and root dentine to material interface assessment of calcium silicate-based root-end filling materials. Clin Oral Investig. 2014;18(5):1437–46.
34. Milutinović-Smiljanić S, Ilić D, Danilović V, Antonijević Đ. Advantages and downsides of Biodentine: satisfactory mechanical properties and radiopacity not meeting ISO standard. Vojnosanit Pregl. 2020:14. https://doi.org/10.2298/VSP191212014M.
35. Al-Sherbiny IM, Farid MH, Abu-Seida AM, Motawea IT, Bastawy HA. Chemico-physical and mechanical evaluation of three calcium silicate-based pulp capping materials. Saudi Dent J. 2020; https://doi.org/10.1016/j.sdentj.2020.02.001.
36. Gandolfi MG, Siboni F, Botero T, Bossù M, Riccitiello F, Prati C. Calcium silicate and calcium hydroxide materials for pulp capping: biointeractivity, porosity, solubility and bioactivity of current formulations. J Appl Biomater Funct Mater. 2015;13(1):43–60.
37. De Souza ET, Nunes Tameirão MD, Roter JM, De Assis JT, De Almeida NA, De-Deus GA. Tridimensional quantitative porosity characterization of three set calcium silicate-based repair cements for endodontic use. Microsc Res Tech. 2013;76(10):1093–8.
38. Guerrero F, Berástegui E. Porosity analysis of MTA and Biodentine cements for use in endodontics by using microcomputed tomography. J Clin Exp Dent. 2018;10(3):e237.
39. Torres FF, Guerreiro-Tanomaru JM, Bosso-Martelo R, Chavez-Andrade GM, Tanomaru FM. Solubility, porosity and fluid uptake of calcium silicate-based cements. J Appl Oral Sci. 2018;26 https://doi.org/10.1590/1678-7757-2017-0465.
40. Cook RA, Hover KC. Mercury porosimetry of hardened cement pastes. Cem Concr Res. 1999;29(6):933–43.
41. Bossa N, Chaurand P, Vicente J, Borschneck D, Levard C, Aguerre-Chariol O, Rose J. Micro- and nano-X-ray computed-tomography: a step forward in the characterization of the pore network of a leached cement paste. Cem Concr Res. 2015;67:138–47.
42. Camilleri J, Sorrentino F, Damidot D. Investigation of the hydration and bioactivity of radiopacified tricalcium silicate cement, Biodentine and MTA Angelus. Dent Mater. 2013;29(5):580–93.
43. Bertolini L, Elsener B, Pedeferri P, Redaelli E, Polder R. Transport processes in concrete. In: Corrosion of steel in concrete: prevention, diagnosis, repair. Weinheim: Wiley-VCH Verlag GmbH & Co; 2013. p. 21–48.

44. Mustafa R, Alshali RZ, Silikas N. The effect of desiccation on water sorption, solubility and hygroscopic volumetric expansion of dentine replacement materials. Dent Mater. 2018;34(8):e205–13.
45. Singh S, Podar R, Dadu S, Kulkarni G, Purba R. Solubility of a new calcium silicate-based root-end filling material. J Conserv Dent. 2015;18(2):149.
46. Atmeh AR. Investigating the effect of bicarbonate ion on the structure and strength of calcium silicate-based dental restorative material—Biodentine. Clin Oral Investig. 2020;26:10.
47. Ochoa-Rodríguez VM, Tanomaru-Filho M, Rodrigues EM, Guerreiro-Tanomaru JM, Spin-Neto R, Faria G. Addition of zirconium oxide to Biodentine increases radiopacity and does not alter its physicochemical and biological properties. J Appl Oral Sci. 2019;27 https://doi.org/10.1590/1678-7757-2018-0429.
48. Song S, Jennings HM. Pore solution chemistry of alkali-activated ground granulated blast-furnace slag. Cem Concr Res. 1999;29(2):159–70.
49. Natale LC, Rodrigues MC, Xavier TA, Simões A, De Souza DN, Braga RR. Ion release and mechanical properties of calcium silicate and calcium hydroxide materials used for pulp capping. Int Endod J. 2015;48(1):89–94.
50. Han L, Okiji T. Bioactivity evaluation of three calcium silicate-based endodontic materials. Int Endod J. 2013;46(9):808–14.
51. Han L, Okiji T. Uptake of calcium and silicon released from calcium silicate-based endodontic materials into root canal dentine. Int Endod J. 2011;44(12):1081–7.
52. Bortoluzzi EA, Broon NJ, Duarte MA, de Oliveira Demarchi AC, Bramante CM. The use of a setting accelerator and its effect on pH and calcium ion release of mineral trioxide aggregate and white Portland cement. J Endod. 2006;32(12):1194–7.
53. Saito T, Toyooka H, Ito S, Crenshaw MA. In vitro study of remineralization of dentin: effects of ions on mineral induction by decalcified dentin matrix. Caries Res. 2003;37(6):445–9.
54. Ramachandran VS. Differential thermal method of estimating calcium hydroxide in calcium silicate and cement pastes. Cem Concr Res. 1979;9(6):677–84.
55. Luo Z, Li D, Kohli MR, Yu Q, Kim S, He WX. Effect of Biodentine™ on the proliferation, migration and adhesion of human dental pulp stem cells. J Dent. 2014;42(4):490–7.
56. Niu LN, Jiao K, Zhang W, Camilleri J, Bergeron BE, Feng HL, Mao J, Chen JH, Pashley DH, Tay FR. A review of the bioactivity of hydraulic calcium silicate cements. J Dent. 2014;42(5):517–33.
57. Qu H, Wei M. The effect of temperature and initial pH on biomimetic apatite coating. J Biomed Mater Res B Appl Biomater. 2008;87:204–12.
58. Kokubo T, Takadama H. How useful is SBF in predicting in vivo bone bioactivity? Biomaterials. 2006;27:2907–15.
59. Kim JR, Nosrat A, Fouad AF. Interfacial characteristics of Biodentine and MTA with dentine in simulated body fluid. J Dent. 2015;43(2):241–7.
60. Fogh-Andersen N, Altura BM, Altura BT, Siggaard-Andersen O. Composition of interstitial fluid. Clin Chem. 1995;41(10):1522–5.
61. Kumar B, Kashyap N, Avinash A, Chevvuri R, Sagar MK, Kumar S. The composition, function and role of saliva in maintaining oral health: a review. Int J Contemp Dent Med Rev. 2017; https://doi.org/10.15713/ins.ijcdmr.121.
62. Rockenbach MI, Marinho SA, Veeck EB, Lindemann L, Shinkai RS. Salivary flow rate, pH, and concentrations of calcium, phosphate, and sIgA in Brazilian pregnant and non-pregnant women. Head Face Med. 2006;2(1):44.
63. Camilleri J. Hydration characteristics of Biodentine and Theracal used as pulp capping materials. Dent Mater. 2014;30(7):709–15.
64. Saghiri MA, Shabani A, Asatourian A, Sheibani N. Storage medium affects the surface porosity of dental cements. J Clin Diagn Res. 2017;11(8):ZC116.
65. Atmeh AR, Chong EZ, Richard G, Boyde A, Festy F, Watson TF. Calcium silicate cement-induced remineralisation of totally demineralised dentine in comparison with glass ionomer cement: tetracycline labelling and two-photon fluorescence microscopy. J Microsc. 2015;257(2):151–60.

66. Matsushita F, Aono Y, Shibata S. Carbonation degree of autoclaved aerated concrete. Cem Concr Res. 2000;30(11):1741–5.
67. Atmeh A. Optical characterisation of the interaction between calcium-silicate based dental restorative materials and dentine. Doctoral dissertation, King's College London, University of London, 2013.
68. Kapusuz D, Ercan B. Calcium phosphate mineralization on calcium carbonate particle incorporated silk-fibroin composites. Celal Bayar Üniversitesi Fen Bilimleri Dergisi. 2019;15(3):301–6.
69. Olah LA, Borbas LA. Properties of calcium carbonate-containing composite scaffolds. Acta Bioeng Biomech. 2008;10(1):61.
70. Matta C, Szűcs-Somogyi C, Kon E, Robinson D, Neufeld T, Altschuler N, Berta A, Hangody L, Veréb Z, Zákány R. Osteogenic differentiation of human bone marrow-derived mesenchymal stem cells is enhanced by an aragonite scaffold. Differentiation. 2019;107:24–34.
71. Elnaghy AM. Influence of acidic environment on properties of Biodentine and white mineral trioxide aggregate: a comparative study. J Endod. 2014;40(7):953–7.
72. Ballal V, Marques JN, Campos CN, Lima CO, Simão RA, Prado M. Effects of chelating agent and acids on Biodentine. Aust Dent J. 2018;63(2):170–6.
73. Deepthi V, Mallikarjun E, Nagesh B, Mandava P. Effect of acidic pH on microhardness and microstructure of Theracal LC, endosequence, mineral trioxide aggregate, and Biodentine when used as root repair material. J Conserv Dent. 2018;21(4):408.
74. Kayahan MB, Nekoofar MH, McCann A, Sunay H, Kaptan RF, Meraji N, Dummer PM. Effect of acid etching procedures on the compressive strength of 4 calcium silicate-based endodontic cements. J Endod. 2013;39(12):1646–8.
75. Agrafioti A, Tzimpoulas N, Chatzitheodoridis E, Kontakiotis EG. Comparative evaluation of sealing ability and microstructure of MTA and Biodentine after exposure to different environments. Clin Oral Investig. 2016;20(7):1535–40.
76. Huang XQ, Camba J, Gu LS, Bergeron BE, Ricucci D, Pashley DH, Tay FR, Niu LN. Mechanism of bioactive molecular extraction from mineralized dentin by calcium hydroxide and tricalcium silicate cement. Dent Mater. 2018;34(2):317–30.
77. Atmeh AR, Chong EZ, Richard G, Festy F, Watson TF. Dentin-cement interfacial interaction: calcium silicates and polyalkenoates. J Dent Res. 2012;91(5):454–9.
78. Guneser MB, Akbulut MB, Eldeniz AU. Effect of various endodontic irrigants on the push-out bond strength of Biodentine and conventional root perforation repair materials. J Endod. 2013;39(3):380–4.
79. Li X, Pongprueksa P, Van Landuyt K, Chen Z, Pedano M, Van Meerbeek B, De Munck J. Correlative micro-Raman/EPMA analysis of the hydraulic calcium silicate cement interface with dentin. Clin Oral Investig. 2016;20(7):1663–73.
80. Reyes-Carmona JF, Felippe MS, Felippe WT. Biomineralization ability and interaction of mineral trioxide aggregate and white Portland cement with dentin in a phosphate-containing fluid. J Endod. 2009;35(5):731–6.
81. Bowes JH. The swelling of collagen in alkaline solutions. 3. Swelling in solutions of bivalent bases. Biochem J. 1950;46(5):530–2.
82. Kemp GD, Tristram GR. The preparation of an alkali-soluble collagen from demineralized bone. Biochem J. 1971;124(5):915–9.
83. Andreasen JO, Farik B, Munksgaard EC. Long-term calcium hydroxide as a root canal dressing may increase risk of root fracture. Dent Traumatol. 2002;18(3):134–7.
84. Hadis M, Wang J, Zhang ZJ, Di Maio A, Camilleri J. Interaction of hydraulic calcium silicate and glass ionomer cements with dentine. Materialia. 2020;9:100515.
85. Daneshpoor N, Pishevar L. Comparative evaluation of bioactive cements on biomimetic remineralization of dentin. J Clin Exp Dent. 2020;12(3):e291.
86. Fathy SM. Remineralization ability of two hydraulic calcium-silicate based dental pulp capping materials: cell-independent model. J Clin Exp Dent. 2019;11(4):e360.

87. Schwendicke F, Al-Abdi A, Moscardó AP, Cascales AF, Sauro S. Remineralization effects of conventional and experimental ion-releasing materials in chemically or bacterially-induced dentin caries lesions. Dent Mater. 2019;35(5):772–9.
88. Watson TF, Atmeh AR, Sajini S, Cook RJ, Festy F. Present and future of glass-ionomers and calcium-silicate cements as bioactive materials in dentistry: biophotonics-based interfacial analyses in health and disease. Dent Mater. 2014;30(1):50–61.
89. Tay FR, Pashley DH. Biomimetic remineralization of resin-bonded acid-etched dentin. J Dent Res. 2009;88(8):719–24.

Biocompatibility and Bioactive Properties of Biodentine™

3

Matthias Widbiller, Charlotte Jeanneau, Kerstin M. Galler, Patrick Laurent, and Imad About

3.1 Introduction

Dental restorative materials are evaluated in vitro and in vivo to ensure their biocompatibility and innocuity to patients. In addition to their biocompatible properties, more and more dental restorative materials are designed to have a bioactive potential, i.e. to influence the host tissue's physiological processes and exploit its regeneration potential [1]. Biodentine™ is a tricalcium silicate-based cement. Its fabrication is based on ultra-pure tricalcium silicate preparation with specific particle size distribution. It contains calcium chloride as a setting accelerator leading to a shortened setting time (12 min) and a superplasticizer as a water-reducing agent to improve its mechanical and handling properties. The biocompatibility and bioactivity of tricalcium silicates, the main core material of Biodentine™, have been extensively evaluated. The effect of Biodentine™ or its released by-products has been evaluated on cell viability, proliferation, migration, differentiation and biomineralization as well as its anti-inflammatory potential. Different tests have been developed using cell lines or primary cell cultures, but one should consider first the target

M. Widbiller · K. M. Galler
Department of Conservative Dentistry and Periodontology, University Hospital Regensburg, Regensburg, Germany
e-mail: matthias.widbiller@ukr.de; kerstin.galler@ukr.de

C. Jeanneau · I. About (✉)
Aix Marseille University, CNRS, ISM, Institute of Movement Science, Marseille, France
e-mail: charlotte.jeanneau@univ-amu.fr; imad.about@univ-amu.fr

P. Laurent
Aix Marseille University, CNRS, ISM, Institute of Movement Science, Marseille, France

Assistance Publique-Hôpitaux de Marseille, Pôle d'Odontologie, Hôpital Timone, Marseille, France
e-mail: patrick.laurent@univ-amu.fr

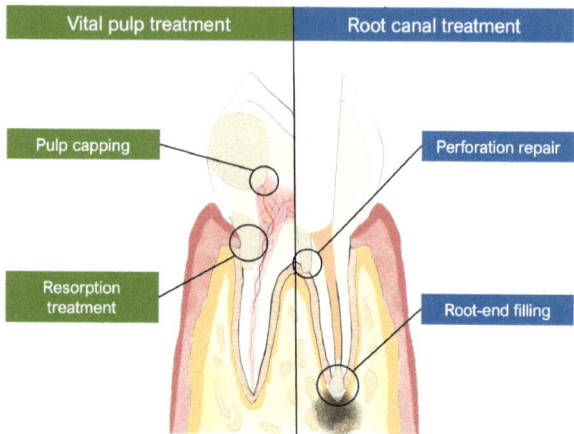

cells of the restorative material and the context of its clinical application. Hence, Biodentine™ can potentially interact with several dental and periodontal tissues and cell types, all along its setting reaction and for a long period after setting. In this chapter, we focus on the interactions between Biodentine™ and dental or periodontal cells following endodontic procedures such as pulp capping, apexification or repair of root perforations (Fig. 3.1).

3.2   Biocompatibility

A wide range of study designs are available to evaluate the biocompatibility of dental materials depending on the cells used, measurement method, and duration and type of contact with unset or set material, which makes them difficult to compare [2]. Since tricalcium silicate cements are widely used in restorative dentistry, their biocompatibility has been investigated using experimental models simulating many clinical applications and cell types. For determining the choice of target cells, one should consider that Biodentine™ interacts with pulp cells during the pulp capping procedures and with cells from the tooth-surrounding tissues in other clinical applications (Table 3.1).

3.2.1   Effects on Target Cells Following Pulp Capping Procedures

In addition to providing a marginal seal to prevent bacterial infiltration, the restorative procedure could modify the pulp microenvironment via released by-products from the material. Upon pulp capping, Biodentine™ may interact with odontoblasts, pulp fibroblasts, dental pulp stem cells (DPSCs) and inflammatory cells, i.e. all cells involved in the dentin e-pulp regenerative process under indirect or direct capping procedures. Biodentine™ biocompatibility has been compared to other biomaterials of the same calcium silicate family, i.e. mineral trioxide aggregate (MTA)-based

Table 3.1 Biodentine™ clinical application and the underlying target tissues/cells

| | Target tissue(s)/cell type(s) | | | | | | | | |
| | Pulp | | | | Apical papilla | Periodontium | | | |
	Odontoblasts	Fibroblasts	DPSCs	Immune cells	SCAP	Gingiva fibroblasts	Periodontal ligament cells	Osteoblasts	Osteoclasts
Indirect pulp capping	×			×					
Direct pulp capping / Pulpotomy		×	×	×					
Resorption treatment	×	×	×	×		×	×	×	×
Perforation repair						×	×	×	×
Apical plug					×				
Root-end filling							×	×	×

DPSCs dental pulp stem cells, *SCAP* stem cells of the apical papilla

cements and derivatives, or to materials used in the same clinical indication, i.e. calcium hydroxide-based and glass ionomer cements. A screening test (MTT assay) is used in most of these studies. This is an enzymatic assay measuring mitochondrial activity which reflects the cell viability. The cell type used is of prime importance to simulate the clinical situation. While in some studies, cell lines, immortalized fibroblasts or odontoblast cells of various origins or species have been extensively used, target cells of human origin should be preferred. Thus, primary culture of human pulp cells is a good choice for pulp capping procedures. Also, the type of interaction between the material and underlying cells needs to be considered. In direct pulp capping, the material interacts directly with the cells, while the presence of a dentine slice or a membrane simulates indirect pulp capping. Finally, biocompatibility studies are performed using either set or unset material. The rationale is that set material provides information on the material behaviour after setting in vivo while use of unset material reflects the clinical condition of the material being directly applied onto the dental tissues and its short-term consequences.

Short-term exposure of human pulp cells to set material for 3 days demonstrated no toxicity to pulp cells incubated with Biodentine™ or ProRoot® MTA. Also, incubating these cells with increasing concentrations of Biodentine™ extracts showed no toxicity when used either with or without dentine slice interposition between the material and the cells [3]. Similar data demonstrated no cytotoxicity of Biodentine™ or ProRoot® MTA cements while calcium hydroxide and TheraCal LC® dramatically decreased cell viability after 3 days [4]. The absence of Biodentine™ toxicity was confirmed on immortalized human dental pulp cell line after a longer incubation period (14 days) [5].

Overall, most of the studies report that Biodentine™ is biocompatible after setting. However, an immediate cytotoxic effect of freshly mixed Biodentine™ was reported. Although this result is not consistent with the vast majority of the studies published so far, it may be due to the high pH of Biodentine™ during the setting reaction [6]. Indeed, an elegant study performed on human DPSCs based on the effect of different calcium silicate cements after ageing cycles or their eluates by placing the materials in transwell inserts revealed that Biodentine™ and MTA Angelus® cements had a low cytotoxicity which further decreased with ageing cycles and use of transwell culture [7].

3.2.2   Interaction with Tooth-Surrounding Tissues

In addition to their application in vital pulp treatment, bioactive cements are used in many other dental procedures. Typical applications include the apical plug in teeth with incomplete root formation, repair of root perforations or resorptive defects of the root surface and retrograde root fillings during apical surgery. In all these situations, the applied material interacts with various cell types and different tissues and affects the biological processes.

If pulp damage and necrosis occur in children and adolescents, root development is arrested, and the morphology of the apex remains as is—depending on the developmental stage at the time point of injury. If wide open, conventional root canal filling is technically impossible. In this case, obturation can only be performed with an apical plug of tricalcium silicate cement (Fig. 3.2a). At the apical end of an immature tooth, the apical papilla can be found as a transient stem cell niche [8], an apical part of the former dental papilla, which gives rise to odontoblasts during the course of tooth development and transforms into the dental pulp. In a healthy state, it is attached loosely to the root apex and separated from the pulp tissue by a cell-rich zone (Fig. 3.2b). Because of its location, the blood supply of these cells is rich

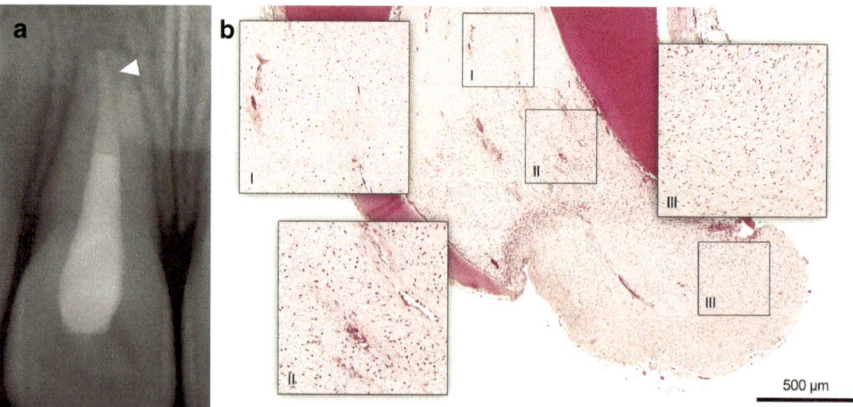

Fig. 3.2 (**a**) Apical plug at an immature incisor with Biodentine™ (white arrowhead). (**b**) Morphology of an apical papilla in H&E staining. The pulp tissue (I) merges into a cell-rich zone (II) that directly adjoins the apical papilla (III)

and allows them to survive pulpal inflammation or necrosis [9]. As described for the dental pulp before, the apical papilla harbours mesenchymal stem cells termed stem cells of the apical papilla (SCAP). These cells were first obtained and described by Sonoyama et al. [10]; they express typical stem cell markers and are able to differentiate into various cell lineages in vitro, e.g. osteogenic, adipogenic or chondrogenic [10, 11]. However, when an immature root canal is filled, tricalcium silicate cements like Biodentine™ come into direct contact with the apical papilla and thus SCAP.

Numerous reports describe the successful clinical application of Biodentine™ for apexification procedures; however, prospective studies are still pending [12–18]. Cell culture experiments, where SCAP were exposed to eluates of Biodentine™, showed an increase of proliferation after 7 days. Furthermore, Biodentine™ induced expression of typical odontogenic marker genes, i.e. dentine matrix acidic phosphoprotein 1 (DMP1), dentine sialophosphoprotein (DSPP) and matrix extracellular phosphoglycoprotein (MEPE), and led to mineralization after 21 days [19]. In another in vitro study, SCAP were seeded on human dentine discs with a central lumen filled with Biodentine™ or other bioactive cements. Besides enhancement of cell viability and proliferation, Biodentine™ promoted expression of alkaline phosphatase (ALP) and DSPP; however, integrin-binding sialoprotein (IBSP) expression was increased with ProRoot® MTA. This led the authors to conclude that Biodentine™ induced an odontogenic phenotype, whereas ProRoot® MTA drove cells rather towards an osteogenic lineage [20]. Furthermore, the culture of SCAP in direct contact with set specimens of Biodentine™ and ProRoot® MTA revealed an increase in the expression of angiogenic genes such as vascular endothelial growth factors A and D (VEGFA and VEGFD). The authors also reported a high secretion of VEGF and inferred a high angiogenic potential by both tricalcium silicate cements [21].

Biodentine™ can also be used within the root canal to repair perforation defects that may either be induced iatrogenically or result from a pathological process such as internal resorption. Furthermore, external resorptions of the tooth root can leave defects that can be filled with Biodentine™ or similar tricalcium silicate cements (Fig. 3.3). Due to its biological and physical properties, Biodentine™ is also suitable for root-end closure during apical surgery. In all these applications, the material

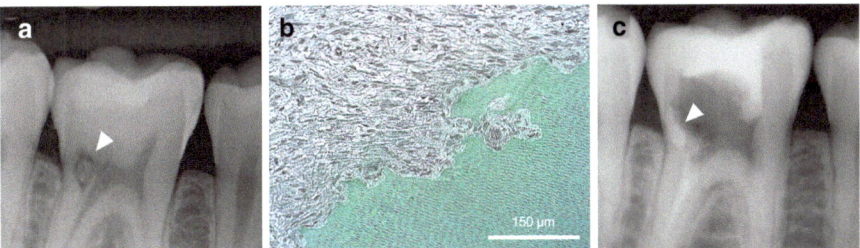

Fig. 3.3 (**a**) Resorptive defect in a lower molar leading to communication between periodontal and pulpal tissue (white arrowhead). (**b**) Invasive fibrous tissue resorbing tubular dentine. (**c**) Reparation of the resorptive perforation with Biodentine™ (white arrowhead)

fulfils the purpose of sealing connections to extraradicular tissue or covering external defects. Hence, the bioactive cement gets in direct contact with the bony tissue, the periodontal ligament or the gingiva.

In the process of bone remodelling, the critical cell types are osteoblasts and osteoclasts. The primary physiological function of osteoblasts is to form bone by first secreting unmineralized osteoid, which subsequently mineralizes by precipitation of calcium phosphates [22]. In vitro studies showed no limitation of osteoblast viability or proliferation by Biodentine™, and cellular attachment to the material's surface could be observed [23–26]. Both Biodentine™ and MTA Angelus® induced high ALP activity and the ability to form calcified nodules in osteoblastic cells; however, the effect of Biodentine™ on mineralization was significantly greater [25]. As antagonists of osteoblasts, the osteoclasts, which arise from the monocyte-macrophage lineage [27], are responsible for bone resorption during physiological and pathological remodelling. In vitro, anti-inflammatory effects of tricalcium silicate cements on osteoclast cell cultures have been described [28]. Biodentine™ and ProRoot® MTA furthermore appeared to inhibit osteoclast differentiation and led to a reduction in tartrate-resistant acid phosphatase (TRAP) of macrophages [28, 29].

Besides bony tissue, cells of the periodontal ligament (PDL) can be confronted with tricalcium silicate cement after the treatment of perforations or root resorption. Similarly to findings on osteoblasts, survival of periodontal ligament cells was not affected in the presence of set Biodentine™ specimens or their eluates [23, 30]. Another in vitro study implicated increased cell adhesion of PDL cells on MTA and Biodentine™ by formation of focal contacts [31]. Adhesion and spreading of periodontal ligament cells on both bioactive cements have also been shown by scanning electron microscopy [32].

If tricalcium silicate cements are placed at the cervical region of the tooth, gingival fibroblasts can be exposed to the material. Again, the viability of human gingiva fibroblasts cultured with extracts of set Biodentine™ or ProRoot® MTA was not affected [33]. Furthermore, gingival cells attached directly onto the bioactive cements and spread onto their surface [26, 33].

3.3 Effects of Biodentine™ on Pulp-Dentine Regeneration Potential

Upon dentine-pulp injury, the underlying pulp response can vary from an upregulation of the odontoblast synthetic activity in case of mild-to-moderate dentine injury to odontoblastic cell differentiation from pulp stem cells in case of pulp exposure or severe pulp injury, which leads to a reparative dentine secretion. Both dentine types provide a dentine-pulp protection that is highly dependent on the severity of the traumatic/carious injury, the pulp capping material used, its sealing ability and the pulp's inflammatory status.

Indeed, the dentine-pulp tissue regeneration is a well-orchestrated process (Fig. 3.4). It requires (1) the resolution of inflammation, (2) neoangiogenesis and innervation, (3) pulp fibroblast proliferation and colonization, (4) proliferation and

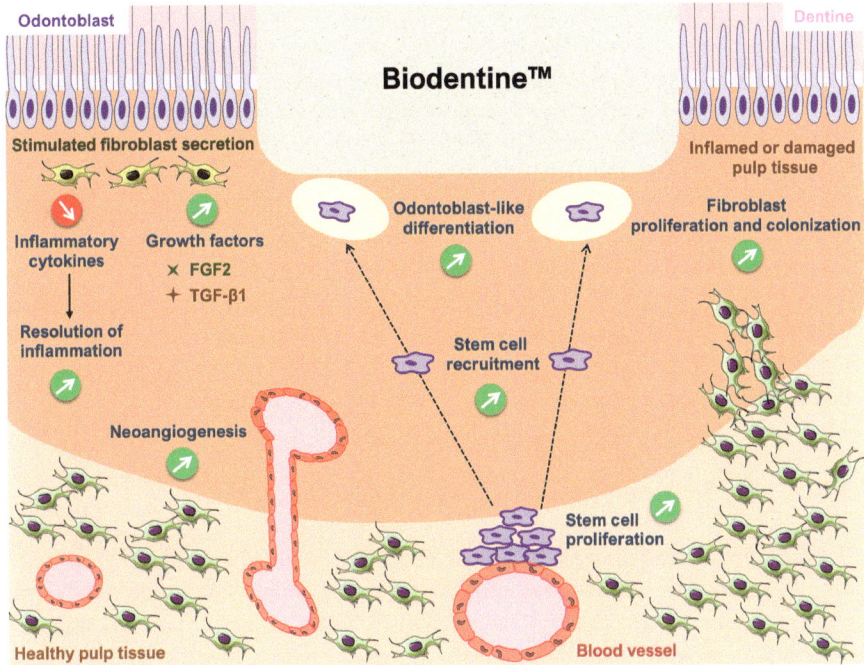

Fig. 3.4 Effects of Biodentine™ on the initial steps of dentine-pulp inflammation and regeneration. Biodentine™ application decreases pro-inflammatory cytokine secretion, which is an important step in the resolution of inflammation. In the course of tissue regeneration, Biodentine™ induces neoangiogenesis and release of growth factors involved in pulp cell proliferation, stem cell recruitment and differentiation

migration of dental pulp stem cells (5) and their differentiation into odontoblast-like cells to synthesize reparative dentine. These steps are regulated by growth factors which are sequestered in the dentine or secreted by pulp cells [34–36]. The release of these factors can be modified by the pulp capping material [3].

3.3.1 Biodentine™ Implication in the Resolution of Inflammation

It is well known that tissue inflammation in response to an injury or infection is essential to eliminate invading pathogens or altered host cells. However, severe inflammation can be detrimental as the pulp is located in a rigid environment, leaving no room for swelling [37]. Thus, upon vital pulp therapy, a rapid resolution of inflammation is a prerequisite and would favour the regenerative process which is key for a successful clinical outcome [38, 39]. Also, applying a material onto the pulp can modulate the balance between inflammation and regeneration. Indeed, recent studies have demonstrated that Biodentine™ has an anti-inflammatory potential in vitro. This has been investigated using Boyden chambers where inflammatory

THP-1 cell migration towards pulp fibroblasts was significantly reduced when fibroblasts were incubated with Biodentine™ extracts [40]. Also, using different experimental models in vitro, when pulp fibroblasts were incubated with lipoteichoic acid (LTA) simulating the presence of gram-positive bacteria, Biodentine™ extracts significantly decreased the recruitment of inflammatory THP-1 cells including their adhesion to the activated endothelial cells, and their migration and activation into macrophage-like cells [41]. This anti-inflammatory potential is confirmed in a recent study investigating the effect of Biodentine™ on THP-1 expression of two enzymes involved in the initial phase of inflammation cyclooxygenase 1 (COX1) and cyclooxygenase 2 (COX2). The results demonstrated a decrease of the expression of COX1 and -2 by THP-1 grown with Biodentine™ as compared to the control. Furthermore, Biodentine™ significantly decreased the secretion of two inflammation mediators: prostaglandin E2 (PGE2) and thromboxane B2 (TXB2) [42].

3.3.2 Biodentine™ Implication in Neoangiogenesis

During pulp capping procedures blood vessels can be destroyed locally. The vascular system ensures not only gas exchange, nutrient supply and waste removal but also pulp inflammatory control and resolution. Thus, an intact vascularization is a determining element for the success of vital pulp therapy. Vascularization is regulated by multiple signals and growth factors. While VEGF is considered as a major angiogenic factor, the process is regulated by many other transcription and growth factors such as fibroblast growth factor 2 (FGF-2), platelet-derived growth factor (PDGF) and transforming growth factor β1 (TGF-β1) [43].

During vital pulp therapy, the material's interaction with dentine or pulp cells can modify the pulp neovascularization potential. Biodentine™ has been shown to upregulate VEGF expression in pulp stem cells and its secretion [21, 44]. Similarly, when Biodentine™ extracts were applied on LTA-stimulated pulp fibroblasts, a significant increase of VEGF secretion was also reported [41].

In addition to investigating angiogenic growth factor secretion, vascular network formation can be studied in vitro, by a well-established endothelial tube formation assay. Using this experimental design, Biodentine™ extract has been shown to enhance the endothelial cell organization into tubular network called "tubes" corresponding to new blood vessels in vitro. When human umbilical vein endothelial cells were cultured with Biodentine™ extract, the number of these tubes significantly increased as compared to the control [45].

3.3.3 Biodentine™ Induces Pulp Fibroblast Proliferation and Recruitment

Fibroblasts represent the most abundant population of the dental pulp. Fibroblasts are irregular shaped cells involved in the synthesis of the extracellular matrix that provides support to tissues [46]. But recent studies demonstrated that they have major roles in regulating the pulp biology and function under normal and pathologic conditions. Indeed, pulp fibroblasts synthesize growth factors and molecules that are involved in re-establishing the vascularization [36, 47], nerve sprouting [48–50] and stem cell recruitment to the injury site [51–53]. Moreover, pulp fibroblasts are also involved in pulp defence against bacterial infection through the secretion and activation of complement proteins [54, 55]. Thus, fibroblast regeneration upon pulp capping is very important to both guarantee tissue integrity and maintain its defensive capacity. Interestingly, Biodentine™ eluates stimulate fibroblast proliferation and induce their recruitment towards LTA-stimulated cells as demonstrated in a scratch assay. This appears to be correlated to an increase of FGF-2 and TGF-β1 secretion from fibroblasts [41].

3.3.4   Biodentine™ Enhances Dental Pulp Stem Cell Recruitment

Following pulp exposure, dentine-pulp regeneration requires DPSC proliferation and their recruitment and differentiation at the injury site. The damaged dentine is then replaced by a reparative dentine secreted by newly differentiated odontoblast-like cells [56]. These processes are orchestrated by growth factors such as TGF-β1, which is known to stimulate odontoblastic differentiation and DPSC recruitment [57], while FGF-2 induces stem cell proliferation [53]. Biodentine™ application has been shown to release growth factors such as TGF-β1 from the dentine [58, 59]. This factor, which diffuses through the dentine tubules, upregulates the odontoblast and underlying pulp cell activity to carry out the tertiary dentine production [60]. Also, when SCAP were grown with Biodentine™ extract [19] or with dentine discs filled with Biodentine™ [20], the latter promoted SCAP proliferation. This appears due to an increased secretion of growth factors. Indeed, Biodentine™ application on injured pulp fibroblasts increased FGF-2 secretion which is known for its role in inducing pulp fibroblast and stem cell proliferation [53]. It also increased TGF-β1 secretion which provides a gradient guiding pulp stem cell recruitment to Biodentine™ application site [3, 53].

3.3.5   Effects on Differentiation and Mineralization

Dental trauma and progressing carious lesions can create defects close to the dental pulp, which is often protected only by a thin layer of remaining dentine. In the most unfavourable scenario, the pulp may be exposed and thus get in direct contact with oral microorganisms. In these cases, the primary therapeutic goal is to keep the pulp vital and thus preserve its sensory, formative and defensive functions [61, 62]. A root canal filling should be avoided to maintain physiological structures and thus improve the chances for tooth survival [63]. Measures to preserve pulp vitality include indirect capping of the dental pulp in deep defects, direct capping of exposed pulp tissue and partial or complete amputation of infected or inflamed tissue (partial or full pulpotomy) [64]. In the case of a dental trauma it must be borne in mind that the pulp tissue is initially healthy and has not been challenged with microorganisms prior to the injury, whereas progressive caries leads to chronic inflammation and irritation of the pulp. Thus, differences in tissue responses as well as success rates after direct or indirect pulp capping by bioactive cements can be anticipated in these two different scenarios. Traditionally, calcium hydroxide preparations were used for vital pulp therapies; however, innovative bioactive materials such as Biodentine™ and MTA represent a promising alternative especially for direct capping or pulpotomy and are routinely used today.

In indirect capping, bioactive agents are applied onto the dentine in areas close to the pulp in order to protect the pulp tissue from external stimuli on the one hand and to induce a biological response on the other. The cements stimulate the underlying odontoblast activity to elaborate a tertiary dentine, which is referred to as reactionary dentine.

However, if the pulp tissue is exposed in deep lesions or after caries excavation, the cells of the odontoblast layer perish. Tricalcium silicate cements can be applied directly on the pulp tissue during direct pulp capping or after pulpotomy. As a result, mesenchymal progenitor cells migrate to the wound area and differentiate into a mineralizing phenotype also known as secondary odontoblasts. These cells deposit hard tissue at the capping site and create a biological closure of the defect, which is called "bridging". The newly formed mineralized tissue is categorized as tertiary dentine and termed reparative dentine.

Therefore, the impact of tricalcium silicate cements like Biodentine™ on the differentiation of human pulp cells and their ability to induce mineralization plays an important role and may modify biological response mechanisms after indirect and direct capping as well as after pulpotomy.

3.3.5.1 In Vitro

The differentiation of pulpal progenitor cells into odontoblast-like cells is subject to complex regulation and generally described by the expression of typical marker genes, which may well differ in vitro and in vivo [65–67].

Multiple in vitro studies investigated the response of human pulp-derived cells cultured either in medium extracts of bioactive dental cements [5–7, 68–70] or in direct contact to set specimens [5–7, 68–70]. Generally, an increased expression of odontoblast marker genes such as DSPP, DMP1, ALP, osteocalcin (OCN) and osteopontin (OPN) has been reported for human pulp cells cultured in monolayers; however, Biodentine™ and MTA triggered differentiation to a similar degree [5–7, 68–70]. The mechanism of differentiation of human pulp cells by Biodentine™ seems to be based on the MAPK and CaMKII pathways as shown repeatedly [68, 69]. Three-dimensional culture methods also revealed positive effects of Biodentine™ on cell differentiation (upregulation of DSPP, DMP1), which were comparable to those of MTA [71]. In this context, a systematic review analysed the impact of tricalcium silicate cements on odontogenic differentiation of both human- and animal-derived pulp cells and reported similar favourable effects by Biodentine™ and MTA [2]. Furthermore, next-generation RNA sequencing was performed after exposure of human dental pulp stem cells to either Biodentine™ or MTA. Despite differences in gene expression, both tricalcium silicate cements showed an effect on important biological processes such as odontoblast differentiation, angiogenesis, neurogenesis, dentinogenesis and tooth mineralization [72].

Once pulpal progenitor cells differentiate in vitro, they acquire a mineralizing phenotype and deposit mineralized nodules under certain culture conditions. Calcification can be detected and quantified by determining the activity of alkaline phosphatase, an enzyme involved in mineralization processes, or by staining with specific dyes such as alizarin red. A number of authors have described pronounced staining with alizarin red after exposure of the cell cultures to Biodentine™ and likewise to MTA [5, 7, 68, 69, 73–75]. Alkaline phosphatase activity was also equally increased by both MTA and Biodentine™ [5, 7, 68, 74, 75]. A study that cultured organoids with Biodentine™ detected mineralized nodules in the scaffolds by micro-computed tomography [71].

In a translational entire tooth culture model, direct pulp capping was performed ex vivo on human molars, which were then maintained in culture for 4 weeks. Histological examination showed that mineralization foci had formed during the incubation period, and the expression of markers of odontoblastic differentiation such as dentine sialoprotein and nestin had increased [3, 76].

3.3.5.2 In Vivo

Responses of the pulp to Biodentine™ were also assessed in vivo in several animal studies. For example, pulps were exposed in rat models followed by direct capping with Biodentine™, MTA or calcium hydroxide. Thorough analysis of the treated teeth by micro-computed tomography and histologic processing showed the reproducible induction of a homogenous dentine bridge by both tricalcium silicate cements [77–80]. In detail, Biodentine™ was described to provoke a particularly thick hard tissue barrier [77]; at the same time only minor local inflammation was observed and the involvement of Wnt/β-catenin signalling was suggested [78]. Similar results were observed for direct pulp capping procedures in dogs, where Biodentine™ and ProRoot® MTA facilitated a complete bridging while the inflammatory response was low compared to calcium hydroxide [81]. Another research group performed pulpotomies as well as direct pulp capping on pig teeth and, again, Biodentine™ and ProRoot® MTA performed equally well and stimulated formation of tertiary dentine in both applications while the local inflammation was mild [82].

Interestingly, several studies evaluated the reaction to Biodentine™ histologically in the course of direct pulp capping as well as pulpotomy in humans. Pulps were exposed cervically and occlusally in permanent premolars as well as third molars scheduled for extraction, and direct pulp capping was conducted with bioactive compounds [83–85]. Histological examination and cone-beam computed tomography (CBCT) imaging showed that the application of both Biodentine™ and MTA on human pulp reliably resulted in the formation of a hard tissue bridge; however, some reported a more extensive bridging with Biodentine™ [83, 84]. Likewise, the application of tricalcium silicate cements for pulpotomy in humans was investigated. Biodentine™ was applied in primary teeth in comparison to an experimental material and revealed minor inflammation and successful hard tissue formation at the amputation site [86]. Similarly, Biodentine™, ProRoot® MTA and TheraCal LC® were used for pulpotomy in third molars, which were examined clinically and histologically after 8 weeks. Whereas teeth treated with Biodentine™ and ProRoot® MTA were asymptomatic, significant pain was reported by patients in the TheraCal LC® group. Moreover, dentine bridge formation was observed most frequently in teeth treated with Biodentine™, followed by ProRoot® MTA; however, it was a rare event when TheraCal LC® was applied [87].

3.3.6 The Role of Hydration By-Products upon Setting

Immediately after carious excavation and Biodentine™ application on the remaining dentine, a direct contact between the cement and injured odontoblastic processes may occur. Also, solubilized by-products after hydration of the material diffuse through dentinal tubules and interact with odontoblast layer and the underlying pulp tissue. However, upon pulp exposure, Biodentine™ interacts directly with the underlying connective tissue while the released hydration by-products modify the local microenvironment and affect the pulp physiological processes required to initiate the tertiary dentine synthesis.

Calcium silicate cements set upon hydration and during this reaction, hydration by-products can be released. Most calcium silicate cements lead to calcium hydroxide formation and leaching of hydroxyl and calcium ions as demonstrated for MTA and Biodentine™, amongst others [88–90]. The released hydroxyl ions increase pH in the underlying tissue providing an antimicrobial activity [91] and leading to the formation of a thin necrotic layer between the remaining vital tissue and the pulp capping agent [92, 93]. This necrotic zone acts as a barrier protecting the underlying vital pulp cells from the material's alkaline pH. The formation of this superficial necrotic layer is followed by tertiary dentine formation by dental pulp stem cells [60].

The hydration also leads to calcium ion release. Calcium acts as a ubiquitous second messenger with multiple physiological roles on intracellular mechanisms such as proliferation and cell differentiation by activating protein kinases. Calcium ions are involved both in odontoblastic differentiation and mineralization processes [94–96]. This explains the fact that calcium ion release from pulp capping materials is investigated in vitro for their potential in inducing odontoblastic differentiation and mineralization [97]. It should be noted that many studies have reported the interest of calcium release for inducing pulp mineralization. However, the required calcium concentrations necessary to achieve these results still need to be determined [98]. Analysis of Biodentine™ after setting by X-ray diffraction demonstrated a significant peak of calcium hydroxide formation [89], which has long been used for pulp capping with a well-demonstrated dentine bridge formation.

The material also contains silicon ions known to stimulate young bone formation by stimulating osteoblasts [99]. In case of direct pulp capping, it is believed that the presence of silicon ions in calcium silicate cements, such as Biodentine™, also promotes mineralization. An ex vivo tooth culture model showed that after pulp capping with Biodentine™, small particles of the material were entrapped in the mineralized nodules suggesting that the material itself is involved in odontoblastic differentiation and mineralization [3, 76]. This effect is frequently demonstrated in vitro by an enhanced expression of biomineralization markers such as dentine sialoprotein, alkaline phosphatase, runt-related transcription factor 2 (RUNX2) and osteopontin (SPP1) [5].

3.4 Osteogenic Potential

As already described in a previous section, Biodentine™ is biocompatible and exerts positive effects on bone cells, in particular osteoblasts and osteoclasts [100]. The proliferation and viability of both cell types do not appear to be affected by tricalcium silicate cements, whereas osteoclast differentiation and activity may be reduced, which could result in positive effects on bone remineralization [28, 29]. This osteoinductive potential might play a major role in clinical applications where tricalcium silicate cements get in contact with bony tissues, such as in the therapy of root perforation or external resorption as well as retrograde root filling.

3.4.1 In Vitro

Some in vitro studies have investigated the effects of Biodentine™ and other bio-active materials on osteogenic differentiation and mineralization of progenitor cells. Murine mesenchymal stem cell exposed to eluates of Biodentine™ and MTA showed an increase of osteogenic gene expression as well as intense staining for alkaline phosphatase compared to controls [101]. Likewise, increased mineralization of a murine osteoblast cell line cultured with tricalcium silicate cements has been shown by alizarin red staining [28]. Furthermore, experiments have been performed with human osteoblastoma cells that were exposed to Biodentine™, MTA Plus™ and experimental cements with different radiopacifiers. All materials induced calcium deposition and increase of alkaline phosphatase activity [24]. Another study focused on BMP-2-transfected human osteoblastoma cells, where Biodentine™ and MTA Angelus® had a stimulatory effect on BMP-2 expression and formation of mineralized nodules; however, Biodentine™ induced more intense calcification and a higher activity of alkaline phosphatase [25]. The osteogenic potential of tricalcium silicate cements has also been tested with human bone marrow-derived mesenchymal stem cells, which were placed in parietal bone defects of neonatal mice ex vivo. Analysis by alkaline phosphatase staining and scanning electron microscopy showed good regeneration by ProRoot® MTA and Biodentine™; however, the latter elicited a slightly higher potential for ex vivo regeneration of the bone defects [102].

3.4.2 In Vivo

In addition to the in vitro observations, a histological evaluation of the osteogenic potential of Biodentine™ was the aim of numerous in vivo studies. In a rat model with furcation perforation, both MTA Angelus® and Biodentine™ proved to induce cementum regeneration and only a mild inflammatory response [103]. Furthermore, immunohistochemical analysis in a similar rat model showed a reduction of immune cell density and narrowing of the periodontal space after perforation repair with Biodentine™ and likewise with MTA Angelus®. The number of osteoclasts was significantly reduced, whereas an increased density of osteoblasts, fibroblasts and collagen was observed [104]. Comparable outcomes were obtained in a dog model where furcation perforations were treated with Biodentine™ and ProRoot® MTA [105]. Hence, another in vivo study in dogs reported that both bioactive cements facilitated bone remineralization at furcation perforations; however, ProRoot® MTA led to a greater thickness of mineralized tissue and more frequently to complete sealing of the defect compared to Biodentine™ [106]. In a follow-up study, the authors found local fibre reinsertion perpendicular to the newly formed mineralized tissue and the induction of OPN and ALP expression by both tricalcium silicate cements, where ProRoot® MTA additionally induced expression of BMP-2, BSP, OCN, CAP and CEMP1 [107]. A study conducted in rabbits, where surgical bone defects in the tibia were filled with various bioactive cements, revealed neoformation of bone without local necrosis or accumulation of osteoclasts after histological imaging and ESEM-EDX [108]. Especially MTA showed a close contact to bone without disintegration of material particles while Biodentine™ led to trabecular bone formation with sparse inclusions of residual material [108].

The clinical suitability of Biodentine™ to repair resorptive defects [12, 109–117] and seal root ends during apicoectomy [118, 119] was described in several case reports. Biodentine™ and ProRoot® MTA were used in a clinical trial to repair lateral perforations of teeth scheduled for extraction. The radiological and histological evaluation proved a good applicability of Biodentine™ with few periodontal destructions; however, according to this study, it fell behind ProRoot® MTA regarding formation of cementum-like tissue [120].

3.5 Conclusions

Studies performed in vitro, in animals and in clinic concluded that Biodentine™ can be applied safely in various restorative and endodontic therapies without compromising the target tissue/cell vitality. Beyond this, it supports the migration of tissue-resident cells such as stem cells or cells of the immune system to the site of injury. As a result, inflammatory changes are resolved, and neoangiogenesis as well as innervation is promoted in both the pulp and the tooth-surrounding tissues. Furthermore, Biodentine™ induces osteogenic and odontogenic differentiation and thus lays the foundation for mineralization processes in the bone or the dental pulp, which are prerequisites for healing. Today, tricalcium silicate cements such as

Biodentine™ represent an indispensable therapeutic tool in daily restorative and endodontic practice.

References

1. Hubbell JA. Bioactive biomaterials. Curr Opin Biotechnol. 1999;10:123–9.
2. Emara R, Elhennawy K, Schwendicke F. Effects of calcium silicate cements on dental pulp cells: a systematic review. J Dent. 2018;77:18–36.
3. Laurent P, Camps J, About I. Biodentine(™) induces TGF-β1 release from human pulp cells and early dental pulp mineralization. Int Endod J. 2012;45:439–48.
4. Poggio C, Ceci M, Dagna A, Beltrami R, Colombo M, Chiesa M. In vitro cytotoxicity evaluation of different pulp capping materials: a comparative study. Arh Hig Rada Toksikol. 2015;66:181–8.
5. Chang SW, Lee S-Y, Ann H-J, Kum K-Y, Kim E-C. Effects of calcium silicate endodontic cements on biocompatibility and mineralization-inducing potentials in human dental pulp cells. J Endod. 2014;40:1194–200.
6. Pedano MS, Li X, Li S, Sun Z, Cokic SM, Putzeys E, et al. Freshly-mixed and setting calcium-silicate cements stimulate human dental pulp cells. Dent Mater. 2018;34:797–808.
7. Bortoluzzi EA, Niu L-N, Palani CD, El-Awady AR, Hammond BD, Pei D-D, et al. Cytotoxicity and osteogenic potential of silicate calcium cements as potential protective materials for pulpal revascularization. Dent Mater. 2015;31:1510–22.
8. Sonoyama W, Liu Y, Yamaza T, Tuan RS, Wang S, Shi S, et al. Characterization of the apical papilla and its residing stem cells from human immature permanent teeth: a pilot study. J Endod. 2008;34:166–71.
9. Huang GT-J, Sonoyama W, Liu Y, Liu H, Wang S, Shi S. The hidden treasure in apical papilla: the potential role in pulp/dentin regeneration and bioroot engineering. J Endod. 2008;34:645–51.
10. Sonoyama W, Liu Y, Fang D, Yamaza T, Seo B-M, Zhang C, et al. Mesenchymal stem cell-mediated functional tooth regeneration in swine. PLoS One. 2006;1:e79.
11. Nagata M, Ono N, Ono W. Unveiling diversity of stem cells in dental pulp and apical papilla using mouse genetic models: a literature review. Cell Tissue Res. 2020;4:45–14.
12. Pruthi PJ, Goel S, Yadav P, Nawal RR, Talwar S. Novel application of a calcium silicate-based cement and platelet-rich fibrin in complex endodontic cases: a case series. Gen Dent. 2020;68:46–9.
13. Songtrakul K, Azarpajouh T, Malek M, Sigurdsson A, Kahler B, Lin LM. Modified apexification procedure for immature permanent teeth with a necrotic pulp/apical periodontitis: a case series. J Endod. 2020;46:116–23.
14. Sharma S, Sharma V, Passi D, Srivastava D, Grover S, Dutta SR. Large periapical or cystic lesions in association with roots having open apices managed nonsurgically using 1-step apexification based on platelet-rich fibrin matrix and Biodentine apical barrier: a case series. J Endod. 2018;44:179–85.
15. Niranjan B, Shashikiran ND, Dubey A, Singla S, Gupta N. Biodentine - a new novel bio-inductive material for treatment of traumatically injured tooth (single visit apexification). J Clin Diagn Res. 2016;10:ZJ03–4.
16. Vidal K, Martin G, Lozano O, Salas M, Trigueros J, Aguilar G. Apical closure in apexification: a review and case report of apexification treatment of an immature permanent tooth with Biodentine. J Endod. 2016;42:730–4.
17. Bajwa NK, Jingarwar MM, Pathak A. Single visit apexification procedure of a traumatically injured tooth with a novel bioinductive material (Biodentine). Int J Clin Pediatr Dent. 2015;8:58–61.

18. Khetarpal A, Chaudhary S, Talwar S, Verma M. Endodontic management of open apex using Biodentine as a novel apical matrix. Indian J Dent Res. 2014;25:513–6.
19. Wongwatanasanti N, Jantarat J, Sritanaudomchai H, Hargreaves KM. Effect of bioceramic materials on proliferation and odontoblast differentiation of human stem cells from the apical papilla. J Endod. 2018;44:1270–5.
20. Miller AA, Takimoto K, Wealleans J, Diogenes AR. Effect of 3 bioceramic materials on stem cells of the apical papilla proliferation and differentiation using a dentin disk model. J Endod. 2018;44:599–603.
21. Peters OA, Galicia J, Arias A, Tolar M, Ng E, Shin SJ. Effects of two calcium silicate cements on cell viability, angiogenic growth factor release, and related gene expression in stem cells from the apical papilla. Int Endod J. 2016;49:1132–40.
22. Kim J-M, Lin C, Stavre Z, Greenblatt MB, Shim J-H. Osteoblast-osteoclast communication and bone homeostasis. Cell. 2020;9:2073.
23. Jung S, Mielert J, Kleinheinz J, Dammaschke T. Human oral cells' response to different endodontic restorative materials: an in vitro study. Head Face Med. 2014;10:55–9.
24. Gomes-Cornélio AL, Rodrigues EM, Salles LP, Mestieri LB, Faria G, Guerreiro-Tanomaru JM, et al. Bioactivity of MTA Plus, Biodentine and an experimental calcium silicate-based cement on human osteoblast-like cells. Int Endod J. 2017;50:39–47.
25. Rodrigues EM, Gomes-Cornélio AL, Soares-Costa A, Salles LP, Velayutham M, Rossa-Junior C, et al. An assessment of the overexpression of BMP-2 in transfected human osteoblast cells stimulated by mineral trioxide aggregate and Biodentine. Int Endod J. 2017;50(Suppl 2):e9–e18.
26. Michel A, Erber R, Frese C, Gehrig H, Saure D, Mente J. In vitro evaluation of different dental materials used for the treatment of extensive cervical root defects using human periodontal cells. Clin Oral Investig. 2017;21:753–61.
27. Roodman GD. Cell biology of the osteoclast. Exp Hematol. 1999;27:1229–41.
28. Kim H-S, Kim S, Ko H, Song M, Kim M. Effects of the cathepsin K inhibitor with mineral trioxide aggregate cements on osteoclastic activity. Restor Dent Endod. 2019;44:e17.
29. Kim M, Kim S, Ko H, Song M. Effect of ProRoot MTA® and Biodentine® on osteoclastic differentiation and activity of mouse bone marrow macrophages. J Appl Oral Sci. 2019;27:e20180150.
30. Akbulut MB, Arpaci PU, Eldeniz AU. Effects of four novel root-end filling materials on the viability of periodontal ligament fibroblasts. Restor Dent Endod. 2018;43:e24.
31. Escobar-García DM, Aguirre-López E, Méndez-González V, Pozos-Guillén A. Cytotoxicity and initial biocompatibility of endodontic biomaterials (MTA and Biodentine™) used as root-end filling materials. Biomed Res Int. 2016;2016:7926961, 7 p.
32. Akbulut MB, Uyar Arpaci P, Unverdi EA. Effects of novel root repair materials on attachment and morphological behaviour of periodontal ligament fibroblasts: scanning electron microscopy observation. Microsc Res Tech. 2016;79:1214–21.
33. Zhou H-M, Shen Y, Wang Z-J, Li L, Zheng Y-F, Häkkinen L, et al. In vitro cytotoxicity evaluation of a novel root repair material. J Endod. 2013;39:478–83.
34. Roberts-Clark DJ, Smith AJ. Angiogenic growth factors in human dentine matrix. Arch Oral Biol. 2000;45:1013–6.
35. Widbiller M, Schweikl H, Bruckmann A, Rosendahl A, Hochmuth E, Lindner SR, et al. Shotgun proteomics of human dentin with different prefractionation methods. Sci Rep. 2019;9:4457.
36. Tran-Hung L, Laurent P, Camps J, About I. Quantification of angiogenic growth factors released by human dental cells after injury. Arch Oral Biol. 2008;53:9–13.
37. Cooper PR, Holder MJ, Smith AJ. Inflammation and regeneration in the dentin-pulp complex: a double-edged sword. J Endod. 2014;40:S46–51.
38. Farges J-C, Alliot-Licht B, Renard E, Ducret M, Gaudin A, Smith AJ, et al. Dental pulp defence and repair mechanisms in dental caries. Mediat Inflamm. 2015;2015:230251, 16 p.
39. Goldberg M, Njeh A, Uzunoglu E. Is pulp inflammation a prerequisite for pulp healing and regeneration? Mediat Inflamm. 2015;2015:347649, 11 p.

40. Giraud T, Jeanneau C, Rombouts C, Bakhtiar H, Laurent P, About I. Pulp capping materials modulate the balance between inflammation and regeneration. Dent Mater. 2019;35:24–35.
41. Giraud T, Jeanneau C, Bergmann M, Laurent P, About I. Tricalcium silicate capping materials modulate pulp healing and inflammatory activity in vitro. J Endod. 2018;44:1686–91.
42. Barczak K, Palczewska-Komsa M, Nowicka A, Chlubek D, Buczkowska-Radlińska J. Analysis of the activity and expression of cyclooxygenases COX1 and COX2 in THP-1 monocytes and macrophages cultured with Biodentine™ silicate cement. Int J Mol Sci. 2020;21:2237.
43. Rombouts C, Giraud T, Jeanneau C, About I. Pulp vascularization during tooth development, regeneration, and therapy. J Dent Res. 2017;96:137–44.
44. Youssef A-R, Emara R, Taher MM, Al-Allaf FA, Almalki M, Almasri MA, et al. Effects of mineral trioxide aggregate, calcium hydroxide, Biodentine and Emdogain on osteogenesis, odontogenesis, angiogenesis and cell viability of dental pulp stem cells. BMC Oral Health. 2019;19:133–9.
45. Olcay K, Taşli PN, Güven EP, Ülker GMY, Öğüt EE, Çiftçioğlu E, et al. Effect of a novel bioceramic root canal sealer on the angiogenesis-enhancing potential of assorted human odontogenic stem cells compared with principal tricalcium silicate-based cements. J Appl Oral Sci. 2020;28:e20190215.
46. Garrett DM, Conrad GW. Fibroblast-like cells from embryonic chick cornea, heart, and skin are antigenically distinct. Dev Biol. 1979;70:50–70.
47. Tran-Hung L, Mathieu S, About I. Role of human pulp fibroblasts in angiogenesis. J Dent Res. 2006;85:819–23.
48. Nosrat IV, Smith CA, Mullally P, Olson L, Nosrat CA. Dental pulp cells provide neurotrophic support for dopaminergic neurons and differentiate into neurons in vitro; implications for tissue engineering and repair in the nervous system. Eur J Neurosci. 2004;19:2388–98.
49. Chmilewsky F, Ayaz W, Appiah J, About I, Chung S-H. Nerve growth factor secretion from pulp fibroblasts is modulated by complement C5a receptor and implied in neurite outgrowth. Sci Rep. 2016;6:31799–10.
50. Chmilewsky F, About I, Chung SH. Pulp fibroblasts control nerve regeneration through complement activation. J Dent Res. 2016;95:913–22.
51. Chmilewsky F, Jeanneau C, Laurent P, About I. Pulp fibroblasts synthesize functional complement proteins involved in initiating dentin-pulp regeneration. Am J Pathol. 2014;184:1991–2000.
52. Howard C, Murray PE, Namerow KN. Dental pulp stem cell migration. J Endod. 2010;36:1963–6.
53. Mathieu S, Jeanneau C, Sheibat-Othman N, Kalaji N, Fessi H, About I. Usefulness of controlled release of growth factors in investigating the early events of dentin-pulp regeneration. J Endod. 2013;39:228–35.
54. Jeanneau C, Rufas P, Rombouts C, Giraud T, Dejou J, About I. Can pulp fibroblasts kill cariogenic bacteria? Role of complement activation. J Dent Res. 2015;94:1765–72.
55. Le Fournis C, Hadjichristou C, Jeanneau C, About I. Human pulp fibroblast implication in phagocytosis via complement activation. J Endod. 2019;45:584–90.
56. Fitzgerald M, Chiego DJ, Heys DR. Autoradiographic analysis of odontoblast replacement following pulp exposure in primate teeth. Arch Oral Biol. 1990;35:707–15.
57. About I. Dentin-pulp regeneration: the primordial role of the microenvironment and its modification by traumatic injuries and bioactive materials. Endod Topics. 2013;28:61–89.
58. Simon S, Smith AJ, Berdal A, Lumley PJ, Cooper PR. The MAP kinase pathway is involved in odontoblast stimulation via p38 phosphorylation. J Endod. 2010;36:256–9.
59. Smith AJ, Scheven BA, Takahashi Y, Ferracane JL, Shelton RM, Cooper PR. Dentine as a bioactive extracellular matrix. Arch Oral Biol. 2012;57:109–21.
60. Schröder U, Sundström B. Transmission electron microscopy of tissue changes following experimental pulpotomy of intact human teeth and capping with calcium hydroxide. Odontol Revy. 1974;25:57–68.

61. Widbiller M, Schmalz G. Endodontic regeneration: hard shell, soft core. Odontology. 2015;2020:230251, 10 p.
62. Goldberg M. The dental pulp. Berlin: Springer; 2014.
63. Caplan DJ, Cai J, Yin G, White BA. Root canal filled versus non-root canal filled teeth: a retrospective comparison of survival times. J Public Health Dent. 2005;65:90–6.
64. Schmalz G, Widbiller M, Galler KM. Clinical perspectives of pulp regeneration. J Endod. 2020;46:S161–74.
65. Widbiller M, Bucchi C, Rosendahl A, Spanier G, Buchalla W, Galler KM. Isolation of primary odontoblasts: expectations and limitations. Aust Endod J. 2019;45:693.
66. Simon S, Smith AJ, Lumley PJ, Berdal A, Smith G, Finney S, et al. Molecular characterization of young and mature odontoblasts. Bone. 2009;45:693–703.
67. Ruch JV, Lesot H, Bègue-Kirn C. Odontoblast differentiation. Int J Dev Biol. 1995;39:51–68.
68. Luo Z, Kohli MR, Yu Q, Kim S, Qu T, He W-X. Biodentine induces human dental pulp stem cell differentiation through mitogen-activated protein kinase and calcium-/calmodulin-dependent protein kinase II pathways. J Endod. 2014;40:937–42.
69. Jung JY, Woo SM, Lee BN, Koh JT, Nör JE, Hwang YC. Effect of Biodentine and Bioaggregate on odontoblastic differentiation via mitogen-activated protein kinase pathway in human dental pulp cells. Int Endod J. 2015;48:177–84.
70. Daltoé MO, Paula-Silva FWG, Faccioli LH, Gatón-Hernández PM, De Rossi A, Bezerra Silva LA. Expression of mineralization markers during pulp response to Biodentine and mineral trioxide aggregate. J Endod. 2016;42:596–603.
71. Jeong SY, Lee S, Choi WH, Jee JH, Kim H-R, Yoo J. Fabrication of dentin-pulp-like organoids using dental-pulp stem cells. Cells. 2020;9:642.
72. Rathinam E, Govindarajan S, Rajasekharan S, Declercq H, Elewaut D, De Coster P, et al. Transcriptomic profiling of human dental pulp cells treated with tricalcium silicate-based cements by RNA sequencing. Clin Oral Investig. 2020;42:915.
73. de Mendonça Petta T, Pedroni ACF, Saavedra DF, Faial KDCF, Marques MM, Couto RSD. The effect of three different pulp capping cements on mineralization of dental pulp stem cells. Dent Mater J. 2020;39:222–8.
74. Kang S. Mineralization-inducing potentials of calcium silicate-based pulp capping materials in human dental pulp cells. Yeungnam Univ J Med. 2020;37:217–25.
75. Kim Y, Lee D, Song D, Kim H-M, Kim S-Y. Biocompatibility and bioactivity of set direct pulp capping materials on human dental pulp stem cells. Materials (Basel). 2020;13:3925.
76. Jeanneau C, Laurent P, Rombouts C, Giraud T, About I. Light-cured tricalcium silicate toxicity to the dental pulp. J Endod. 2017;43:2074–80.
77. Kim J, Song Y-S, Min K-S, Kim S-H, Koh J-T, Lee B-N, et al. Evaluation of reparative dentin formation of ProRoot MTA, Biodentine and BioAggregate using micro-CT and immunohistochemistry. Restor Dent Endod. 2016;41:29–36.
78. Yaemkleebbua K, Osathanon T, Nowwarote N, Limjeerajarus CN, Sukarawan W. Analysis of hard tissue regeneration and Wnt signalling in dental pulp tissues after direct pulp capping with different materials. Int Endod J. 2019;52:1605–16.
79. Amin LE, Montaser M. Comparative evaluation of pulpal repair after direct pulp capping using stem cell therapy and biodentine: an animal study. Aust Endod J. 2020;21:763.
80. Chicarelli LPG, Webber MBF, Amorim JPA, Rangel ALCA, Camilotti V, Sinhoreti MAC, et al. Effect of tricalcium silicate on direct pulp capping: experimental study in rats. Eur J Dent. 2020;100:S102.
81. Zaen El-Din AM, Hamama HH, Abo El-Elaa MA, Grawish ME, Mahmoud SH, Neelakantan P. The effect of four materials on direct pulp capping: an animal study. Aust Endod J. 2020;46:249–56.
82. Shayegan A, Jurysta C, Atash R, Petein M, Abbeele AV. Biodentine used as a pulp-capping agent in primary pig teeth. Pediatr Dent. 2012;34:e202–8.
83. Hoseinifar R, Eskandarizadeh A, Parirokh M, Torabi M, Safarian F, Rahmanian E. Histological evaluation of human pulp response to direct pulp capping with MTA, CEM cement, and Biodentine. J Dent (Shiraz). 2020;21:177–83.

84. Nowicka A, Wilk G, Lipski M, Kołecki J, Buczkowska-Radlińska J. Tomographic evaluation of reparative dentin formation after direct pulp capping with Ca(OH)2, MTA, Biodentine, and dentin bonding system in human teeth. J Endod. 2015;41:1234–40.

85. Jalan A, Warhadpande M, Dakshindas D. A comparison of human dental pulp response to calcium hydroxide and Biodentine as direct pulp-capping agents. J Conserv Dent. 2017;20:129.

86. Elhamouly Y, El Backly RM, Talaat DM, Omar SS, El Tantawi M, Dowidar KML. Tailored 70S30C bioactive glass induces severe inflammation as pulpotomy agent in primary teeth: an interim analysis of a randomised controlled trial. Clin Oral Investig. 2021. (Online ahead of print); https://doi.org/10.1007/s00784-020-03707-5.

87. Bakhtiar H, Nekoofar MH, Aminishakib P, Abedi F, Naghi Moosavi F, Esnaashari E, et al. Human pulp responses to partial pulpotomy treatment with TheraCal as compared with Biodentine and ProRoot MTA: a clinical trial. J Endod. 2017;43:1786–91.

88. Camilleri J, Sorrentino F, Damidot D. Investigation of the hydration and bioactivity of radiopacified tricalcium silicate cement, Biodentine and MTA Angelus. Dent Mater. 2013;29:580–93.

89. Camilleri J. Hydration characteristics of Biodentine and Theracal used as pulp capping materials. Dent Mater. 2014;30:709–15.

90. Natale LC, Rodrigues MC, Xavier TA, Simões A, de Souza DN, Braga RR. Ion release and mechanical properties of calcium silicate and calcium hydroxide materials used for pulp capping. Int Endod J. 2015;48:89–94.

91. Torabinejad M, Hong CU, McDonald F, Pitt Ford TR. Physical and chemical properties of a new root-end filling material. J Endod. 1995;21:349–53.

92. Téclès O, Laurent P, Aubut V, About I. Human tooth culture: a study model for reparative dentinogenesis and direct pulp capping materials biocompatibility. J Biomed Mater Res. 2008;85:180–7.

93. Aeinehchi M, Eslami B, Ghanbariha M, Saffar AS. Mineral trioxide aggregate (MTA) and calcium hydroxide as pulp-capping agents in human teeth: a preliminary report. Int Endod J. 2003;36:225–31.

94. Ghilotti J, Sanz JL, López-García S, Guerrero-Gironés J, Pecci-Lloret MP, Lozano A, et al. Comparative surface morphology, chemical composition, and cytocompatibility of Bio-C repair, Biodentine, and ProRoot MTA on hDPCs. Materials (Basel). 2020;13:2189.

95. Okabe T, Sakamoto M, Takeuchi H, Matsushima K. Effects of pH on mineralization ability of human dental pulp cells. J Endod. 2006;32:198–201.

96. Zanini M, Sautier JM, Berdal A, Simon S. Biodentine induces immortalized murine pulp cell differentiation into odontoblast-like cells and stimulates biomineralization. J Endod. 2012;38:1220–6.

97. An S. The emerging role of extracellular Ca2+ in osteo/odontogenic differentiation and the involvement of intracellular Ca2+ signaling: from osteoblastic cells to dental pulp cells and odontoblasts. J Cell Physiol. 2019;234:2169–93.

98. Braga RR, About I. How far do calcium release measurements properly reflect its multiple roles in dental tissue mineralization? Clin Oral Investig. 2019;23:501–11.

99. Bielby RC, Christodoulou IS, Pryce RS, Radford WJP, Hench LL, Polak JM. Time- and concentration-dependent effects of dissolution products of 58S sol-gel bioactive glass on proliferation and differentiation of murine and human osteoblasts. Tissue Eng. 2004;10:1018–26.

100. Mori GG, Teixeira LM, de Oliveira DL, Jacomini LM, da Silva SR. Biocompatibility evaluation of Biodentine in subcutaneous tissue of rats. J Endod. 2014;40:1485–8.

101. Lee B-N, Lee K-N, Koh J-T, Min K-S, Chang H-S, Hwang I-N, et al. Effects of 3 endodontic bioactive cements on osteogenic differentiation in mesenchymal stem cells. J Endod. 2014;40:1217–22.

102. Costa F, Sousa Gomes P, Fernandes MH. Osteogenic and angiogenic response to calcium silicate-based endodontic sealers. J Endod. 2016;42:113–9.

103. de Sousa RM, Scarparo RK, Steier L, de Figueiredo JAP. Periradicular inflammatory response, bone resorption, and cementum repair after sealing of furcation perforation with mineral trioxide aggregate (MTA Angelus™) or Biodentine™. Clin Oral Investig. 2019;23:4019–27.

104. da Fonseca TS, Silva GF, Guerreiro-Tanomaru JM, Delfino MM, Sasso-Cerri E, Tanomaru-Filho M, et al. Biodentine and MTA modulate immunoinflammatory response favoring bone formation in sealing of furcation perforations in rat molars. Clin Oral Investig. 2019;23:1237–52.
105. Cardoso M, Dos Anjos Pires M, Correlo V, Reis R, Paulo M, Viegas C. Biodentine for furcation perforation repair: an animal study with histological, radiographic and micro-computed tomographic assessment. Iran Endod J. 2018;13:323–30.
106. Silva LAB, Pieroni KAMG, Nelson-Filho P, Silva RAB, Hernandéz-Gatón P, Lucisano MP, et al. Furcation perforation: periradicular tissue response to Biodentine as a repair material by histopathologic and indirect immunofluorescence analyses. J Endod. 2017;43:1137–42.
107. Silva RAB, Borges ATN, Hernandéz-Gatón P, de Queiroz AM, Arzate H, Romualdo PC, et al. Histopathological, histoenzymological, immunohistochemical and immunofluorescence analysis of tissue response to sealing materials after furcation perforation. Int Endod J. 2019;52:1489–500.
108. Gandolfi MG, Iezzi G, Piattelli A, Prati C, Scarano A. Osteoinductive potential and bone-bonding ability of ProRoot MTA, MTA Plus and Biodentine in rabbit intramedullary model: microchemical characterization and histological analysis. Dent Mater. 2017;33:e221–38.
109. Borkar S, de Noronha de Ataide I. Management of a massive resorptive lesion with multiple perforations in a molar: case report. J Endod. 2015;41:753–8.
110. Umashetty G, Hoshing U, Patil S, Ajgaonkar N. Management of inflammatory internal root resorption with Biodentine and thermoplasticised gutta-percha. Case Rep Dent. 2015;2015:452609, 4 p.
111. Salzano S, Tirone F. Conservative nonsurgical treatment of class 4 invasive cervical resorption: a case series. J Endod. 2015;41:1907–12.
112. Pruthi PJ, Dharmani U, Roongta R, Talwar S. Management of external perforating root resorption by intentional replantation followed by Biodentine restoration. Dent Res J. 2015;12:488–93.
113. Karypidou A, Chatzinikolaou I-D, Kouros P, Koulaouzidou E, Economides N. Management of bilateral invasive cervical resorption lesions in maxillary incisors using a novel calcium silicate-based cement: a case report. Quintessence Int. 2016;47:637–42.
114. Baranwal AK. Management of external invasive cervical resorption of tooth with Biodentine: a case report. J Conserv Dent. 2016;19:296–9.
115. Ambu E, Fimiani M, Vigna M, Grandini S. Use of bioactive materials and limited FOV CBCT in the treatment of a replanted permanent tooth affected by inflammatory external root resorption: a case report. Eur J Paediatr Dent. 2017;18:51–5.
116. Eftekhar L, Ashraf H, Jabbari S. Management of invasive cervical root resorption in a mandibular canine using Biodentine as a restorative material: a case report. Iran Endod J. 2017;12:386–9.
117. Karunakar P, Soloman RV, Anusha B, Nagarjun M. Endodontic management of invasive cervical resorption: report of two cases. J Conserv Dent. 2018;21:578–81.
118. Pawar AM, Kokate SR, Shah RA. Management of a large periapical lesion using Biodentine(™) as retrograde restoration with eighteen months evident follow up. J Conserv Dent. 2013;16:573–5.
119. Caron G, Azérad J, Faure M-O, Machtou P, Boucher Y. Use of a new retrograde filling material (Biodentine) for endodontic surgery: two case reports. Int J Oral Sci. 2014;6:250–3.
120. Tirone F, Salzano S, Piattelli A, Perrotti V, Iezzi G. Response of periodontium to mineral trioxide aggregate and Biodentine: a pilot histological study on humans. Aust Dent J. 2018;63:231–41.

Biodentine™ in Inflammation and Pain Control

4

Fionnuala T. Lundy, Thomas Giraud, Ikhlas A. El-Karim, and Imad About

4.1 Introduction

The dental pulp is extensively innervated by nerve fibres of the peripheral nervous system [1, 2]. The majority of these are sensory trigeminal afferent nerves (transmitting signals towards the brain), with the remainder being characterised as autonomic efferents (transmitting signals away from the brain). The sensory nerve fibres detect noxious stimuli in the local environment and respond by transmitting nerve impulses from the tooth to the central nervous system, where interpretation and/or modulation of these impulses occurs, giving rise to the sensation of pain. Indeed, there is evidence that neuroplasticity in both the central and peripheral nervous systems, following dental pulp injury, can contribute to the development of chronic pain [3].

The autonomic (sympathetic and parasympathetic) nerves transmit signals from the brain to the dental pulp and have been studied in much less detail. It is currently understood that the sympathetic nerves contribute to the regulation of pulpal blood flow and undoubtedly influence sensory function, particularly when the dental pulp is inflamed [4]. Indeed, intact sympathetic innervation is important for the recruitment and migration of inflammatory cells in the dental pulp [5]. There is incomplete

F. T. Lundy (✉) · I. A. El-Karim
The Wellcome-Wolfson Institute for Experimental Medicine, School of Medicine, Dentistry and Biomedical Sciences, Queen's University Belfast, Belfast, UK
e-mail: F.Lundy@qub.ac.uk; i.elkarim@qub.ac.uk

T. Giraud
Aix Marseille University, CNRS, ISM, Institute of Movement Science, Marseille, France

Assistance Publique-Hôpitaux de Marseille, Pôle Odontologie, Hôpital Timone, Marseille, France

I. About
Aix Marseille University, CNRS, ISM, Institute of Movement Science, Marseille, France
e-mail: imad.about@univ-amu.fr

© Springer Nature Switzerland AG 2022
I. About (ed.), *Biodentine™*, https://doi.org/10.1007/978-3-030-80932-4_4

evidence for parasympathetic innervation of the dental pulp, although the neuropeptide, vasoactive intestinal polypeptide (VIP), considered a marker for parasympathetic nerves, has been detected within the human dental pulp tissue [6–9]. While there is no current consensus on parasympathetic innervation in pulpal physiology, a potential role for parasympathetic innervation may yet be elucidated.

4.2   The Physiology of Pulpal Pain

It is well documented that pain of dental origin is prevalent globally in both adults and children [10]. Pain is defined as an unpleasant sensory and emotional experience associated with actual or potential tissue damage or described in terms of such damage [11]. The sensation of pain alerts the brain to potential danger and although it is perceived as unpleasant and unwanted, its ultimate purpose is protective.

Dental pain is experienced when sensory nerve fibres innervating the dental pulp detect the presence of noxious stimuli. Sensory nerve fibres are generally classified based on their diameters and conduction velocities; 'A fibres' are myelinated nerves with large diameters and high conduction velocities, whereas 'C fibres' are unmyelinated with smaller diameters and lower conduction velocities. The trigeminal afferent sensory axons that innervate the dental pulp include both A fibres and C fibres, with approximately 13% of the pulpal sensory nerves classified as myelinated A fibres (93% Aδ and 7% Aβ) and the remaining 87% classed as unmyelinated C fibres [12, 13]. Somewhat surprisingly, it is reported that although the vast majority of pulpal nerves are unmyelinated, the parent axons entering the tooth through the apical foramen tend to be myelinated. Immunohistological studies by Henry et al. [14] support the view that unmyelinated dental pulp axons have phenotypic similarities with myelinated axons, such as their expression of neurofilament. It is now recognised that many myelinated nerves lose their myelin sheath on entering the dental pulp or as they course and branch from the radicular to the coronal pulp tissue [15].

4.2.1   Nerves

Nerve fibres can perceive a wide variety of noxious stimuli in the dental pulp, including thermal, chemical and mechanical stimuli (Table 4.1).

Although pulpal sensory neurons are generally classified based on their morphology and speed of conduction, they can also be classified based on their neurochemistry (expression of receptors/channels and neurotransmitters). The expression of various receptors and channels, such as transient receptor potential (TRP) channels, as well as acid-sensing ion channels (ASIC), potassium (K^+), sodium (Na^+) and ligand-gated ion channels on both A- and C-fibre neurones, plays a vital role in noxious stimuli detection. The TRP family of ion channels are nonselective cation channels that respond to a wide range of thermal, chemical and mechanical stimuli [17]. Based on their sequence homology, there are six mammalian TRP subfamilies:

Table 4.1 Location of nerve fibre types within the dental pulp, stimuli that they respond to and the resulting pain sensation perceived [16]

Nerve fibre type	Mechanical threshold	Pulpal location	Stimulus	Pain sensation
Aβ fibres	Low	Peripheral pulp; inner dentine	Air puff; vibration	Innocuous 'pre-pain' sensations; sharp, short-lasting pain
Aδ fibres	High	Peripheral pulp; inner dentine	Heat/cold; mechanical sensations (drilling, probing)	Sharp, short-lasting pain
C fibres	High	Pulp proper	Inflammatory mediators; heat; mechanical injury	Dull, throbbing ache; longer lasting pain

vanilloid (TRPV), ankyrin (TRPA), melastatin (TRPM), canonical/classical (TRPC), polycystin (TRPP) and mucolipin (TRPML). The TRPV, TRPA and TRPM families have been widely studied as the nociceptive TRP channels. The TRPV, TRPA and TRPM families contain members that are thermo-sensitive ion channels, responding to hot (TRPV1 >43 °C), cold (TRPA1 <17 °C) and cool (TRPM8 <27 °C) bodily temperatures, respectively (discussed in detail below). TRP channels are classified as polymodal ion channels, responding to both chemical [18] and mechanical stimuli [19]. TRPV1, TRPM8, TRPA1 [20] and TRPV4 [21] are expressed by human dental primary afferent neurons.

Many of the TRP channels are also expressed on odontoblasts and pulp cells and therefore sensory perception within the dental pulp is unlikely to be exclusive to pulpal nerves.

4.2.2 Odontoblasts

It is not surprising that the odontoblast layer, with its strategic anatomical location subjacent to the dentine layer, has been proposed to have a sensory role within the dental pulp. The identification of functional K^+ channels [22, 23], Na^+ channels [22, 24] and TRP channels [25] on human odontoblasts supports their roles in detecting external stimuli and potentially mediating pain sensation. The finding that odontoblasts are capable of generating action potentials [24] provides further support for their role in the initiation of pain transmission. Action potential in odontoblasts could induce depolarisation beyond the neuronal threshold potential and allow propagation of signals from the odontoblast to the nerve, and ultimately along the nerve fibre. Alternatively, extracellular ATP could act as a signalling molecule between odontoblasts and nerves [26]. Odontoblasts have been shown to release ATP via pannexin-3 [27] and this extracellular ATP could act on the P2X3 channels expressed on peripheral nerves. The identification and functionality of TRP channels on odontoblasts allow physiologically relevant pain sensations, such as hot and cold, to be detected and these are discussed in further detail below.

4.3 Odontoblasts and Pulp Cells Express Functional Hot and Cold Receptors

Amongst the nociceptors identified in the dental pulp, much interest has been focused on the TRP channels, and in particular the thermo-sensitive TRPV, TRPA and TRPM families. The TRPV1 channel is renowned for its sensitivity to capsaicin (8-methyl-N-vanillyl-trans-6-nonenamide), the pungent ingredient of hot chilli peppers. In line with its polymodal properties, TRPV1 is also responsive to temperature (>43 °C) and acidic pH (<pH 5.5). Of particular interest is the finding that the sensitivity of TRPV1 to noxious heat can be enhanced by inflammation, which could provide a mechanism through which tissue injury can produce thermal hypersensitivity [28]. The TRPV2, TRPV3 and TRPV4 channels also respond to increased temperature, with various activation thresholds [29–31]. Moreover, TRPV2 and TRPV4 have been shown to respond to mechanical or osmotic stimuli [32, 33].

TRPA1 is the only known member of the TRPA family and it has been shown to be activated by painfully cold (<17 °C) temperatures [34], whereas the TRPM8 channel responds to cool (<27 °C) temperatures [35, 36]. Like the heat-sensing TRPV channels, the TRPA1 and TRPM8 channels are polymodal and display chemosensitivity to a range of natural ligands. TRPA1 is activated by natural isothiocyanate-containing compounds, such as horseradish, mustard oil and wasabi [37], whereas TRPM8 is activated by menthol [35, 36], which is recognised to elicit a cooling sensation in the mouth.

Although the physiological relevance of thermosensitive TRPs is often questioned in medical research fields, it is conceivable that high temperatures could be reached near the dental pulp during cavity preparation, and that cold temperatures could be reached if dentine is exposed to frozen foodstuffs. In human odontoblasts, the expression of thermosensitive TRPs equips these cells with specific channels to facilitate direct responses to environmental hot and cold temperatures. Thermosensitive TRP channels have been identified in native human odontoblasts and in cultured odontoblast-like cells, the latter being used for in vitro experiments as native odontoblasts are terminally differentiated and cannot be passaged in culture. Our research group initially demonstrated functional TRPV1, TRPA1 and TRPM8 channels in human odontoblasts and odontoblast-like cells [25], supporting the idea that TRP channels play a role in mediating thermal sensation in teeth. Further studies provided evidence for functional TRPV4 [38], and gene and protein expression of TRPV2 and TRPV3 [39] in human odontoblast-like cells. TRPM8 functionality in freshly isolated native human odontoblasts has also been corroborated [40].

Despite the TRP channel research field largely focusing on 'sensory' cells, mammalian TRP channel expression was first identified in mouse fibroblast (COS) cells [41]. Moreover, several TRP channel family members have been studied in dental pulp fibroblasts. TRPM2 (closely related to TRPM8) is expressed in dental pulp fibroblasts, with increased expression in irreversible pulpitis [42]. Furthermore, functional TRPA1 and TRPM8 channels have been reported in dental pulpal fibroblasts, suggesting a possible role for fibroblasts in mediating cold/cool sensations in dental pulp tissue [43].

4.4   Pulpal Pain and Inflammation

Dental caries and trauma are the leading causes of pulp inflammation. This inflammation is initiated as soon as bacteria or their toxins reach the dental pulp through the dentine tubules. Upon detection of bacteria or their toxins, pulp cells release defence molecules aimed at initiating an inflammatory reaction to eliminate the invading bacteria. Depending on caries depth, different cell populations recognise bacteria and release cytokines to initiate an inflammatory reaction.

Odontoblasts play a significant role as a first defence line as they secrete antimicrobial peptides (β-defensins) and express surface molecules such as Toll-like receptors (TLRs), and nucleotide-oligomerisation-binding domains (NODs), which recognise pathogen-associated molecular patterns (PAMPs) on bacteria. It has been shown that TLR and NOD activation by invading bacteria/toxins activates mitogen-activated protein kinases and nuclear factor kappa-B ligand (NF-κB) which control transcription of DNA and subsequent cytokine production [44].

When bacteria reach the dental pulp, odontoblasts and other resident immune cells, such as macrophages, secrete pro-inflammatory cytokines, which play a role in immune cell recruitment. Furthermore, recent data have demonstrated that pulp fibroblasts secrete pro-inflammatory cytokines such as interleukin-6 (IL-6), interleukin-8 (IL-8), complement bioactive molecules and angiogenic growth factors, such as vascular endothelial growth factor (VEGF) [45]. IL-6 and -8 are considered as potent cytokines involved in the acute inflammatory process [46]. IL-6 is responsible for stimulating acute-phase protein synthesis, as well as the production of neutrophils in the bone marrow, while IL-8 is known as a neutrophil chemotactic factor. VEGF acts on vascular permeability during initiation of inflammation [47].

Pulp fibroblasts also express and synthesise complement active molecules which play multiple roles in the initiation and control of inflammation [48]. Indeed, complement C3a and C5a are known as anaphylatoxins. They induce vascular permeability and provide a chemotactic gradient to direct phagocytic cell recruitment to the injury site. C3b opsonises pathogens and enhances their phagocytosis by the recruited phagocytes while a complex structure of several complement molecules known as the membrane attack complex (MAC) allows direct lysis of pathogens.

Moreover, nerve fibres in the dental pulp contain neuropeptides [49–52] which are released into the local tissue by an axonal reflex following activation of sensory neurons by both external and internal stimuli. The locally released neuropeptides orchestrate the inflammatory response via increased vascular permeability, plasma extravasation and oedema formation [52]. The subsequent recruitment and infiltration of immune and inflammatory cells facilitate increased levels of master inflammatory cytokines, such as tumour necrosis factor-alpha (TNF-α), IL-1β, IL-8 and neurotrophic factors, such as nerve growth factor (NGF) [28], that modulate nociceptive TRP channels and cause increased nociceptive excitation and prolonged nociceptor firing [53], characteristic of inflammatory pain conditions. Many studies reported a direct correlation between the level of neuropeptides, TRP channel expression and pulpal pain [38, 49, 54]. Therefore, modulation of neuronal excitability and TRP channel sensitisation is likely to result in effective pain relief.

4.5   Biodentine Sealing and Antibacterial Potentials

In restorative dentistry, bacterial infiltration is one of the main factors affecting restoration success. Indeed, a retrospective study performed on 317 class V cavities to determine the factors influencing pulpal response to cavity restorations demonstrated that, in most cases, the presence of bacteria on the cavity walls was associated with severe pulp inflammation [55]. This explains why a special attention is given to the material sealing and its antibacterial potential to eliminate both residual and infiltrating bacteria.

The antimicrobial potential of Biodentine has been evaluated in numerous studies and compared to other capping materials. When freshly mixed Biodentine was tested on *Streptococcus mutans*, *Enterococcus faecalis*, *Escherichia coli* and *Candida albicans*, it showed a higher antibacterial effect ($p < 0.05$) than mineral trioxide aggregate (ProRoot® MTA, Dentsply) and a glass ionomer cement [56]. However, the outcome of comparative studies varies from one to another depending on the experimental protocol and tested bacterial strains and whether these are isolated bacteria or organised in a biofilm. Overall, hydroxyl ions released upon hydration of Biodentine lead to an alkaline pH in the surrounding environment with antimicrobial effects. This alkaline pH is also produced with other capping materials such as MTA or calcium hydroxide. Thus, given the fact that the antibacterial mechanism is the same, comparative experimental data should be interpreted with caution.

According to the manufacturer, Biodentine can be used as a permanent bulk dentine substitute and as a temporary enamel substitute for up to 6 months. Given its wide range of applications in restorative dentistry and endodontics and in order to protect the underlying tissues, an intimate interaction of Biodentine with hard and soft tissues is essential in restorative dentistry and endodontic applications. This should lead to a hermetic marginal seal to prevent bacterial infiltration and to provide pulp protection. Experimental work using third molar teeth was exploited to investigate Biodentine marginal sealing either alone or in combination of other resin-based materials in Class II cavities [57]. No marginal leakage was observed at the Biodentine/dentine interface nor at the enamel/Biodentine interface when the whole cavity was filled with Biodentine as a bulk restorative material, replacing dentine and enamel without any prior conditioning treatment. Additionally, no leakage was observed when Biodentine surface was prepared with the total-etch technique and resin composite application. The sealing with Biodentine was similar to that of resin-modified glass ionomer cement (Fuji II LC, GC) considered as a reference material in this type of indications [57]. An interesting study compared the shear bond strengths of different adhesive systems to Biodentine [58]. Adhesive systems such as Prime&Bond NT (Dentsply): etch-and-rinse adhesive system, Clearfil SE Bond (Kuraray): 2-step self-etch adhesive system and Clearfil S3 Bond (Kuraray): 1-step self-etch adhesive system were applied onto Biodentine discs for 12 min or 24 h and then a composite material (Clearfil Majesty, Kuraray) was applied. Data showed that the shear bond strengths were the same for different adhesive systems to Biodentine [58]. This confirms that different restorative materials can be overlaid successfully on the material's surface [57, 58].

Biodentine marginal sealing was also evaluated as root-end filling material in endodontic surgery, perforation repair or apical plug. Experimental work was conducted on extracted teeth to evaluate this property by simulating root-end resection and filling and comparing Biodentine to ProRoot® MTA and IRM® (Dentsply). After resection, root canals were filled with 3 mm of Biodentine. After setting, *E. faecalis* was then cultured on the coronal part of the teeth. Bacterial colonisation was evaluated by confocal microscopy using live/dead assay. Results showed no difference in maximal colonisation depth; however, more viable bacteria were found on ProRoot® MTA group as compared to IRM® or Biodentine. This reduction in viable bacteria could lead to a reduced periapical tissue inflammation [59]. In the same manner after perforation repair of extracted teeth with MTA Angelus® or Biodentine and infection with E. faecalis, less viable bacteria were detected at the perforation margins with both materials. However, a higher dead/live bacterial ratio was obtained with Biodentine [60]. Finally, when applied as an apical plug and compared to various MTA and bioceramic formulations, Biodentine was efficient against *E. faecalis* bacterial leakage, regardless of the material thickness [61]. Thus, in addition to its antibacterial potential due to the alkaline pH, Biodentine provides a hermetic sealing both at the coronal and radicular levels.

4.6   Modulation of Pulpal Pain and Inflammation by Biodentine: Evidence from In Vitro Studies

Pulp capping procedures are performed by applying the biomaterial on inflamed/injured pulp. The ideal pulp capping material should have anti-inflammatory properties to control the acute inflammatory response and to facilitate healing and repair. Adequate control of inflammation is also important to effectively relieve acute pain and prevent development of chronic pain conditions.

4.6.1   Biodentine Modulation of Pro- and Anti-inflammatory Molecules

Many studies have shown that Biodentine exerts anti-inflammatory effects by modulating inflammatory cytokine secretion such as IL-6, IL-8, TNF-α, VEGF and IL-1β [62, 63]. The role of these cytokines in neuronal sensitisation and inflammatory pain is well documented [64]; therefore reduction of these cytokines by Biodentine might be one of the mechanisms by which the material alleviates pain when used in managing teeth with symptomatic pulpitis. Furthermore, Biodentine was shown to directly downregulate the expression of pain receptors such as TRPA1 that are upregulated by inflammatory cytokine TNFα in human odontoblasts [65], supporting further a role for this material in the modulation of pain signalling under inflammatory conditions.

Interestingly, the combined pro- and anti-inflammatory effects of Biodentine were investigated in cultures of human periapical lesion cells. Biodentine decreased TNF-α, IL-1β, IL-6, IL-8 and monocyte chemoattractant protein-1 (MCP-1) secretion and inhibited the production of osteolytic receptor activator of nuclear factor kappa-B ligand. This study also demonstrated that Biodentine stimulated the production of IL-10 anti-inflammatory cytokine [66]. Similarly, Biodentine has been shown to induce anti-inflammatory TGF-β1 synthesis from cultured pulp cells [67].

4.6.2 Modulation of Inflammatory Cell Recruitment

The dental pulp contains resident immune surveillance cells, such as macrophages. In case of infection, they detect invading pathogens and initiate the inflammation by producing multiple pro-inflammatory cytokines. The production of pro-inflammatory cytokines has been reported from other pulp cells, such as fibroblasts and odontoblasts [68]. The production of these molecules induces vascular modifications and allows inflammatory cell recruitment at the inflammation site. This follows a well-orchestrated and well-investigated process which starts by inducing vascular modifications with blood vessel dilatation, and production of inflammatory signals which direct inflammatory cell recruitment [69] at the inflammation/injury and induce their activation. This immune cell recruitment implies immune cell adhesion to endothelial cells, their diapedesis through vascular walls and migration to the inflammatory site and their activation to carry out pathogen phagocytosis. Vascular wall modifications by vasodilatation, decreased blood flow and endothelial cell expression of P- and E-selectin, represent an important step for immune cell initial adhesion on endothelial cells. Immune cell integrins strengthen this adhesion by binding to intercellular adhesion molecule-1 and vascular cell adhesion molecule-1 on endothelial cells. Cytoskeleton modifications allow immune cell polarisation [70] and migration from blood vessel to the inflammatory site. The cell recruitment is guided by chemotactic gradients and their subsequent activation at the inflammatory site allows pathogen phagocytosis and inflammation control.

The effects of Biodentine on immune cell recruitment were studied by investigating its effects on pro-inflammatory signal production by pulp fibroblasts and on all above-mentioned inflammatory cell recruitment steps. These effects were compared to those of an adhesive resinous material Xeno®III (Dentsply). The materials' extracts were applied on physically injured and lipoteichoic acid (LTA)-stimulated pulp fibroblasts, simulating an infection with Gram-positive bacteria. Macrophages (THP-1) were used to study immune cell adhesion on human umbilical vein endothelial cells [62]. Fluorescein-labelled macrophage cells were added onto endothelial cell monolayer, under gentle agitation. Fluorescent microscopy showed that Biodentine decreased the number of adhering cells as compared to the control and

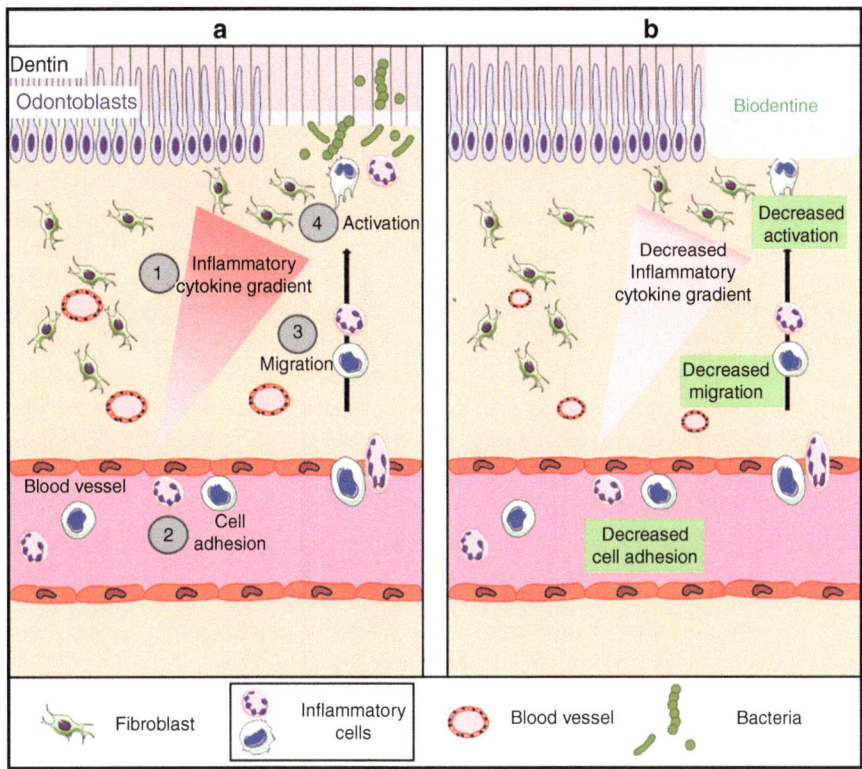

Fig. 4.1 Pro-inflammatory molecule secretion and inflammatory cell recruitment. (**a**) Tissue injury or infection induces release of pro-inflammatory factors from multiple cell types including odontoblasts, fibroblasts and resident macrophages. Inflammatory cells respond to pro-inflammatory signals by adhering to blood vessel walls. Then, they migrate to the inflammation site where they are activated. (**b**) Biodentine™ application decreases pro-inflammatory molecule synthesis and significantly decreases inflammatory cell recruitment by decreasing their adhesion to endothelial cells, migration to the infection site and activation

Xeno®III [62]. The migration step was evaluated using Boyden Chambers. Macrophages were placed in the upper chamber while LTA-stimulated and injured fibroblasts were cultured in the lower chamber with the material extracts. Biodentine induced a significant decrease ($p < 0.05$) of THP-1 cell migration towards LTA-treated fibroblasts as compared to the control and Xeno®III [62]. Finally, the activation step was investigated by incubating macrophages with fibroblast supernatants and detecting adherent immune cells. Biodentine significantly decreased ($p < 0.05$) immune cell activation [62] (Fig. 4.1).

Overall, these experimental data clearly demonstrate that Biodentine modulates the inflammatory response by decreasing the pro-inflammatory signals' release and the subsequent inflammatory cell recruitment and activation in vitro.

4.7   Modulation of Inflammation: Evidence from In Vivo Studies

In line with these findings, the effect of Biodentine on the inflammatory response was investigated in vivo after furcation perforation sealing in rats and compared to ProRoot® White MTA [71]. The histologic analysis was followed at different time periods and demonstrated an initial high value of IL-6-labelled immune cells and osteoclasts at day 7 with both materials. A significant reduction ($p \leq 0.05$) of inflammatory cell density, IL-6 expression and osteoclasts was observed from 7 to 60 days with the two materials. At all time periods, the number of IL-6-labelled immune cells, osteoclasts and periodontal space was higher in the control than in Biodentine and MTA groups. At 60 days, no significant differences in inflammatory cell density, periodontal ligament space, osteoclasts or osteoblasts were found between Biodentine and MTA, while the number of osteoblasts was higher in Biodentine and MTA groups than in the control [71]. A similar study investigated the periradicular tissue response after sealing of furcation perforations with Biodentine, ProRoot® White MTA and gutta-percha as a positive control in dog teeth. Biodentine and MTA exhibited no bone resorption in the furcation region and fewer inflammatory cells and induced new mineralized tissue formation [72].

Similarly, the effect of Biodentine and ProRoot® White MTA on pulp inflammation was investigated after vital pulp therapy of mechanically exposed intact human molars. Histological analysis of teeth extracted after 6 weeks demonstrated the absence or presence of a mild inflammation with no significant differences between the materials. Complete dentine bridge formation was also obtained with both groups [73]. This has also been confirmed recently after direct pulp capping of human teeth where pulps of fully erupted premolars scheduled to be extracted for orthodontic reasons were mechanically exposed in the middle of the cavity floor and treated with MTA, Biodentine or treated dentine matrix hydrogel. Histological analysis demonstrated a mild-to-moderate inflammatory reaction after 2 weeks. A resolution of this inflammatory reaction was observed after 2 months and a complete dentine bridge formed with no significant differences between the three groups [74].

Overall, these data obtained both in vitro and in vivo demonstrate that tri-calcium silicate-based materials such as Biodentine and MTA dampen the inflammatory reaction shortly after application and set adequate conditions for the tissue regeneration.

4.8   Modulation of Pulpal Pain by Biodentine: Evidence from Clinical Studies

The evidence from in vitro studies of the potential role of Biodentine in reducing pain is further supported by human clinical studies in which the material is used for managing the cariously exposed pulp. In teeth with deep caries and limited degree of pulp inflammation as evident from symptoms of mild pain and transient sensitivity to thermal stimuli, a clinical diagnosis of reversible pulpitis is usually made [75]. However, when the pulp is cariously exposed and bacteria gain access to the pulp space, more severe inflammation characterised by spontaneous severe pain develops leading to irreversible pulpitis [75]. Traditionally the treatment of the deep carious lesion involves removal of all carious dentine and/or diseased pulp; however, the emerging body of evidence suggests that such teeth can now be treated more conservatively with vital pulp treatments (VPT) [76] using novel biomaterials including Biodentine.

The success of Biodentine in VPT is documented in Chap. 5 of this book, and we will therefore discuss here its effect on pain relief in these studies, with emphasis on post-operative pain. Pioneer case reports on treatment of symptomatic pulpitis using Biodentine showed that application of this material provided effective pain relief [77]. Following studies including prospective and randomised control trial further confirmed this pain-relieving effect for Biodentine. In teeth with deep caries and exposed pulp, direct pulp capping with Biodentine led to pain relief in all teeth (100%) at 1-week follow-up [78], while Hegde et al. [79] reported post-operative pain relief in 83% of those receiving direct pulp capping with Biodentine.

In adult teeth with clinical diagnosis of irreversible pulpitis treated with complete pulpotomy using Biodentine, pain relief was reported by 93.8% of the subjects 2 days post-operatively [80]. In young permanent teeth with irreversible pulpitis, Biodentine application in pulpotomy was effective in pain relief in 100% of subjects after 2 post-operative days [81]. In a clinical trial investigating Biodentine, ProRoot® MTA and TheraCal® LC (Bisco) as partial pulpotomy agents, none of the participants in Biodentine or MTA arm of the study reported pain at post-operative day 7 [82].

In conclusion, the evidence from clinical studies supports a pain-relieving effect for Biodentine in asymptomatic and symptomatic pulpitis, which is in line with its in vitro anti-inflammatory action.

The following scenario can be envisioned after vital pulp therapy for teeth with pulpitis using Biodentine: In caries-induced pulpitis, recruitment of inflammatory cells and vasodilatation associated with the inflammatory response result in an increase in intra-pulpal pressure and subsequent pain. An expected decrease in intra-pulpal pressure during operative procedure and opening of pulp space coupled with anti-inflammatory effect of Biodentine (Fig. 4.2) contribute to effective pain relief observed in vital pulp therapies.

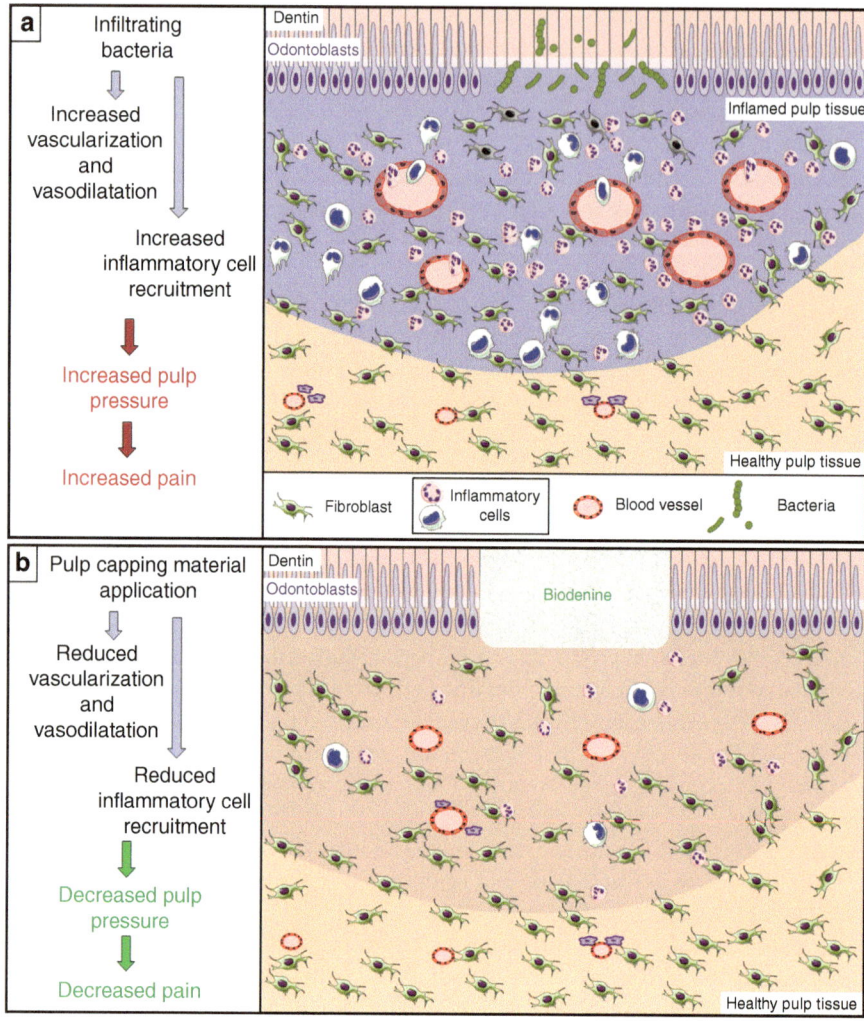

Fig. 4.2 Schematic drawing showing the inflammatory pulp state during pulpitis and after caries removal and application of Biodentine. (**a**) Inflamed pulp is highly vascularised and contains numerous inflammatory cells leading to a high intra-pulpal pressure and pain. (**b**) Applying Biodentine decreases pro-inflammatory molecule secretion and inflammatory cell recruitment. This leads to a decreased pulp pressure and subsequently decreased pain

References

1. Cadden SW, Lisney SJW, Matthews B. Thresholds to electrical stimulation of nerves in cat canine tooth-pulp with Aβ-, Aδ- and C-fibre conduction velocities. Brain Res. 1983;261:31–41.
2. Reader A, Foreman DW. An ultrastructural qualitative investigation of human intradental innervation. J Endod. 1981;7:161–8.

3. Lee C, Ramsey A, De Brito-Gariepy H, Michot B, Podborits E, Melnyk J, Gibbs JL. Molecular, cellular and behavioral changes associated with pathological pain signaling occur after dental pulp injury. Mol Pain. 2017;13:1744806917715173.
4. Olgart L. Neural control of pulpal blood flow. Crit Rev Oral Biol Med. 1996;7:159–71.
5. Haug SR, Heyeraas KJ. Modulation of dental inflammation by the sympathetic nervous system. J Dent Res. 2006;85:488–95.
6. Caviedes-Bucheli J, Muñoz HR, Azuero-Holguín MM, Ulate E. Neuropeptides in dental pulp: the silent protagonists. J Endod. 2008;34:773–88.
7. El Karim IA, Lamey P-J, Ardill J, Linden GJ, Lundy FT. Vasoactive intestinal polypeptide (VIP) and VPAC1 receptor in adult human dental pulp in relation to caries. Arch Oral Biol. 2006;51:849–55.
8. Luthman J, Luthman D, Hökfelt T. Occurrence and distribution of different neurochemical markers in the human dental pulp. Arch Oral Biol. 1992;37:193–208.
9. Rodd HD, Boissonade FM. Comparative immunohistochemical analysis of the peptidergic innervation of human primary and permanent tooth pulp. Arch Oral Biol. 2002;47:375–85.
10. Lipton JA, Ship JA, Larach-Robinson D. Estimated prevalence and distribution of reported orofacial pain in the United States. J Am Dent Assoc. 1993;1939(124):115–21.
11. Merskey H, Bogduk N. IASP taxonomy. Update from pain terms, a curr list with defin notes usage. Classif chronic pain. 2nd ed. IASP Task Force Taxon; 2012. pp. 209–14.
12. Nair PNR, Schroeder HE. Number and size spectra of non-myelinated axons of human premolars. Anat Embryol (Berl). 1995;192:35–41.
13. Nair PN, Luder HU, Schroeder HE. Number and size-spectra of myelinated nerve fibers of human premolars. Anat Embryol (Berl). 1992;186:563–71.
14. Henry MA, Luo S, Levinson SR. Unmyelinated nerve fibers in the human dental pulp express markers for myelinated fibers and show sodium channel accumulations. BMC Neurosci. 2012;13:29.
15. Bae YC, Yoshida A. Ultrastructural basis for craniofacial sensory processing in the brainstem. Int Rev Neurobiol. 2011;97:99–141.
16. Närhi M, Bjørndal L, Pigg M, Fristad I, Haug S. Acute dental pain I: pulpal and dentinal pain. Nor Tannlegeforen Tid. 2016;126:10–8.
17. Ramsey IS, Delling M, Clapham DE. An introduction to TRP channels. Annu Rev Physiol. 2006;68:619–47.
18. Voets T, Nilius B. TRPs make sense. J Membr Biol. 2003;192:1–8.
19. Corey DP, García-Añoveros J, Holt JR, Kwan KY, Lin S-Y, Vollrath MA, Amalfitano A, Cheung EL-M, Derfler BH, Duggan A, et al. TRPA1 is a candidate for the mechanosensitive transduction channel of vertebrate hair cells. Nature. 2004;432:723–30.
20. Park C-K, Kim MS, Fang Z, Li HY, Jung SJ, Choi S-Y, Lee SJ, Park K, Kim JS, Oh SB. Functional expression of thermo-transient receptor potential channels in dental primary afferent neurons: implication for tooth pain. J Biol Chem. 2006;281:17304–11.
21. Bakri MM, Yahya F, Munawar KMM, Kitagawa J, Hossain MZ. Transient receptor potential vanilloid 4 (TRPV4) expression on the nerve fibers of human dental pulp is upregulated under inflammatory condition. Arch Oral Biol. 2018;89:94–8.
22. Ichikawa H, Kim H-J, Shuprisha A, Shikano T, Tsumura M, Shibukawa Y, Tazaki M. Voltage-dependent sodium channels and calcium-activated potassium channels in human odontoblasts in vitro. J Endod. 2012;38:1355–62.
23. Magloire H, Lesage F, Couble ML, Lazdunski M, Bleicher F. Expression and localization of TREK-1 K+ channels in human odontoblasts. J Dent Res. 2003;82:542–5.
24. Allard B, Magloire H, Couble ML, Maurin JC, Bleicher F. Voltage-gated sodium channels confer excitability to human odontoblasts: possible role in tooth pain transmission. J Biol Chem. 2006;281:29002–10.
25. El Karim IA, Linden GJ, Curtis TM, About I, McGahon MK, Irwin CR, Lundy FT. Human odontoblasts express functional thermo-sensitive TRP channels: implications for dentin sensitivity. Pain. 2011;152:2211–23.

26. Shibukawa Y, Sato M, Kimura M, Sobhan U, Shimada M, Nishiyama A, Kawaguchi A, Soya M, Kuroda H, Katakura A, et al. Odontoblasts as sensory receptors: transient receptor potential channels, pannexin-1, and ionotropic ATP receptors mediate intercellular odontoblast-neuron signal transduction. Pflugers Arch. 2015;467:843–63.

27. Magloire H, Maurin JC, Couble ML, Shibukawa Y, Tsumura M, Thivichon-Prince B, Bleicher F. Topical review. Dental pain and odontoblasts: facts and hypotheses. J Orofac Pain. 2010;24:335–49.

28. Julius D, Basbaum AI. Molecular mechanisms of nociception. Nature. 2001;413:203–10.

29. Caterina MJ, Rosen TA, Tominaga M, Brake AJ, Julius D. A capsaicin-receptor homologue with a high threshold for noxious heat. Nature. 1999;398:436–41.

30. Güler AD, Lee H, Iida T, Shimizu I, Tominaga M, Caterina M. Heat-evoked activation of the ion channel, TRPV4. J Neurosci. 2002;22:6408–14.

31. Smith GD, Gunthorpe MJ, Kelsell RE, Hayes PD, Reilly P, Facer P, Wright JE, Jerman JC, Walhin J-P, Ooi L, et al. TRPV3 is a temperature-sensitive vanilloid receptor-like protein. Nature. 2002;418:186–90.

32. Liedtke W, Choe Y, Martí-Renom MA, Bell AM, Denis CS, Sali A, Hudspeth AJ, Friedman JM, Heller S. Vanilloid receptor-related osmotically activated channel (VR-OAC), a candidate vertebrate osmoreceptor. Cell. 2000;103:525–35.

33. Muraki K, Shigekawa M, Imaizumi Y. Chapter 28: A new insight into the function of TRPV2 in circulatory organs. In: Liedtke WB, Heller S, editors. TRP ion channel function in sensory transduction and cellular signaling cascades. Boca Raton, FL: CRC Press/Taylor & Francis; 2007.

34. Story GM, Peier AM, Reeve AJ, Eid SR, Mosbacher J, Hricik TR, Earley TJ, Hergarden AC, Andersson DA, Hwang SW, et al. ANKTM1, a TRP-like channel expressed in nociceptive neurons, is activated by cold temperatures. Cell. 2003;112:819–29.

35. McKemy DD, Neuhausser WM, Julius D. Identification of a cold receptor reveals a general role for TRP channels in thermosensation. Nature. 2002;416:52–8.

36. Peier AM, Moqrich A, Hergarden AC, Reeve AJ, Andersson DA, Story GM, Earley TJ, Dragoni I, McIntyre P, Bevan S, et al. A TRP channel that senses cold stimuli and menthol. Cell. 2002;108:705–15.

37. Jordt S-E, Bautista DM, Chuang H-H, McKemy DD, Zygmunt PM, Högestätt ED, Meng ID, Julius D. Mustard oils and cannabinoids excite sensory nerve fibres through the TRP channel ANKTM1. Nature. 2004;427:260–5.

38. El Karim I, McCrudden MTC, Linden GJ, Abdullah H, Curtis TM, McGahon M, About I, Irwin C, Lundy FT. TNF-α-induced p38MAPK activation regulates TRPA1 and TRPV4 activity in odontoblast-like cells. Am J Pathol. 2015;185:2994–3002.

39. Wen W, Que K, Zang C, Wen J, Sun G, Zhao Z, Li Y. Expression and distribution of three transient receptor potential vanilloid (TRPV) channel proteins in human odontoblast-like cells. J Mol Histol. 2017;48:367–77.

40. Tazawa K, Ikeda H, Kawashima N, Okiji T. Transient receptor potential melastatin (TRPM) 8 is expressed in freshly isolated native human odontoblasts. Arch Oral Biol. 2017;75:55–61.

41. Zhu X, Jiang M, Peyton M, Boulay G, Hurst R, Stefani E, Birnbaumer L. Trp, a novel mammalian gene family essential for agonist-activated capacitative Ca2+ entry. Cell. 1996;85:661–71.

42. Rowland KC, Kanive CB, Wells JE, Hatton JF. TRPM2 immunoreactivity is increased in fibroblasts, but not nerves, of symptomatic human dental pulp. J Endod. 2007;33:245–8.

43. El Karim IA, Linden GJ, Curtis TM, About I, McGahon MK, Irwin CR, Killough SA, Lundy FT. Human dental pulp fibroblasts express the "cold-sensing" transient receptor potential channels TRPA1 and TRPM8. J Endod. 2011;37:473–8.

44. Yumoto H, Hirao K, Hosokawa Y, Kuramoto H, Takegawa D, Nakanishi T, Matsuo T. The roles of odontoblasts in dental pulp innate immunity. Jpn Dent Sci Rev. 2018;54:105–17.

45. El Karim IA, Linden GJ, Irwin CR, Lundy FT. Neuropeptides regulate expression of angiogenic growth factors in human dental pulp fibroblasts. J Endod. 2009;35:829–33.

46. Heinrich PC, Castell JV, Andus T. Interleukin-6 and the acute phase response. Biochem J. 1990;265:621–36.

47. Hippenstiel S, Krüll M, Ikemann A, Risau W, Clauss M, Suttorp N. VEGF induces hyperpermeability by a direct action on endothelial cells. Am J Phys. 1998;274:L678–84.
48. Chmilewsky F, Jeanneau C, Laurent P, About I. Pulp fibroblasts synthesize functional complement proteins involved in initiating dentin-pulp regeneration. Am J Pathol. 2014;184:1991–2000.
49. Awawdeh L, Lundy FT, Shaw C, Lamey PJ, Linden GJ, Kennedy JG. Quantitative analysis of substance P, neurokinin A and calcitonin gene-related peptide in pulp tissue from painful and healthy human teeth. Int Endod J. 2002;35:30–6.
50. Byers MR, Taylor PE, Khayat BG, Kimberly CL. Effects of injury and inflammation on pulpal and periapical nerves. J Endod. 1990;16:78–84.
51. El Karim IA, Lamey P-J, Linden GJ, Awawdeh LA, Lundy FT. Caries-induced changes in the expression of pulpal neuropeptide Y. Eur J Oral Sci. 2006;114:133–7.
52. Lundy FT, Linden GJ. Neuropeptides and neurogenic mechanisms in oral and periodontal inflammation. Crit Rev Oral Biol Med. 2004;15:82–98.
53. Mickle AD, Shepherd AJ, Mohapatra DP. Nociceptive TRP channels: sensory detectors and transducers in multiple pain pathologies. Pharmaceuticals (Basel). 2016;9:72.
54. Chung M-K, Lee J, Duraes G, Ro JY. Lipopolysaccharide-induced pulpitis up-regulates TRPV1 in trigeminal ganglia. J Dent Res. 2011;90:1103–7.
55. Camps J, Déjou J, Rémusat M, About I. Factors influencing pulpal response to cavity restorations. Dent Mater. 2000;16:432–40.
56. Bhavana V, Chaitanya KP, Gandi P, Patil J, Dola B, Reddy RB. Evaluation of antibacterial and antifungal activity of new calcium-based cement (Biodentine) compared to MTA and glass ionomer cement. J Conserv Dent. 2015;18:44–6.
57. Raskin A, Eschrich G, Dejou J, About I. In vitro microleakage of Biodentine as a dentin substitute compared to Fuji II LC in cervical lining restorations. J Adhes Dent. 2012;14:535–42.
58. Odabaş ME, Bani M, Tirali RE. Shear bond strengths of different adhesive systems to Biodentine. Sci World J. 2013;2013:626103.
59. Tsesis I, Elbahary S, Venezia NB, Rosen E. Bacterial colonization in the apical part of extracted human teeth following root-end resection and filling: a confocal laser scanning microscopy study. Clin Oral Investig. 2018;22:267–74.
60. Elbahary S, Haj Yahya S, Koç C, Shemesh H, Rosen E, Tsesis I. Bacterial Colonization and Proliferation in Furcal Perforations Repaired by Different Materials: A Confocal Laser Scanning Microscopy Study. Applied Sciences. 2021;11(8):3403.
61. Lertmalapong P, Jantarat J, Srisatjaluk RL, Komoltri C. Bacterial leakage and marginal adaptation of various bioceramics as apical plug in open apex model. J Investig Clin Dent. 2019;10:e12371.
62. Giraud T, Jeanneau C, Bergmann M, Laurent P, About I. Tricalcium silicate capping materials modulate pulp healing and inflammatory activity in vitro. J Endod. 2018;44:1686–91.
63. Jeanneau C, Laurent P, Rombouts C, Giraud T, About I. Light-cured tricalcium silicate toxicity to the dental pulp. J Endod. 2017;43:2074–80.
64. Sommer C, Kress M. Recent findings on how proinflammatory cytokines cause pain: peripheral mechanisms in inflammatory and neuropathic hyperalgesia. Neurosci Lett. 2004;361:184–7.
65. El Karim IA, McCrudden MTC, McGahon MK, Curtis TM, Jeanneau C, Giraud T, Irwin CR, Linden GJ, Lundy FT, About I. Biodentine reduces tumor necrosis factor alpha-induced TRPA1 expression in odontoblast like cells. J Endod. 2016;42:589–95.
66. Eraković M, Duka M, Bekić M, Tomić S, Ismaili B, Vučević D, Čolić M. Anti-inflammatory and immunomodulatory effects of Biodentine on human periapical lesion cells in culture. Int Endod J. 2020;53:1398–412.
67. Laurent P, Camps J, About I. Biodentine(™) induces TGF-β1 release from human pulp cells and early dental pulp mineralization. Int Endod J. 2012;45:439–48.
68. Cooper PR, Holder MJ, Smith AJ. Inflammation and regeneration in the dentin-pulp complex: a double-edged sword. J Endod. 2014;40:S46–51.
69. Witko-Sarsat V, Rieu P, Descamps-Latscha B, Lesavre P, Halbwachs-Mecarelli L. Neutrophils: molecules, functions and pathophysiological aspects. Lab Investig. 2000;80:617.

70. Niggli V. Signaling to migration in neutrophils: importance of localized pathways. Int J Biochem Cell Biol. 2003;35:1619–38.
71. da Fonseca TS, Silva GF, Guerreiro-Tanomaru JM, Delfino MM, Sasso-Cerri E, Tanomaru-Filho M, Cerri PS. Biodentine and MTA modulate immunoinflammatory response favoring bone formation in sealing of furcation perforations in rat molars. Clin Oral Investig. 2019;23:1237–52.
72. Silva LAB, Pieroni KAMG, Nelson-Filho P, Silva RAB, Hernandéz-Gatón P, Lucisano MP, Paula-Silva FWG, de Queiroz AM. Furcation perforation: periradicular tissue response to Biodentine as a repair material by histopathologic and indirect immunofluorescence analyses. J Endod. 2017;43:1137–42.
73. Nowicka A, Lipski M, Parafiniuk M, Sporniak-Tutak K, Lichota D, Kosierkiewicz A, Kaczmarek W, Buczkowska-Radlińska J. Response of human dental pulp capped with Biodentine and mineral trioxide aggregate. J Endod. 2013;39:743–7.
74. Holiel AA, Mahmoud EM, Abdel-Fattah WM, Kawana KY. Histological evaluation of the regenerative potential of a novel treated dentin matrix hydrogel in direct pulp capping. Clin Oral Investig. 2021;25:2101–12.
75. Glickman GN, Schweitzer JL. Endodontic diagnosis. Chicago, IL: American Association of Endodontists; 2013.
76. Duncan HF, Galler KM, Tomson PL, Simon S, El-Karim I, Kundzina R, Krastl G, Dammaschke T, Fransson H, Markvart M, et al. European Society of Endodontology position statement: management of deep caries and the exposed pulp. Int Endod J. 2019;52:923–34.
77. Villat C, Grosgogeat B, Seux D, Farge P. Conservative approach of a symptomatic carious immature permanent tooth using a tricalcium silicate cement (Biodentine): a case report. Restor Dent Endod. 2013;38:258–62.
78. Brizuela C, Ormeño A, Cabrera C, Cabezas R, Silva CI, Ramírez V, Mercade M. Direct pulp capping with calcium hydroxide, mineral trioxide aggregate, and Biodentine in permanent young teeth with caries: a randomized clinical trial. J Endod. 2017;43:1776–80.
79. Hegde S, Sowmya B, Mathew S, Bhandi SH, Nagaraja S, Dinesh K. Clinical evaluation of mineral trioxide aggregate and Biodentine as direct pulp capping agents in carious teeth. J Conserv Dent. 2017;20:91–5.
80. Taha NA, Abdelkhader SZ. Outcome of full pulpotomy using Biodentine in adult patients with symptoms indicative of irreversible pulpitis. Int Endod J. 2018;51:819–28.
81. Taha NA, Abdulkhader SZ. Full pulpotomy with Biodentine in symptomatic young permanent teeth with carious exposure. J Endod. 2018;44:932–7.
82. Bakhtiar H, Nekoofar MH, Aminishakib P, Abedi F, Naghi Moosavi F, Esnaashari E, Azizi A, Esmailian S, Ellini MR, Mesgarzadeh V, et al. Human pulp responses to partial pulpotomy treatment with TheraCal as compared with Biodentine and ProRoot MTA: a clinical trial. J Endod. 2017;43:1786–91.

Biodentine™ Clinical Applications in Vital Pulp Therapy in Permanent Teeth

5

Avijit Banerjee and Montse Mercadé

5.1 Introduction

One of the major challenges in contemporary minimally invasive (MI) operative dentistry is to enhance the remineralisation/repair process of the retained hypomineralised deep caries-affected dentine after carrying out selective carious tissue removal in an attempt to preserve tooth structure and maintain pulp sensibility and vitality in the long term. Conventional complete carious tissue removal in deep lesions results in a significant increase in pulp exposure and ultimately pulp death [1, 2]. The minimally invasive (MI) approach to the operative caries management of deep, active, cavitated carious lesions encourages the selective removal of only the superficial, highly bacterially contaminated and denatured zone of tissue that is clinically wet, soft and sticky—the caries-infected (or contaminated) dentine. The remaining deeper caries-affected (demineralised) tissues can be healed and repaired by the dentine-pulp complex and therefore can be retained and sealed off using bioactive/bio-interactive restorative materials. This MI intervention preserves more dental tissue and ultimately improves the long-term survival of the dentine-pulp complex [3].

Direct and indirect pulp protection (or capping), using various biocompatible and bioactive restorative materials with specific clinical management protocols

A. Banerjee (✉)
Cariology and Operative Dentistry, Centre for Oral Clinical Translational Sciences, Faculty of Dentistry, Oral and Craniofacial Sciences, King's College London/Guy's and St. Thomas' Hospitals Trust, London, UK
e-mail: avijit.banerjee@kcl.ac.uk

M. Mercadé
Department of Dentistry, Universitat de Barcelona, Barcelona, Spain

Researcher at IDIBELL Institute, Barcelona, Spain

Private Practice Limited to Endodontics and Dental Traumatology in Barcelona, Barcelona, Spain
e-mail: montsemercade@ub.edu

© Springer Nature Switzerland AG 2022
I. About (ed.), *Biodentine™*, https://doi.org/10.1007/978-3-030-80932-4_5

(Table 5.1), has been used to protect and preserve pulp sensibility and induce pulp cells to form protective hard tissues (reactionary/tertiary dentine) [4]. Direct pulp protection is necessary when the vital pulp is visibly exposed due to trauma, iatrogenic cause or exposure during deep carious lesion management. Indirect pulp protection can be considered as an adjunct to selective carious tissue removal in deep carious lesions with a vital pulp and no direct pulp exposure [2, 5]. The ultimate objectives of any pulp protection material should be to (Table 5.2):

- Arrest bacterial activity within the lesion (bactericidal/bacteriostatic)
- Promote protective hard-tissue deposition by stimulating odontoblasts to form tertiary dentine
- Maintain pulp vitality/sensibility
- Adhere to dentine and overlying restorative material
- Provide a biocompatible and durable seal that protects the dentine-pulp complex from further bacterial and noxious agent ingress over time

The success of both direct and indirect pulp protection depends upon the pre-existing vitality and sensibility of the dentine-pulp complex, the bio-interactivity of the materials used and their precise clinical application in obtaining an adequate peripheral seal and adhesion [2, 5]. It is important to note that more contemporary restorative materials exhibit many of the above properties, hence reducing, or even eliminating, the need for individual "liners", "bases" and "capping" materials to be placed separately.

5.2   Histopathology of Carious Dentine

In contemporary MI dentistry, it is important to consider the dentine-pulp complex as one entity since the physiological processes during tooth development, homeostasis, pathology and repair are interlinked and reliant upon one another. The pulp and dentine form a complex network via the dentine tubules and the odontoblast processes. This structural unit consists of the dentine tubules being fluid filled throughout their entire length. This fluid plays an important role as a channel for communication. The primary pulp response to the caries process is activated by bacterial acids, lipopolysaccharides (LPS) and soluble plaque metabolic products. These diffuse towards the pulp against the natural direction of pulp tissue fluid movement. The initial pulp response includes an increased secretory activity by the odontoblasts, leading to tertiary reactionary dentine formation [1]. The most superficial part of the exposed carious dentine begins to decompose and denature by the action of acids and proteolytic enzymes produced by the bacteria and endogenously, respectively [3, 6]. Clinically, this tissue appears as the soft, wet and sticky zone of the lesion. It is often, but not always, darkly stained and discoloured. This caries-infected/contaminated dentine is grossly demineralised with denatured collagen, infiltrated with the highest concentrations of bacteria and irreparably damaged. However, the inner caries-affected layer closer towards the pulp is also

Table 5.1 Pulp protection/capping materials with their main indication, composition, advantages, disadvantages with commercial examples at the time of publication

Material	Main indication	General composition	Advantages	Disadvantages	Commercial examples	References
Calcium hydroxide	Direct/indirect pulp capping, pulpotomy	Base paste: Titanium dioxide, calcium tungstate, 1,3-butylene glycol disalicylate Catalyst paste: Calcium hydroxide, zinc oxide, zinc stearate, ethyl toluene sulfonamide	– Antibacterial properties – Low cytotoxicity	– Highly soluble in oral fluid – Dissolution over time – Lack of adhesion	Dycal (Dentsply, USA), Life (Kerr, USA)	[20, 21]
Mineral trioxide aggregate (MTA)	Direct/indirect pulp capping, pulpotomy, root perforation and resorption, retro-end apicectomy	Powder: Tricalcium silicate, dicalcium silicate, tricalcium aluminate Liquid: Distilled water	– Biocompatibility – Absence of pulp inflammation	– Cost – Poor handling characterisation – Higher solubility – The presence of iron in the grey MTA formulation may darken the tooth	MTA Angelus (Angelus, Brazil) MTA ProRoot (Dentsply, USA) MM-MTA (Micro-Mega, France) RetroMTA (BioMTA, Korea) OrthoMTA (BioMTA, Korea) NeoMTA Plus (Avalon Biomed, USA) CEM (Bionique Dent, Iran) Totalfill BC RRM (FKG Dentaire, Switzerland)	[20–22]

(continued)

Table 5.1 (continued)

Material	Main indication	General composition	Advantages	Disadvantages	Commercial examples	References
Calcium silicate-based	Direct/indirect pulp capping, pulpotomy, root perforation and resorption, retro-end apicectomy	Powder: Tricalcium silicate, dicalcium silicate, calcium carbonate, zirconium dioxide Liquid: Water, calcium chloride, modified polycarboxylate (super-plasticising agent)	– Biocompatible – Antimicrobial activity – Stimulating tertiary dentine formation	– It needs ideally a minimum of 1 week before overlaying with resin composite [23]	Biodentine (Septodont, France)	[20, 22, 24]
Calcium phosphate-based	Direct/indirect pulp capping, pulpotomy, root perforation and resorption, retro-end apicectomy	Powder: Calcium compounds such as calcium oxide, calcium phosphate, calcium carbonate, calcium silicate, calcium sulphate, calcium hydroxide, calcium chloride Liquid: Distilled water	– Good physical properties – Absence of pulp inflammation	– Insufficient clinical trials	Calcium-enriched mixture (CEM) cement (Bionique-Dent, Iran)	[20, 21]
Dentine bonding agents	Indirect pulp capping	Primer: 10-Methacryloyloxydecyl dihydrogen phosphate (MDP), dimethacrylate monomer, hydroxyethyl methacrylate (HEMA), silica, N,N-diethanol-p-toluidine, camphorquinone Bond: Hydroxy ethyl methacrylate (HEMA), dimethacrylate monomer, bisphenol A glycidyl methacrylate (Bis-GMA), N,N-diethanol-p-toluidine silica, camphorquinone	– Superior adhesion to hard tissue – Effective seal ageist microleakage	– Cytotoxic effect – Absence of calcific bridge formation	Clearfil SE Bond (Kuraray Medical, Japan), Optibond S (Kerr, USA), Prime & Bond 2.1 (Dentsply, USA)	[20, 21]
Zinc oxide-eugenol	Indirect pulp capping	Powder: Zinc oxide, poly-methyl methacrylate (PMMA) pigment Liquid: Eugenol, acetic acid	– Reduces inflammations	– Lack of calcific bridge formation – Demonstrates interfacial leakage	IRM (Dentsply, USA), Temp Bond (Kerr, USA), Relix Tempo (3M, USA)	[20, 21]

Material	Clinical application	Composition	Advantages	Disadvantages	Product	References
Bioactive materials (containing bioactive proteins)	Direct/indirect pulp capping, pulpotomy	Enamel matrix proteins, water, propylene glycol alginate	– Promote odontoblast differentiation	– Insufficient clinical studies – Incomplete dentine bridge even inferior to that of calcium hydroxide	Emdogain (Straumann, Switzerland)	[20, 21]
Glass-ionomer/ resin-modified glass-ionomer cement	Indirect pulp capping	Polymeric water-soluble acid, basic (ion-leachable) glass, and water/for RMGIC + monomer component and associated initiator system	– Good bacterial seal – Fluoride release – Bond to enamel and dentine – Biocompatibility	– Causes chronic inflammation – Lack of dentine bridge formation – Cytotoxic when in direct cell contact – Poor physical properties, high solubility and slow setting rate – RMGIC is more cytotoxic than conventional GIC	GC Fuji (GC America)	[20, 25, 26]

Table 5.2 Laboratory and clinical comparison of Biodentine (BD) with other pulp protection materials (adopted from Careddu and Duncan, 2018 [27])

Ideal property	Comparative results	References
Stimulates tertiary dentine formation (direct pulp protection)	– Clinical trial, histological ex vivo studies. Tested calcium hydroxide (CH), single bond universal + resin-bonded composite (RBC), ProRoot MTA (PrMTA), BD. Both PrMTA and BD materials induced a similar hard-tissue bridge formation. The bridge (BD and MTA) was homogeneous with no tunnel defects. MTA, BD and CH showed a thicker dentine bridge than RBC – The dentine bridges in the Biodentine samples showed the highest average and maximum volumes compared to mineral trioxide aggregate (MTA) and Single Bond Universal (3M ESPE, Seefeld, Germany) – Clinical trial, Biodentine and MTA performed better than TheraCal (TCal) when used as partial pulpotomy agent and presented the best clinical outcomes – Similar results for BD and PrMTA (lack of inflammation and good tissue organisation); however, BD group showed complete dentine bridge formation in all teeth with TCal (11%) and PrMTA (67%), respectively – Randomised clinical trial. Tested CH, BD and PrMTA. No significant difference between the materials, selected failures in PrMTA and CH groups, but BD had a success rate of 100%	[27–30]
Maintain pulp vitality/sensibility	– PrMTA and BD maintain pulp vitality in "sound" teeth over the duration of the 6-week period of the study – Biodentine had a similar efficacy in the clinical setting and may be considered an interesting alternative to MTA in pulp capping treatment during vital pulp therapy – Both PrMTA and BD maintain pulp vitality. Even if no statistically significant MTA showed one case of failure	[28, 30, 31]
Bactericidal/ bacteriostatic	– PrMTA, BD and glass-ionomer cement (GIC) tested against *S. mutans*, *E. faecalis*, *E. coli* and *C. albicans*. All materials tested showed antimicrobial activity against the tested strains except for GIC on Candida. Biodentine created larger inhibition zones than MTA and GIC – PrMTA, MTA and IRM showed better results against *S. mutans* and *S. salivarius*. BD showed better results against *S. sanguis*, but was not active against *S. mutans*	[32, 33]
Adhesion to dentine	– Tested by push-out strength test BD, PrMTA, immediate replacement material (IRM), Amalgam, Dyract AP. BD demonstrated greater adherence to dentine than PrMTA. The statistical ranking of push-out bond strength values was as follows: Dyract AP > amalgam ≥ IRM ≥ Biodentine > MTA. The push-out bond strength of Dyract AP, amalgam, IRM, and Biodentine was not significantly different when immersed in NaOCl and saline solutions, whereas MTA lost strength – Compared PrMTA and BD by push-out strength testing. BD better adhesion to dentine	[34, 35]

Table 5.2 (continued)

Ideal property	Comparative results	References
Adhesion to restorative material	– Shear bond strength study compared flowable composite (X-tra base; Voco GmbH, Cuxhaven, Germany) to mineral trioxide aggregate (MTA), Biodentine and calcium-enriched mixture (CEM; Yektazist Dandan, Tehran, Iran). BD showed the weakest adhesion to flowable composites	[23, 36]
Provide seal against bacterial ingress	– Both PrMTA and BD did not allow bacterial infiltration – BD, PrMTA, IRM. Allow bacterial colonisation at the interface material/dentine, but more live bacteria showed the more viability in MTA samples compared with BD and IRM	[37]

demineralised (but to a lesser extent) with its collagen microstructure still partly intact. With a significantly reduced bacterial load, it still has the potential for remineralisation and repair [7–10].

5.3   Indirect Pulp Protection

The indirect pulp protection (or capping (IPC)) procedure is used during deep carious dentine management, with or without excavation of the carious dentine tissues in close proximity to the pulp, but where the pulp is not directly exposed clinically or radiographically [2, 11]. According to the 2019 European Society of Endodontology (ESE)-approved definitions and terminology [12], alongside other published consensus guidelines [13–16], indirect pulp protection after removal of both soft (caries-infected) and firm, leathery caries-affected dentine until hard, sound dentine is reached [12, 17, 18], is now considered aggressive and acknowledged as unnecessary overtreatment. There are two appropriate contemporary clinical approaches of using indirect pulp protection as part of MI operative intervention:

5.3.1   One-Step Approach

All or most of the caries-infected dentine is removed and an indirect pulp capping material is placed in closest approximation to, but not in direct contact with the pulp and the final restoration is applied, all in the same appointment [4]. Several bioactive restorative materials (e.g. Biodentine™) have the relevant pulp protection properties themselves which therefore precludes the need for a separate "lining" to be placed. Indeed, the terminology of "base" and "lining" is now considered historical and should not be used [19].

5.3.2 Two-Step Approach

With two-stage or "stepwise" carious lesion management, all carious dentine is removed from the lesion periphery in the first appointment. A layer of deeper carious dentine may be left on the pulp floor of the preparation to prevent unnecessary iatrogenic pulp exposure. A setting calcium hydroxide base material is applied and the cavity is restored and sealed, traditionally with a zinc phosphate-based cement, but nowadays a high-viscosity glass-ionomer cement (GIC) is advocated. In the second appointment, between 3 and 9 months later, the restoration is removed and the underlying dentine is reassessed. Classically, the remaining dark-stained and dry dentine was further excavated until removed, a base material placed and the final cavity restored [1, 2, 4]. This second appointment is now not necessary in the contemporary era of minimally invasive caries management, where the recommended restoration placed (high-viscosity GIC) will provide an adequate seal, adhesion and physical properties to both arrest the caries process and create a functional medium-term restoration.

5.3.3 Materials Used for Indirect Pulp Protection

There are different types of bioactive/bio-interactive restorative materials that can be used for pulp protection (Table 5.1). The complete removal of all carious substrate is no longer considered mandatory and is deemed overtreatment. Indirect pulp protection following selective, partial carious tissue removal has been supported in clinical studies. By leaving the deepest layer of caries-affected dentine in closest proximity to the pulp undisturbed, the risk of pulp exposure and post-operative pulp symptoms is significantly reduced and favourable clinical results have been reported with residual dentine remineralisation [20, 21].

Historically, setting calcium hydroxide cement ($Ca(OH)_2$) has been considered the gold standard material for pulp protection. Calcium hydroxide was the main material evaluated for indirect pulp protection because it has important biological and antimicrobial characteristics. Despite its wide use, this material creates a poor seal to dentine, does not adhere to tooth substrate and is soluble over time. Thus, in an attempt to overcome these drawbacks, several other materials have been introduced to be used for this purpose [2].

5.4 Biodentine™

Preservation and protection of the vitality and sensibility of the pulp tissue with emphasis on inducing dentine regeneration are the ultimate goals of any indirect pulp protection treatment strategy. The use of a hydraulic calcium silicate cement has numerous advantages when used for pulp protection. These include stimulating pulp cell recruitment and differentiation [38], up-regulating gene expression and release of growth factors [39] and promoting dentinogenesis [40]. Hydraulic calcium silicate-based cements are considered bioactive, showing a dynamic and direct biological ionic interaction with dentine and pulp tissue interfaces [5, 41]. Improved calcium silicate-based materials have gained significant attention in recent years due to their resemblance to mineral trioxide aggregate (MTA) and their biocompatibility and applicability in cases where MTA is indicated. Although various calcium silicate-based products have been launched to the market, Biodentine has been the focus of attention and the topic of a variety of investigations, since it first became commercially available in 2009 [42].

Biodentine™ (Septodont Ltd., Saint-Maur-des-Fossés, France) is a tricalcium silicate (Ca_3SiO_5)-based inorganic restorative cement. It has a wide range of applications including endodontic repair (root perforations, apexification, resorptive lesions, retrograde filling material in endodontic apical surgery) and pulp protection/capping and can be used as a temporary/provisional direct restorative material in conservative dentistry [41].

5.4.1   Pulp Protection and Dentine Replacement (Table 5.2)

Biodentine releases calcium ions effectively [43, 44]. Dentine bridge formation occurs when it is used for direct pulp protection [45]. A clinical trial reported its success in maintaining pulp sensibility and restoration of function over a 2-year follow-up period when used as indirect pulp protection in vital teeth with deep carious lesions and clinical signs and symptoms of reversible pulpitis. Indeed, in the trial there were some cases reported that presented initially with radiographic signs of periapical periodontitis, observed using cone beam computer tomography (CBCT) with all other signs and symptoms indicating positive pulp vitality, but with CBCT apical resolution post-1-year treatment with Biodentine [46, 47]. The pulp response to Biodentine is similar to other calcium silicate-based materials including MTA [48], with favourable cell proliferation and increased alkaline phosphatase activity of human dental pulp cells [49]. This reaction was observed when testing leachates of Biodentine [50]. The calcium-releasing ability also contributes towards the antimicrobial properties of Biodentine, which is relevant since dental caries is a bacterially mediated disease [50]. The antimicrobial properties of $Ca(OH)_2$ were associated with higher cytotoxicity [51] compared to Biodentine.

Furthermore, the physical properties of Biodentine allow it to be used as a temporary/provisional bulk restorative material, thus avoiding unnecessary layering procedures, where interfaces created on restoration placement that can cause medium- to long-term micro-leakage and ultimate failure of the tooth-restoration complex. Biodentine shows less micro-leakage than resin-based dentine replacement materials [52]. Placing the definitive restorative material over Biodentine can be challenging due to its moisture content. Thus, ideally, the final restoration should be delayed for at least 1 week to allow maturation of the material [23]. Both total-etch and self-etch dental adhesives can then be used to adhere to an overlying resin composite layer [23]. Biodentine was shown to be able to restore teeth provisionally for up to 6 months and then overlaid with a resin composite [53]. Resin-based tricalcium silicate-based pulp capping materials have an advantage as they can be layered more readily with a resin composite providing a stronger bond [54]. However, the effects on the pulp are adverse [55]. The calcium ion release from such materials has been shown to be low and no crystalline $Ca(OH)_2$ is formed [43]. A model using extracted teeth kept in media for 15 days showed limited hydration of the resin-based tricalcium silicate [43]. Also, in agreement with previous published work, in-vitro and in-vivo studies [29, 56] showed that resin-based tricalcium silicate-conditioned media significantly decreased pulp fibroblast proliferation and induced proinflammatory interleukin-8 release from cultured pulp fibroblasts [56].

Sluyk and colleagues showed that MTA required a setting time of 72 h to resist displacement and dislodgement from dentine walls of a cavity preparation [57]. An evaluation comparing Biodentine to two commercially available liner/base materials, Fuji IX (GC America) and VitreBond (3M) in their resistance to compressive deflection when covered with a restorative resin composite, demonstrated that after a 10-min setting time all three materials supported the resin composite at clinically relevant loads (Table 5.3).

5.5   Direct Pulp Protection

Treatment options after a carious or traumatic pulp exposure include direct pulp capping and pulpotomy (partial and full).

Direct pulp capping protection is defined according to the ESE [12] as the application of a biomaterial directly onto the exposed pulp, prior to immediate placement of a definitive restoration, with preservation of an aseptic working field as a prerequisite. It is classified into two classes.

- Class I: No preoperative presence of a deep carious lesion. Pulp exposure judged clinically to be through sound dentine with an expectation that the underlying pulp tissue is healthy (for example, exposure due to a traumatic injury to the tooth or an iatrogenic exposure due to overtreatment).
- Class II: Preoperative presence of a deep carious lesion. Pulp exposure judged clinically to be through a zone of bacterial contamination with an expectation that the underlying pulp tissue is inflamed histologically. An enhanced operative protocol might be recommended (aseptic procedure using magnification, disinfectant and application of a hydraulic calcium silicate cement).

Partial pulpotomy is defined as the removal of a small portion of coronal pulp tissue immediately subjacent to the exposure, followed by application of a biomaterial directly onto the remaining pulp tissue prior to placement of an overlying definitive restoration.

Full pulpotomy is defined as the complete removal of the coronal pulp and application of a biomaterial directly onto the pulp tissue at the level of the root canal orifice(s), prior to placement of a definitive restoration [12].

Table 5.3 A summary of clinical studies using Biodentine as pulp protection material in permanent teeth

Study type	No. of teeth	Follow-up (months)	References	Comments
RCT	72	12	[46]	Biodentine™ and Fuji IX are clinically effective when used as IPC materials in teeth with reversible pulpitis. CBCT demonstrated a statistically significant difference between the two materials. The majority of teeth with healing/healed lesions identified using CBCT had received Biodentine.
RCT	72	24	[47]	Biodentine™ and Fuji IX™ were clinically effective when used as IPC materials in teeth with reversible pulpitis after 24 months. Resin composite restorations overlying both materials performed well after 24 months.
RCT	50	6	[58]	The success rates in the MTA Angelus and Biodentine groups were 95.5% (21/23 teeth) and 96% (23/24 teeth), respectively. No statistically significant difference was found between the groups.
RCT	397 cases	6	[53]	– When Biodentine was retained as a dentine substitute after pulp vitality control, it was covered routinely with resin composite Z100®. This procedure yielded restorations that were clinically sound and symptom free. – Biodentine is able to restore posterior teeth for up to 6 months (trial duration). When subsequently covered with Z100®, it is a convenient, efficient and well-tolerated dentine substitute. – Biodentine as a dentine substitute can be used under a resin composite for posterior restorations.
Case report	1	12	[59]	– Single-visit indirect pulp cap using Biodentine. – The patient was reviewed 1 year later. The tooth was asymptomatic. Clinically and radiographically there were no signs of endodontic disease.
Case report	1	24	[60]	Biodentine seems to be a promising material for the treatment of invasive cervical resorption lesions.
Case report	1	6	[61]	Indirect pulp capping treatment was performed with Biodentine. Following 6 months of the treatment, the clinical symptoms were resolved and a calcific bridge was found.

RCT randomized controlled clinical trial

5.5.1 Direct Pulp Protection: Clinical Procedure

Using the principles of minimally invasive operative dentistry described above, pulp exposures should be minimised/avoided where possible. However, there are some situations where pulp protection is still necessary. The dental pulp might be exposed for three reasons: during the operative management of a deep carious lesion, dental trauma and an iatrogenic "error". In the clinical scenario involving a clinically healthy pulp or one with signs and symptoms of reversible pulpitis, vital pulp therapy is recommended (direct pulp capping or partial/full pulpotomy). The clinical procedure includes the following steps:

– Suitable anaesthesia.
– Dental rubber dam isolation.
– Peripheral carious tissue removal with a sterile rotary bur in a low-speed handpiece. Due to the COVID-19 pandemic, avoidance of aerosol-generating procedures is recommended whenever possible. If aerosol-generating procedures are necessary for operative care, it is advisable to use four-handed dentistry with appropriate personal protective equipment, high vacuum suction, a reduced water output through rotary handpieces or micromotors without irrigation, to minimise droplet splatter and aerosols.
– Once the pulp is exposed (1 mm size approximately) after changing to a new sterile bur, disinfection of the pulp tissue using 2.5% sodium hypochlorite or 2% chlorhexidine for 1–2 min is advocated.
– Once haemostasis is achieved, the use of a calcium silicate restorative cement is recommended.

5.5.2 Partial/Full Pulpotomy: Clinical Procedure

In contrast to direct pulp capping procedure, which does not involve any pulp tissue removal, partial pulpotomy removes 2–3 mm of the pulp tissue subjacent to the site of exposure [12]. In practice this technique is used for removing the superficial layer of infected soft pulp tissue in cases of carious pulp exposure or when pulp has been exposed to the oral environment. It has been suggested that partial pulpotomy, compared with full/cervical pulpotomy, has many advantages including preservation of the cell-rich coronal pulp tissue, a necessary element for better healing [62] and the physiologic apposition of dentine in the coronal area. In cases of traumatised teeth, studies reported that the amount of coronal pulp removed did not affect the outcome [63]. In carious exposures, it is more difficult to determine the amount of pulp that is infected and needs to be removed [64]. Full pulpotomy may be successful in cases where there is partial irreversible pulpitis in the coronal pulp and there are some studies published with excellent results. However, the clinical diagnosis of this situation is fraught with difficulty due to the variations in signs and symptoms [65]; however, better long-term prospective randomised clinical data are required before this becomes the treatment of choice.

The pulpotomy procedure includes partial or full pulpotomy. The extension of the pulpotomy will be dependent on the ability to obtain haemostasis. Haemostasis and disinfection should be achieved using cotton pellets soaked with sodium hypochlorite (0.5–5%) or chlorhexidine (0.2–2%) [66–68]. If haemostasis cannot be controlled after 5 min, further pulp tissue should be removed (partial or full pulpotomy) and the wound surface rinsed as before [12].

When encountering a carious exposure, it is difficult to assess the condition of the pulp, which plays a critical role in the outcome of the pulp therapy [64]. Signs and symptoms do not always correlate well with the histologic status [69]. Observing the degree of pulp bleeding rather than relying on preoperative clinical signs and symptoms has been suggested [70]. Therefore, profuse bleeding that is difficult to stop indicates severe pulp inflammation.

5.5.3 Materials Used for Direct Pulp Protection

A pulp protection/capping agent is defined as the material used as a protective layer to an exposed dental pulp to allow the tissue to recover and maintain its normal function, sensibility and vitality.

Pulp capping/protection materials should be not only inert, in the sense that they should not be toxic to pulp cells, but also "bioactive" towards the tissues by stimulating migration, proliferation and osteogenic differentiation of the cells [71, 72].

Until the introduction of MTA, $Ca(OH)_2$ was the gold standard material for pulp capping, despite its high solubility causing a gap to form over time between the pulp tissue and the restorative material provoking a low-quality dentine bridge [73]. MTA is now the gold standard, but it also has several drawbacks, namely its prolonged setting time, technique sensitivity, lack of adhesion to dentine and potential for discoloration [74–77]. Several new products have been introduced on the market in the last few years in an attempt to mitigate these disadvantages. However, besides the required physical properties, direct pulp protection materials also require suitable biological properties, given their direct contact with vital pulp tissue [78]. Among all the calcium silicate-based materials used for direct pulp capping procedures, Biodentine (BD) stands out for the following reasons [78–81]:

- Approximate 12 min mixing/setting time
- No discoloration
- Adhesion to dentine
- Relatively ease of handling
- High biocompatibility

Biodentine, compared with the previous gold standard material, $Ca(OH)_2$, is mechanically stronger and less soluble and produces a higher quality histological seal to dentine [82].

Pedano et al. [83], in a recent systematic review, compared direct pulp capping agents, including resin-based materials. The results of this systematic review regarding the in-vivo inflammatory effect of the different direct pulp capping agents did not reveal any differences among the materials tested. However, one of the limitations of this review was that only studies including vital pulp therapy on sound teeth were used. This is not the most common clinical situation for the direct pulp capping procedure. Dentists often deal with carious teeth in a bacterium-contaminated environment close to the pulp.

Table 5.4 Clinical studies evaluating Biodentine as direct pulp capping/pulpotomy agent in carious teeth of permanent dentition

Study type	No. of teeth	Follow-up (months)	References	Comments
In vivo, carious teeth	24	6	[84]	Direct pulp capping. – Follow-up = 6 months. MTA and Biodentine showed 91.7% and 83.3% success rate
In vivo, carious teeth	169	12	[30]	Direct pulp capping. – Follow-up = 1 week. The patients showed 100% clinical success – Follow-up = 3 months. 1 failure in the CH group – Follow-up = 6 months. 4 new failures (1 in the CH group and 3 in the MTA group) – Follow-up = 1 year. 1 new failure in the CH group. There were no statistically significant differences among the experimental groups. Biodentine had a 100% success; both the CH and MTA groups had 13.64% accumulated failures
In vivo, carious teeth	58	12	[45]	Direct pulp capping. – Follow-up = 6 and 12 months. 100% success rate with both Biodentine and MTA. Radiographically, dentine bridge formation was evident after 6- and 12-month follow-up
In vivo, carious teeth	20	12	[85]	Pulpotomies with Biodentine. 70% of teeth had clinical signs and symptoms suggestive of irreversible pulpitis – Follow-up = 1 year. Clinical success 100%. Radiographic success 95%)
In vivo, carious teeth	68	36	[86]	Pulpotomies: – Follow-up = 6 months. Success rate was 93.3% (Biodentine = 93.1% and MTA = 93.5%) – Follow-up = 12 months. Success rate was 96.2% (Biodentine = 96.0% and MTA = 100%) – Follow-up = 24 months. Success rate was 100% at 2 years – Follow-up = 36 months. Success rate was 93.8% (Biodentine = 91.7% and MTA = 96.0%) There were no significant differences in the overall success rate between Biodentine and MTA
In vivo, carious teeth	86	12–18 (mean = 14.7)	[87]	Direct pulp capping with Biodentine Overall success rate was 82.6%

Table 5.4 (continued)

Study type	No. of teeth	Follow-up (months)	References	Comments
In vivo, carious teeth	55	6–54 (mean = 18.9 ± 12.9)	[88]	Direct pulp capping Success rate was 94.5% (ProRoot MTA = 92.6% and Biodentine = 96.4%)
In vivo, carious teeth	69	7–69 (mean = 32.2 ± 17.9)	[89]	Pulpotomy: 6–18-year-old patients with signs and symptoms indicative of irreversible pulpitis Overall success was 90% (ProRoot MTA = 92% and Biodentine = 87% ($P = 0.487$))
In vivo, carious teeth	245	2–88 (mean = 27.06)	[68]	Direct pulp capping with Biodentine: – Follow-up = 2.3 years. Overall success was 86.0% – Follow-up = 7.4 years. Overall success was 83.4%
In vivo, non-carious teeth	51	1–24 (mean = 13)	[63]	Pulpotomies with Biodentine: – Follow-up = 24 months. Survival rate of 100%. Success rate of 91%
In vivo, non-carious teeth	50	18	[90]	Pulpotomies: – Follow-up = 6 months. Success rate of 100% (Biodentine) and 100% (ProRoot MTA) – Follow-up = 12 months. Success rate of 84% (Biodentine) and 88% (ProRoot MTA) – Follow-up = 18 months. 80% (Biodentine) and 80% (ProRoot MTA) No significant statistical difference was observed in the radiographic outcomes between MTA and Biodentine. There was no statistically significant difference between survival times for the two groups
In vivo, carious teeth	52	12–60 (mean = 36)	[91]	Pulpotomies with Biodentine. Overall pulp survival was 90.2%

Several studies have evaluated the success of Biodentine in vital pulp therapy when applied in carious and non-carious teeth, obtaining positive results (Table 5.4).

In conclusion, as discussed in this chapter, it is clear that there is a burgeoning evidence base, both through in-vitro and in-vivo studies using Biodentine, that it can be used successfully as both an indirect and direct pulp protection material to maintain pulp vitality and sensibility. As it can also be considered a provisional restorative material, its use can remove the need for separate pulp protection "lining and base" placement, hence simplifying the clinical operative procedures. As is always the case, more clinical studies with long-term recalls are needed to reinforce these findings and to evaluate any future developments of the material.

References

1. Bjørndal L, Simon S, Tomson PL, Duncan HF. Management of deep caries and the exposed pulp. Int Endod J. 2019;52:949–73.
2. Kunert M, Lukomska-Szymanska M. Bio-inductive materials in direct and indirect pulp capping—a review. Materials (Basel). 2020;13(5):1204. Available from: https://pubmed.ncbi.nlm.nih.gov/32155997.
3. Banerjee A. Selective removal of carious dentin. In: Schwendicke F, editor. Management of deep carious lesions. Cham: Springer International Publishing; 2018. p. 55–70.
4. Alex G. Direct and indirect pulp capping: a brief history, material innovations, and clinical case report. Compend Contin Educ dent. 2018;39(3):182–9. Available from: http://www.ncbi.nlm.nih.gov/pubmed/29493248.
5. Rajasekharan S, Martens LC, Cauwels RGEC, Anthonappa RP. Biodentine™ material characteristics and clinical applications: a 3 year literature review and update. Eur Arch Paediatr Dent. 2018;19(1):1–22.
6. Schwendicke F. Removing carious tissue: why and how? Monogr Oral Sci. 2018;27:56–67.
7. Banerjee A, Watson TF, Kidd EA. Dentine caries: take it or leave it? Dent Update. 2000;27(6):272–6.
8. Banerjee A, Yasseri M, Munson M. A method for the detection and quantification of bacteria in human carious dentine using fluorescent in situ hybridisation. J Dent. 2002;30(7–8):359–63.
9. Kidd EAM. How "clean" must a cavity be before restoration? Caries Res. 2004;38:305–13.
10. Munson MA, Banerjee A, Watson TF, Wade WG. Molecular analysis of the microflora associated with dental caries. J Clin Microbiol. 2004;42(7):3023–9.
11. De Souza Costa CA, Hebling J, Hanks CT. Current status of pulp capping with dentin adhesive systems: a review. Dent Mater. 2000;16(3):188–97.
12. Duncan HF, Galler KM, Tomson PL, Simon S, El-Karim I, Kundzina R, et al. European Society of Endodontology position statement: management of deep caries and the exposed pulp. Int Endod J. 2019;52(7):923–34.
13. Schwendicke F, Frencken JE, Bjørndal L, Maltz M, Manton DJ, Ricketts D, et al. Managing carious lesions: consensus recommendations on carious tissue removal. Adv Dent Res. 2016;28:58–67.
14. Schwendicke F, Splieth C, Breschi L, Banerjee A, Fontana M, Paris S, et al. When to intervene in the caries process? An expert Delphi consensus statement. Clin Oral Investig. 2019;23(10):3691–703.
15. Martignon S, Pitts NB, Goffin G, Mazevet M, Douglas GVA, Newton JT, et al. CariesCare practice guide: consensus on evidence into practice. Br Dent J. 2019;227(5):353–62.
16. Askar H, Krois J, Göstemeyer G, Bottenberg P, Zero D, Banerjee A, et al. Secondary caries: what is it, and how it can be controlled, detected, and managed? Clin Oral Investig. 2020;24(5):1869–76.
17. Innes NPT, Frencken JE, Bjørndal L, Maltz M, Manton DJ, Ricketts D, et al. Managing carious lesions: consensus recommendations on terminology. Adv Dent Res. 2016;28(2):49–57.
18. Schwendicke F, Leal S, Schlattmann P, Paris S, Dias Ribeiro AP, Gomes Marques M, et al. Selective carious tissue removal using subjective criteria or polymer bur: study protocol for a randomised controlled trial (SelecCT). BMJ Open. 2018;8(12):e022952.
19. Stone S, Whitworth J, Wassell R. Preserving pulp vitality. In: Barnes J, editor. The principles of endodontics. Oxford: OUP; 2019. p. 93–8.
20. Hilton TJ. Keys to clinical success with pulp capping: a review of the literature. Oper Dent. 2009;34(5):615–25.
21. da Rosa WLO, Cocco AR, da Silva TM, Mesquita LC, Galarça AD, da Silva AF, et al. Current trends and future perspectives of dental pulp capping materials: a systematic review. J Biomed Mater Res B Appl Biomater. 2018;106:1358–68.
22. Macwan C, Deshpande A. Mineral trioxide aggregate (MTA) in dentistry: a review of literature. J Oral Res Rev. 2014;6(2):71.

23. Hashem DF, Foxton R, Manoharan A, Watson TF, Banerjee A. The physical characteristics of resin composite-calcium silicate interface as part of a layered/laminate adhesive restoration. Dent Mater. 2014;30(3):343–9.
24. Saghiri MA, Orangi J, Asatourian A, Gutmann JL, Garcia-Godoy F, Lotfi M, et al. Calcium silicate-based cements and functional impacts of various constituents. Dent Mater J. 2017;36:8–18.
25. Qureshi A, Soujanya E, Kumar N, Kumar P, Hivarao S. Recent advances in pulp capping materials: an overview. J Clin Diagn Res. 2014;8(1):316–21.
26. Sidhu S, Nicholson J. A review of glass-ionomer cements for clinical dentistry. J Funct Biomater. 2016;7(3):16.
27. Careddu R, Duncan HF. How does the pulpal response to Biodentine and proroot mineral trioxide aggregate compare in the laboratory and clinic? Br Dent J. 2018;225(8):743–9.
28. Nowicka A, Wilk G, Lipski M, Kołecki J, Buczkowska-Radlińska J. Tomographic evaluation of reparative dentin formation after direct pulp capping with ca(OH)2, MTA, Biodentine, and dentin bonding system in human teeth. J Endod. 2015;41(8):1234–40.
29. Bakhtiar H, Nekoofar MH, Aminishakib P, Abedi F, Naghi Moosavi F, Esnaashari E, et al. Human pulp responses to partial Pulpotomy treatment with TheraCal as compared with Biodentine and ProRoot MTA: a clinical trial. J Endod. 2017;43(11):1786–91.
30. Brizuela C, Ormeño A, Cabrera C, Cabezas R, Silva CI, Ramírez V, et al. Direct pulp capping with calcium hydroxide, mineral trioxide aggregate, and Biodentine in permanent young teeth with caries: a randomized clinical trial. J Endod. 2017;43(11):1776–80.
31. Nowicka A, Lipski M, Parafiniuk M, Sporniak-Tutak K, Lichota D, Kosierkiewicz A, et al. Response of human dental pulp capped with Biodentine and mineral trioxide aggregate. J Endod. 2013;39(6):743–7.
32. Bhavana V, Chaitanya KP, Gandi P, Patil J, Dola B, Reddy RB. Evaluation of antibacterial and antifungal activity of new calcium-based cement (Biodentine) compared to MTA and glass ionomer cement. J Conserv Dent. 2015;18(1):44–6.
33. Ceci M, Beltrami R, Chiesa M, Colombo M, Poggio C. Biological and chemical-physical properties of root-end filling materials: a comparative study. J Conserv Dent. 2015;18(2):94–9.
34. Guneser MB, Akbulut MB, Eldeniz AU. Effect of various endodontic irrigants on the push-out bond strength of Biodentine and conventional root perforation repair materials. J Endod. 2013;39(3):380–4.
35. Nagas E, Cehreli ZC, Uyanik MO, Vallittu PK, Lassila LVJ. Effect of several intracanal medicaments on the push-out bond strength of ProRoot MTA and Biodentine. Int Endod J. 2016;49(2):184–8.
36. Altunsoy M, Tanriver M, Ok E, Kucukyilmaz E. Shear bond strength of a self-adhering flowable composite and a flowable base composite to mineral trioxide aggregate, calcium-enriched mixture cement, and Biodentine. J Endod. 2015;41(10):1691–5.
37. Tsesis I, Elbahary S, Venezia NB, Rosen E. Bacterial colonization in the apical part of extracted human teeth following root-end resection and filling: a confocal laser scanning microscopy study. Clin Oral Investig. 2018;22(1):267–74.
38. Costa F, Sousa Gomes P, Fernandes MH. Osteogenic and angiogenic response to calcium silicate-based endodontic sealers. J Endod. 2016;42(1):113–9.
39. Lee BN, Lee KN, Koh JT, Min KS, Chang HS, Hwang IN, et al. Effects of 3 endodontic bioactive cements on osteogenic differentiation in mesenchymal stem cells. J Endod. 2014;40(8):1217–22.
40. Luo Z, Li D, Kohli MR, Yu Q, Kim S, He WX. Effect of Biodentine™ on the proliferation, migration and adhesion of human dental pulp stem cells. J Dent. 2014;42(4):490–7.
41. Rajasekharan S, Martens LC, Cauwels RGEC, Verbeeck RMH. Biodentine material characteristics and clinical applications: a review of the literature. Eur Arch Paediatr Dent. 2014;15(3):147–58.
42. Malkondu Ö, Kazandağ MK, Kazazoğlu E. A review on Biodentine, a contemporary dentine replacement and repair material. BioMed Res Int. 2014;2014:160951.

43. Camilleri J. Hydration characteristics of Biodentine and Theracal used as pulp capping materials. Dent Mater. 2014;30(7):709–15.
44. Aksoy MK, Oz FT, Orhan K. Evaluation of calcium (Ca2+) and hydroxide (OH−) ion diffusion rates of indirect pulp capping materials. Int J Artif Organs. 2017;40(11):641–6.
45. Katge FA, Patil DP. Comparative analysis of 2 calcium silicate-based cements (Biodentine and mineral trioxide aggregate) as direct pulp-capping agent in young permanent molars: a split mouth study. J Endod. 2017;43(4):507–13.
46. Hashem D, Mannocci F, Patel S, Manoharan A, Brown JE, Watson TF, et al. Clinical and radiographic assessment of the efficacy of calcium silicate indirect pulp capping: a randomized controlled clinical trial. J Dent Res. 2015;94(4):562–8.
47. Hashem D, Mannocci F, Patel S, Manoharan A, Watson TF, Banerjee A. Evaluation of the efficacy of calcium silicate vs. glass ionomer cement indirect pulp capping and restoration assessment criteria: a randomised controlled clinical trial-2-year results. Clin Oral Investig. 2019;23(4):1931–9.
48. Chang SW, Lee SY, Ann HJ, Kum KY, Kim EC. Effects of calcium silicate endodontic cements on biocompatibility and mineralization-inducing potentials in human dental pulp cells. J Endod. 2014;40(8):1194–200.
49. Luo Z, Kohli MR, Yu Q, Kim S, Qu T, He WX. Biodentine induces human dental pulp stem cell differentiation through mitogen-activated protein kinase and calcium-/calmodulin-dependent protein kinase II pathways. J Endod. 2014;40(7):937–42.
50. Arias-Moliz MT, Farrugia C, Lung CYK, Wismayer PS, Camilleri J. Antimicrobial and biological activity of leachate from light curable pulp capping materials. J Dent. 2017;64:45–51.
51. Poggio C, Arciola CR, Beltrami R, Monaco A, Dagna A, Lombardini M, et al. Cytocompatibility and antibacterial properties of capping materials. Sci World J. 2014;2014:181945.
52. Abdelmegid FY, Salama FS, Al-Mutairi WM, Al-Mutairi SK, Baghazal SO. Effect of different intermediary bases on microleakage of a restorative material in class II box cavities of primary teeth. Int J Artif Organs. 2017;40(2):82–7.
53. Koubi G, Colon P, Franquin J-C, Hartmann A, Richard G, Faure M-O, et al. Clinical evaluation of the performance and safety of a new dentine substitute, Biodentine, in the restoration of posterior teeth—a prospective study. Clin Oral Investig. 2013;17(1):243–9.
54. Meraji N, Camilleri J. Bonding over dentin replacement materials. J Endod. 2017;43(8):1343–9.
55. Hebling J, Lessa FCR, Nogueira I, De Carvalho RM, De Costa CAS. Cytotoxicity of resin-based light-cured liners. Am J Dent. 2009;22(3):137–42.
56. Jeanneau C, Laurent P, Rombouts C, Giraud T, About I. Light-cured tricalcium silicate toxicity to the dental pulp. J Endod. 2017;43(12):2074–80.
57. Chauhan A, Dua P, Saini S, Mangla R, Butail A, Ahluwalia S. In vivo outcomes of indirect pulp treatment in primary posterior teeth: 6 months' follow-up. Contemp Clin Dent. 2018;9(5):S69–73.
58. Song M, Kang M, Kim HC, Kim E. A randomized controlled study of the use of proroot mineral trioxide aggregate and endocem as direct pulp capping materials. J Endod. 2015;41(1):11–5.
59. Patel S, Vincer L. Case report: single visit indirect pulp cap using Biodentine. Dent Update. 2017;44(2):141–5.
60. Karypidou A, Chatzinikolaou ID, Kouros P, Koulaouzidou E, Economides N. Management of bilateral invasive cervical resorption lesions in maxillary incisors using a novel calcium silicate-based cement: a case report. Quintessence Int (Berl). 2016;47(8):637–42.
61. Sultana R, Alam MS. Conduction of reparative dentin: a pulp protecting approach by indirect pulp capping in deep carious lesion with Biodentine. Bangabandhu Sheikh Mujib Med Univ J. 2016;9(4):227.
62. Fong CD, Davis MJ. Partial pulpotomy for immature permanent teeth, its present and fixture. Pediatr Dent. 2002;24:29–32.
63. Haikal L, Ferraz dos Santos B, Vu DD, Braniste M, Dabbagh B. Biodentine pulpotomies on permanent traumatized teeth with complicated crown fractures. J Endod. 2020, in press. pii: S0099-2399(20)30393-9.

64. Chailertvanitkul P, Paphangkorakit J, Sooksantisakoonchai N, Pumas N, Pairojamornyoot W, Leela-apiradee N, et al. Randomized control trial comparing calcium hydroxide and mineral trioxide aggregate for partial pulpotomies in cariously exposed pulps of permanent molars. Int Endod J. 2014;47(9):835–42.
65. Zafar K, Nazeer M, Ghafoor R, Khan F. Success of pulpotomy in mature permanent teeth with irreversible pulpitis: a systematic review. J Conserv Dent. 2020;23:121–5.
66. Mente J, Hufnagel S, Leo M, Michel A, Gehrig H, Panagidis D, et al. Treatment outcome of mineral trioxide aggregate or calcium hydroxide direct pulp capping: long-term results. J Endod. 2014;40(11):1746–51.
67. Kundzina R, Stangvaltaite L, Eriksen HM, Kerosuo E. Capping carious exposures in adults: a randomized controlled trial investigating mineral trioxide aggregate versus calcium hydroxide. Int Endod J. 2017;50(10):924–32.
68. Harms CS, Schäfer E, Dammaschke T. Clinical evaluation of direct pulp capping using a calcium silicate cement—treatment outcomes over an average period of 2.3 years. Clin Oral Investig. 2019;23(9):3491–9.
69. Mejàre IA, Axelsson S, Davidson T, Frisk F, Hakeberg M, Kvist T, et al. Diagnosis of the condition of the dental pulp: a systematic review. Int Endod J. 2012;45(7):597–613.
70. Matsuo T, Nakanishi T, Shimizu H, Ebisu S. A clinical study of direct pulp capping applied to carious-exposed pulps. J Endod. 1996;22(10):551–6.
71. Schröder U. Effects of calcium hydroxide-containing pulp-capping agents on pulp cell migration, proliferation, and differentiation. J Dent Res. 1985;64 Spec No:541–8.
72. About I. Dentin regeneration in vitro: the pivotal role of supportive cells. Adv Dent Res. 2011;23:320–4.
73. Sangwan P, Sangwan A, Duhan J, Rohilla A. Tertiary dentinogenesis with calcium hydroxide: a review of proposed mechanisms. Int Endod J. 2013;46(1):3–19.
74. Vallés M, Mercadé M, Duran-Sindreu F, Bourdelande JL, Roig M. Color stability of white mineral trioxide aggregate. Clin Oral Investig. 2013;17(4):1155–9.
75. Parirokh M, Torabinejad M. Mineral trioxide aggregate: a comprehensive literature review-part I: chemical, physical, and antibacterial properties. J Endod. 2010;36:16–27.
76. Marciano MA, Costa RM, Camilleri J, Mondelli RFL, Guimarães BM, Duarte MAH. Assessment of color stability of white mineral trioxide aggregate angelus and bismuth oxide in contact with tooth structure. J Endod. 2014;40:1235–40.
77. Camilleri J. Mineral trioxide aggregate: present and future developments. Endod Top. 2015;32(1):31–46.
78. Giraud T, Jeanneau C, Rombouts C, Bakhtiar H, Laurent P, About I. Pulp capping materials modulate the balance between inflammation and regeneration. Dent Mater. 2019;35:24–35.
79. Vallés M, Roig M, Duran-Sindreu F, Martínez S, Mercadé M. Color stability of teeth restored with Biodentine: a 6-month in vitro study. J Endod. 2015;41(7):1157–60.
80. Vallés M, Mercadé M, Duran-Sindreu F, Bourdelande JL, Roig M. Influence of light and oxygen on the color stability of five calcium silicate-based materials. J Endod. 2013;39(4):525–8.
81. Wang Z. Bioceramic materials in endodontics. Endod Top. 2015;32(1):3–30.
82. About I. Biodentine: dalle proprietà biochimiche e bioattive alle applicazioni cliniche. G Ital Endod. 2016;30(2):81–8.
83. Pedano MS, Li X, Yoshihara K, Van Landuyt K, Van Meerbeek B. Cytotoxicity and bioactivity of dental pulp-capping agents towards human tooth-pulp cells: a systematic review of in-vitro studies and meta-analysis of randomized and controlled clinical trials. Materials (Basel). 2020;13(12):2670.
84. Hegde S, Sowmya B, Mathew S, Bhandi SH, Nagaraja S, Dinesh K. Clinical evaluation of mineral trioxide aggregate and Biodentine as direct pulp capping agents in carious teeth. J Conserv Dent. 2017;20(2):91–5.
85. Taha NA, Abdulkhader SZ. Full pulpotomy with Biodentine in symptomatic young permanent teeth with carious exposure. J Endod. 2018;44(6):932–7.

86. Awawdeh L, Al-Qudah A, Hamouri H, Chakra RJ. Outcomes of vital pulp therapy using mineral trioxide aggregate or Biodentine: a prospective randomized clinical trial. J Endod. 2018;44(11):1603–9.

87. Lipski M, Nowicka A, Kot K, Postek-Stefańska L, Wysoczańska-Jankowicz I, Borkowski L, et al. Factors affecting the outcomes of direct pulp capping using Biodentine. Clin Oral Investig. 2018;22(5):2021–9.

88. Parinyaprom N, Nirunsittirat A, Chuveera P, Na Lampang S, Srisuwan T, Sastraruji T, et al. Outcomes of direct pulp capping by using either ProRoot mineral trioxide aggregate or Biodentine in permanent teeth with carious pulp exposure in 6- to 18-year-old patients: a randomized controlled trial. J Endod. 2018;44(3):341–8.

89. Uesrichai N, Nirunsittirat A, Chuveera P, Srisuwan T, Sastraruji T, Chompu-inwai P. Partial pulpotomy with two bioactive cements in permanent teeth of 6- to 18-year-old patients with signs and symptoms indicative of irreversible pulpitis: a noninferiority randomized controlled trial. Int Endod J. 2019;52(6):749–59.

90. Abuelniel GM, Duggal MS, Kabel N. A comparison of MTA and Biodentine as medicaments for pulpotomy in traumatized anterior immature permanent teeth: a randomized clinical trial. Dent Traumatol. 2020;36(4):400–10.

91. Tan SY, Yu VSH, Lim KC, Tan BCK, Neo CLJ, Shen L, et al. Long-term pulpal and restorative outcomes of pulpotomy in mature permanent teeth. J Endod. 2020;46(3):383–90.

Biodentine™: Applications in Pulpotomy of Deciduous Teeth

6

Sivaprakash Rajasekharan

6.1   Introduction

Dental care for children is established on the principle of retaining the complete deciduous dentition in a healthy state until exfoliation, thereby enabling the natural eruption pattern of the permanent dentition. Unfortunately, dental caries with pulpal involvement is seen in several children before the intended time of exfoliation. In such cases, pulpotomy helps preserve the integrity of the dental arch by avoiding early extraction of extensively decayed teeth and consequently allows for a smoother transition from deciduous to permanent dentition. Pulpotomy is the most commonly used vital pulp therapy technique for the treatment of deciduous teeth with pulp exposure.

Pulpotomy is based on the rationale that inflammation and diminished vascularity caused by the traumatic or carious injury would be limited to the coronal pulp, while the radicular pulp would remain unaffected. According to the American Academy of Paediatric Dentistry (AAPD), pulpotomy is defined as the ablation of infected or affected pulp tissues leaving the residual vital pulp tissues intact, thus preserving the vitality and function (totally or partially) of the radicular pulp, and the remaining pulp stump is covered with a pulp medicament. The primary objective of pulpotomy is to retain a tooth in its functional state (allowing mastication, phonation, swallowing and aesthetics) to fulfil its role as a significant component of the deciduous and mixed dentition.

S. Rajasekharan (✉)
Department of Paediatric Dentistry and Special Care, PAECOMEDIS Research Cluster, Ghent University, Ghent University Hospital, Ghent, Belgium

© Springer Nature Switzerland AG 2022   87
I. About (ed.), *Biodentine™*, https://doi.org/10.1007/978-3-030-80932-4_6

6.2   Pulpotomy in Deciduous Teeth

Treatment of deciduous teeth with inflamed pulp presents a unique challenge. Pulp diagnosis in the primary dentition is imprecise as child behaviour compromises the reliability of pain as an indicator of the extent of pulpal inflammation. Moreover, clinical symptoms do not correlate well with histologic pulpal status. Proper diagnosis is essential to ensure that pulpal inflammation is limited to the coronal pulp and reversible. Radiographic examinations are imperative to confirm the need for pulpotomy in deciduous teeth. Bitewings and periradicular radiographs help assess the depth of caries and determine the condition of the periradicular tissues. Pulpotomy in deciduous dentition is advantageous over other alternatives such as pulp capping, pulpectomy or extraction. Due to the high cellular content of pulp tissue in primary teeth, pulp capping is considered less beneficial. The complicated anatomy of the root canals in primary teeth, the number of accessory canals which can be assessed, the proximity of the permanent tooth germ and the difficulties in finding a root-canal filling material compatible with physiological root resorption make pulpectomy a tedious procedure [1]. Moreover, pulpotomy is the choice of treatment for cariously exposed primary teeth when retention is more advantageous than extraction and replacement with a space maintainer.

6.3   Deciduous vs. Permanent Tooth Pulp

No histological differences exist between deciduous and permanent pulp tissue except for the presence of a cap-like zone of reticular and collagenous fibres in the primary coronal pulp. However, deciduous and permanent teeth differ in their cellular responses to irritation, trauma and medication [2]. Pulp healing in deciduous teeth is influenced by high coronal cellularity and apical vascularity. The abundant blood supply attributed to the enlarged apical foramen leads to a more typical inflammatory response in deciduous teeth whereas the reduced blood supply in permanent teeth favours calcific response and healing [3]. However, the incidence of reparative dentine formation beneath carious lesions is more extensive in deciduous than in permanent teeth.

6.4   Regenerative Potential of Dental Pulp

The principal function of dental pulp is to produce primary dentine during early tooth development, secondary dentine throughout the entire lifespan of the tooth and tertiary dentine under pathogenic stimuli. Consistently, the pulp is primarily connective tissue and has considerable healing potential but injured dental pulp has limited potential for self-recovery. In case of mild or slowly progressing stimuli, such as in mild caries, superficial fracture, erosion or moderate attrition, odontoblasts can usually survive and continue to produce the dentine barrier beneath the injury, allowing the underlying soft pulp tissue to retain its function. On the other hand, when the stimuli are strong and/or rapidly progressing, such as in deep dentine caries, fracture or severe abrasion, the primary odontoblasts will be destroyed due to severity of the injury. In these cases, the postmitotic terminally differentiated odontoblasts lack the ability to proliferate to replace injured odontoblasts, or to produce new dentine. In such rapidly progressing circumstances, undifferentiated mesenchymal cells within the dental pulp can differentiate into odontoblasts and secrete reparative dentine. Undifferentiated mesenchymal cells within the pulp also have the potential to differentiate into other cell types, including fibroblasts, to repair the damaged soft pulp tissue. The ability to stimulate the stem cell to differentiate into odontoblast-like cells, rather than fibroblasts, is vital in dentine repair [4].

The recruitment and differentiation of odontoblast-like cells from within the pulp are not well defined. What is known is that this process occurs differently than during development, where cells require the presence of epithelium to signal differentiation. Studies suggest that certain molecules are expressed that participate in the signalling process to begin this differentiation [5]. Recent studies have quantified the release of non-collagenous proteins and glycosaminoglycans from dentine and have also confirmed that growth factors, such as the TGF-β, show effects related to odontoblast-like cell differentiation [6]. Experiments suggest that Notch 1 protein, a component of an important cell signalling pathway involved in odontogenesis, has been found in some pulp cells close to injury sites [7]. The key to understanding the entire dentine repair process must be pursued at the molecular level to develop materials or procedures that can stimulate it under controlled and regulated conditions.

6.5 Interaction of Pulpotomy Materials with Dentine–Pulp Complex

The interaction between a dental material and tooth tissue is critical in terms of biocompatibility and the ability of the material to modulate the response of the tissue. This interaction is influenced by many factors, including the chemistry and composition of the material, and any of its eluted components, degradation products and the manner in which the tissue responds to these agents. Theoretically, the ideal material would interact with the dentine–pulp complex to repair the damage caused by demineralisation from the caries attack, mechanical destruction from the cavity preparation and chemical irritation from components of the material itself. Previous literature on the interaction between materials and pulp was principally aimed at identifying toxic effects of materials on cells but recent investigations focus on specific cellular responses that help understand how the materials themselves actually may contribute to regenerative processes in the tooth, an area of study with exciting potential [8, 9].

Certain materials are truly inert, and their placement within the dynamic tissue environment of the dentine–pulp complex may potentially give rise to a wide spectrum of physico-chemical and biological effects. Such effects may differ, dependent upon whether the tissue is healthy or carious, because bacterial infection, inflammation and pulpal cell responses may dramatically modify the tissue environment in caries. The pulpotomy medicaments that are recently used have demonstrated the solubilisation of proteins such as TGF-β1 from exposed dentine with the subsequent modulation by these proteins of gene expression in odontoblast-like cells. The release of these molecules may stimulate the natural healing process of the tooth, either by direct stimulation of existing cells to produce extracellular matrix for the deposition of new mineral through the process of reactionary dentinogenesis or by recruitment of new cells with their subsequent differentiation into odontoblast-like cells that produce new mineral through reparative dentinogenesis [8].

6.6   Materials Used in Pulpotomy

An ideal pulpotomy medicament must be bactericidal, promote healing of the radicular pulp, be biocompatible, offer the dentine–pulp complex a relatively stable environment, support the regeneration of dentine–pulp complex and not interfere with the physiological process of root resorption [4]. The search for the appropriate material for pulpotomy has continued from the beginning of dentistry to the present. Throughout the ages, dentistry has depended to a great degree on material science and this relationship continues. Pulp therapy for primary teeth and the materials to be used have historically been subject to change but a better understanding of the reactions of the pulp and dentine to the recent medicaments has developed over time, primarily through improvements in histologic techniques.

6.7   Classification of Pulpotomy Medicaments

Pulpotomy entails the removal of the coronal pulp and maintenance of the radicular pulp. There are three main approaches to this technique:

1. Rendering the radicular pulp inert
2. Preserving the radicular pulp in a healthy state
3. Stimulating tissue regeneration and healing at the site of radicular pulp amputation

The medicaments used for pulpotomy can also be classified on the basis of the same principle.

Devitalisation was the first approach to be used with the intention of treating radicular pulp tissue to be inert, sterilised, metabolically suppressed and incapable of autolysis [1]. Widely known medicament in this category is formocresol which has been used as gold standard in the comparison of pulpotomy medicaments due to its high success rate over a long period of time. It is the intent of the formocresol pulpotomy that pulp remains in a metastable condition until the tooth is exfoliated [10]. Concerns have been raised about formocresol due to its toxicity and potential carcinogenicity [11].

Preservation approach involved medicaments and techniques that provide minimal insult to the orifice tissue and maintain the vitality and normal histologic appearance of the entire radicular pulp. Most common pharmacotherapeutic agents included in this category are glutaraldehyde and ferric sulphate. Non-pharmacotherapeutic techniques in this category include electrosurgical and laser pulpotomies. Recently, with improvement of medicaments, that are not only bio-compatible, but also bio-inductive, the focus has been directed from preservation and conservation to regeneration of the remaining pulp tissue.

Regeneration approach includes pulpotomy agents that have cell-inductive capacity to either replace lost cells or induce existent cells to differentiate into hard tissue-forming elements. The ultimate goal of regenerative treatment strategy is to reconstitute lost tissues, and to improve altered tissue functions. Historically, calcium hydroxide was the first medicament to be used in a "regenerative" capacity because of its ability to stimulate hard-tissue barrier formation. Calcium hydroxide is considerably less harsh on pulp tissue than formocresol and for a time, calcium hydroxide was touted as an alternative to formocresol for pulpotomy in deciduous teeth, but was observed to stimulate internal resorption rather than dentine formation, and its popularity has waned. The calcium hydroxide pulpotomy is predicated on the healing of pulp tissue beneath the overlying dentine bridge. Recently, its regenerative capacity has been questioned because calcium hydroxide tissue response is more reactive than inductive. Other regenerative materials that are widely used in pulpotomy procedures are calcium hydroxide-related materials such as calcium-enriched mixture (CEM), Portland cement, mineral trioxide aggregate (MTA) and Biodentine.

6.8   Efficacy of Biodentine as a Pulpotomy Medicament in Deciduous Teeth

Two single tooth case reports [12, 13] and two case series with 8 [14] and 122 [15] deciduous molars have reported high clinical and radiographic success with Biodentine as a pulpotomy medicament in primary molar. Biodentine pulpotomy of 35 deciduous molars with physiologic root resorption (stage 3) showed 100% clinical and radiographic success indicating that the material is ideal to be used in deciduous molars with physiological root resorption [16]. The most commonly observed radiographic finding was pulp canal obliteration (PCO) in 25.7% of the treated teeth after 12-month follow-up. In a similar study with 75 mature primary molars (stage 2) Biodentine showed 100% radiographic success and 98.7% clinical success [17]. Interestingly, PCO was radiographically observed in 54% of the teeth after 12-month follow-up period. The increase in the incidence of PCO in this study could be attributed to the higher healing potential of the pulp in stage 2 deciduous molars compared to stage 3 deciduous molars with physiologic root resorption. The authors hypothesised that the younger the patient, the higher the chance of PCO following Biodentine pulpotomies. Table 6.1 summarises the clinical and radiographic success of Biodentine pulpotomies in deciduous teeth (case reports and case series).

Table 6.1 Summary of case series and case reports showing the clinical and radiographic success of Biodentine in deciduous teeth pulpotomy

Author [reference]	Year	Study design	Age range of patients (years)	No. of teeth treated	Follow-up period (months)	Clinical success (%)	Radiographic success (%)
Akhtar et al. [15]	2016	CS	4–12	122	3	95.9	94.26
Poornima et al. [14]	2017	CS	5–8	8	9	100	87.5
Nasrallah et al. [17]	2018	CS	5–8	75	12	98.7	100
Nasseh et al. [16]	2018	CS	8–11	35	12	100	100
Sultana et al. [12]	2015	CR	6	1	12	100	100
Sheikh et al. [13]	2017	CR	7	1	12	100	100

Legend: *CS* case series, *CR* case report

Pulp canal obliteration (PCO) has been a controversial radiographic outcome with different schools of thought. Few authors [18] categorise PCO as a radiographic failure since it demonstrates a deviation from normal-appearing pulp. According to these authors, PCO is the result of extensive activity of odontoblast-like cells and reactionary dentine is formed when teeth experience an injury as an attempted repair process within the pulpal tissue. Waterhouse et al. postulated that after an initial attempt by the pulp tissue to "wall off" the bacterial and inflammatory insult, the protective processes fail and result in clinical failures [18]. On the other hand, some other authors [19–21] argue that the extensive activity of odontoblast-like cells demonstrates that the tooth has retained some degree of vitality and hence PCO should be considered as a success.

6.9   Biodentine vs. Formocresol

Formocresol has long been the gold standard material for pulpotomy owing to its high success rate in deciduous dentition, availability and cost-effectiveness. However, the use of formocresol has been debated due to its possible mutagenic, carcinogenic and toxic effects. In June 2004 the International Agency for Research on Cancer classified medicaments containing formaldehyde as carcinogenic which should not be used for humans [22]. Furthermore, all countries within the European Union have withdrawn all dental products containing formaldehyde from the dental market.

Findings from ten randomised controlled trials (RCTs) showed that Biodentine was a suitable alternative to the use of formocresol in pulpotomy of deciduous molars. Of the ten studies, three studies reported that Biodentine showed significantly higher radiographic success [23–25] while one study revealed significantly higher clinical success than formocresol pulpotomy of deciduous molars [26]. In all other studies, Biodentine demonstrated better clinical and radiographic results than formocresol in deciduous teeth pulpotomy but the difference was not statistically significant [27–32].

Radiographic failures after formocresol pulpotomy were mostly due to internal root resorption, furcal/periapical radiolucency and external pathological resorption of the root. These failures could be a result of the fixative effect of formocresol and also due to the continuous irritation from vapours of the liquid that escape via the apical foramen. Histological comparison showed that formocresol-pulpotomised teeth revealed zones of atrophy, inflammation and fibrosis but after Biodentine pulpotomy, a dentine bridge was formed with odontoblast and odontoblast-like cells in the adjacent area. In the Biodentine group, the occurrence of PCO was higher than in the formocresol group and was observed to be 17.9% [28], 45.5% [24] or 68.9% [30] compared to 12.5% [28], 13.4% [24] and 0% [30]. This could be a result of vigorous odontoblastic activity in the teeth treated with Biodentine.

6.10   Biodentine vs. MTA

The search for nontoxic pulp therapy materials as an alternative to formocresol revealed tricalcium silicate-based materials to be an ideal candidate. The US Food and Drug Administration (FDA) approved MTA in 1998 as a therapeutic endodontic material for humans [33] and the first study suggesting the use of MTA in pulpotomy of primary molars was by Rocha et al. in the year 1999 [34] comparing the success rate of MTA with calcium hydroxide. Since then there have been numerous studies comparing the clinical success of MTA in primary molars with other pulpotomy medicaments such as formocresol, calcium hydroxide, ferric sulphate, calcium-enriched cement, Portland cement and Biodentine. Ng et al. published an evidence-based systematic assessment, where all studies comparing MTA with either calcium hydroxide, formocresol or ferric sulphate were analysed. The study concluded that, in comparison with formocresol, ferric sulphate and calcium hydroxide, MTA resulted in significantly higher clinical and radiographic successes in all time periods up to exfoliation [35, 36].

Non-randomised cohort studies comparing Biodentine vs. MTA pulpotomy in deciduous molars showed high success with both materials (100% and 95.5%) and no significant difference was observed between the two groups [37, 38]. In the study by Ramanandvignesh et al., Biodentine showed higher clinical and radiographic success rates (100% and 94.1%, respectively) compared to MTA (82.3% and 82.3%, respectively), but the difference was not statistically significant [39]. Table 6.2 summarises the clinical and radiographic success of Biodentine pulpotomies in deciduous teeth compared to other medicaments (non-randomised trials).

Findings from 14 RCTs showed that there was no significant difference in the clinical and radiographic outcomes of deciduous molar pulpotomies between Biodentine and MTA (Table 6.2). Only the study by Rajasekharan et al. demonstrated that Biodentine group exhibited significantly more PCO when compared to the ProRoot WMTA group after 6-month ($p = 0.008$) and 18-month ($p = 0.003$) follow-up [40].

Table 6.2 Clinical and radiographic success rate of Biodentine compared to other materials as a pulpotomy medicament in deciduous molars

Author [reference]	Year	Study design	Age range of patients (years)	Follow-up period (months)	Material compared with	No. of teeth treated	Clinical success percentile	Radiographic success percentile	Overall success
El Meligy et al. [28]	2016	RCT	4–8	6	Biodentine	56	100	100	
					FC	56	100	100	
Rubanenko et al. [31]	2019	RCT	2–10	48	Biodentine	37			97.3
					FC	35			91.4
Chotitanmapong et al. [24]	2019	RCT	4–8	12	Biodentine	25	100	95.5[a]	
					FC	25	100	73.9[b]	
Khatab and Deraz [29]	2019	RCT	4–8	12	Biodentine	30	90	86.6	
					FC	30	80	73.3	
El Meligy et al. [27]	2019	RCT	4–8	12	Biodentine	56	100	100	
					FC	56	100	98.1	
El Aziem Elbardissy and El Sayed [25]	2019	RCT	4–6	12	Biodentine	41	100	100[a]	
					FC	41	95.1	78[b]	
Verma et al. [32]	2019	RCT	4–9	6	Biodentine	30	100	100	
					FC	30	100	96.7	
					Pulpotec	30	100	100	
Juneja and Kulkarni [26]	2017	RCT	5–9	18	Biodentine	17	100[a]	86.6[a]	
					MTA	17	100[a]	100[a,c]	
					FC	17	73.3[b]	73.3[a]	
Musale et al. [30]	2018	RCT	4–8	12	Biodentine	30	100	92.9	
					WMTA	30	100	92.9	
					FC	30	100	75	
Ahuja et al. [23]	2020	RCT	4–7	9	Biodentine	20	100	95[a]	
					MTA	20	95	60[b]	
					FC	20	70	25[c]	
Fouad and Youssef [37]	2013	Cohort	3–7	6	Biodentine	27	100	100	
					MTA	25	100	100	
Cuadros-Fernandez et al. [48]	2016	RCT	4–9	12	Biodentine	45	97	95	
					MTA	45	92	97	

Study	Year	Type	Age	Follow-up	Material	n		
Carti and Oznurha [49]	2017	RCT	5–9	12	Biodentine	25	96	60
					MTA	25	96	80
Fouad and Abd Al Gawad [50]	2019	RCT	3–7	12	Biodentine	42	100	100
					MTA	42	100	100
Kamboj et al. [51]	2019	RCT	4–9	6	Biodentine	1	100	93.3
					MTA	15	100	86.7
Celik et al. [52]	2019	RCT	5–9	24	Biodentine	20	89.4	89.4
					MTA	24	100	100
El Habashy [53]	2020	RCT	2–6	12	Biodentine	15	100	73.3
					MTA	15	100	86.6
Rajasekharan et al. [40]	2017	RCT	3–8	18	Biodentine	25	95.24	94.4
					MTA	29	100	90.9
					Tempophore	27	95.65	82.4
Mythraiye et al. [47]	2019	RCT	5–9	6	Biodentine	28	100	90
					MTA	28	96	96
					Pulpotec	28	100	100
Kusum et al. [43]	2015	RCT	3–10	9	Biodentine	25	100[a]	80
					MTA	25	100[a]	82
					Propolis	25	84[b]	72
Niranjani et al. [46]	2015	RCT	5–9	6	Biodentine	20	90	90
					MTA	20	100	100
					Diode laser	20	90	90
Togaru et al. [38]	2016	Cohort	4–9	12	Biodentine	45	95.5	95.5
					MTA	45	95.5	95.5
					Er,Cr:YSGG laser	18	81.2	81.2

(continued)

Table 6.2 (continued)

Author [reference]	Year	Study design	Age range of patients (years)	Follow-up period (months)	Material compared with	No. of teeth treated	Clinical success percentile	Radiographic success percentile	Overall success
Guven et al. [45]	2017	RCT	5–7	24	Biodentine	29			82.75
					PR-MTA	29			86.2
					MTA-Plus	29			93.1
					FS	29			75.86
Sirohi et al. [44]	2017	RCT	4–8	9	Biodentine	25	100	92	
					FS	25	96	84	
Grewal et al. [42]	2016	RCT	5–10	12	Biodentine	20	100		
					CH	20	93.3		
Afroz et al. [41]	2019	RCT	6–9	12	Biodentine	50	92		92
					CH	50	84		84
Caruso et al. [54]	2018	Retrospective	5–9	18	Biodentine	200			89.5[a]
					CH	200			79.5[b]

Legend: Different superscript alphabets indicate statistical significance ($p < 0.05$)

FC formocresol, *MTA* mineral trioxide aggregate, *PR-MTA* ProRoot MTA, *WMTA* white MTA, *CH* calcium hydroxide, *FS* ferric sulphate, *Er,Cr:YSGG* erbium, chromium-doped yttrium, scandium, gallium

6.11   Biodentine vs. Other Pulpotomy Materials

In a retrospective study, comparing Biodentine and calcium hydroxide pulpotomy in 400 deciduous molars, Biodentine exhibited a significantly higher clinical and radiographic success rate compared to calcium hydroxide after 18-month follow-up. Clinically, after 18 months, pain, sensitivity to percussion and swelling were significantly ($p < 0.05$) higher in the calcium hydroxide group compared to the Biodentine group [41]. Results of two RCTs revealed that calcium hydroxide showed lesser success than Biodentine in pulpotomy of deciduous teeth but the results were not statistically significant [41, 42]. However, in the study by Afroz et al., 12-month follow-up of 100 teeth treated with either Biodentine ($n = 50$) or calcium hydroxide ($n = 50$) revealed that Biodentine showed significantly increased dentine bridge formation compared to calcium hydroxide ($p < 0.05$).

Teeth treated with Biodentine showed more favourable clinical and radiographic success as compared to propolis after 9-month follow-up [43]. No significant difference in the clinical and radiographic outcomes was seen between Biodentine and ferric sulphate [44, 45] Er,Cr:YSGG (erbium, chromium-doped yttrium, scandium, gallium and garnet) laser [39], diode laser [46], pulpotec [32, 47] or tempophore [40] in pulpotomy-treated teeth.

6.12   Pulpotomy Procedure with Biodentine

The intervention design for performing pulpotomy includes caries removal and coronal access with a high-speed cylindrical diamond bur with ample water spray. The coronal pulp is removed with a sterile spoon excavator. The pulp should appear bright red in colour to indicate a vital pulp. Normal haemostasis is obtained after removal of carious pulp by application of light pressure with a cotton pellet (Fig. 6.1). If haemostasis is not obtained after few minutes, pulp tissue in the canal is assumed to be infected and an alternative treatment plan should be executed. In case of normal haemostasis achievement, a minimum of 2 mm layer of Biodentine is placed above the pulp followed by a permanent restoration. However, Biodentine can also be used as a temporary restoration up to the occlusal level (Fig. 6.2).

In a multicentric, randomised, 3-year prospective study by Koubi et al., 146 class I and II posterior restorations and 24 direct pulp capping cases showed no clinical complications after 6 months. Upon further follow-up for up to 3 years, deterioration of anatomic form, marginal adaptation and proximal contact was observed but all the teeth maintained vitality. These results indicated that Biodentine could be used as a dentine substitute for definitive dentinal treatment of posterior teeth for up to 6 months [55]. This could be an advantage while treating paediatric patients in the clinical setting as it shortens the procedure time, eliminating the need to place a separate restoration.

Fig. 6.1 Pulpotomy in carious second primary molar (tooth 85) showing bright red pulp and complete haemostasis. (Image courtesy of Lieselotte Hillaert, Ghent University)

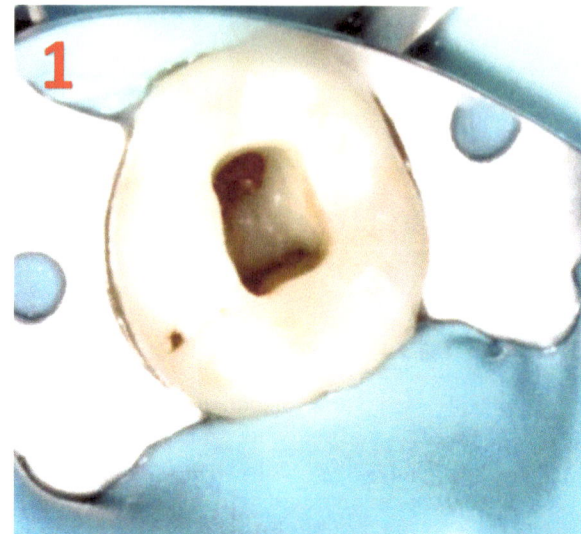

Fig. 6.2 Biodentine used a temporary restoration up to the occlusal level after pulpotomy in carious second primary molar (tooth 85). (Image courtesy of Lieselotte Hillaert, Ghent University)

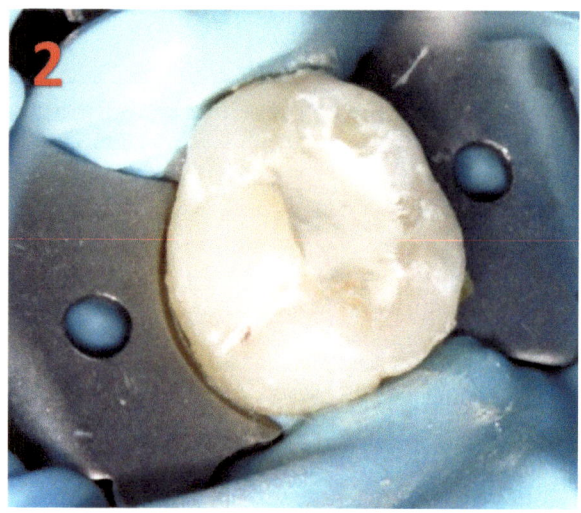

If permanent restoration is desired in the same visit, a stainless steel crown loaded with glass-ionomer cement (GIC) is well suitable for immediate permanent restoration after pulpotomy. The stainless steel crown could be placed on unset Biodentine after the third minute of mixing in pulpotomy-treated tooth [56]. Results of shear bond strength analysis revealed that in contrast to MTA, bonding procedures directly on top of Biodentine can be performed immediately (after 12 min) with resin-based flowable composite, GIC [57, 58], light-cured GIC or amalgam [59] as a restorative material.

6.13   Conclusion

Biodentine showed a significantly higher clinical and radiographic success rate compared to formocresol, calcium hydroxide and propolis in pulpotomy of carious deciduous molars. There was no significant difference in the clinical and radiographic outcomes of deciduous molar pulpotomies between Biodentine and ferric sulphate, tempophore or MTA. However, faster setting time, increased mechanical properties, absence of discoloration and ability to be used as a temporary restorative material make Biodentine an advantageous alternative to other pulpotomy medicaments for use in paediatric endodontics.

References

1. Ranly DM. Pulpotomy therapy in primary teeth: new modalities for old rationales. Pediatr Dent. 1994;16(6):403–9.
2. Benzer G, Bevelander S. Morphology and incidence of secondary dentin in human teeth. J Am Dent Assoc. 1943;30:1075.
3. Massler M. Preventive endodontics: vital pulp therapy. Dent Clin N Am. 1967:663–73.
4. Zhang W, Yelick PC. Vital pulp therapy-current progress of dental pulp regeneration and revascularization. Int J Dent. 2010;2010:856087. https://doi.org/10.1155/2010/856087.
5. Li Y, Lu X, Sun X, Bai S, Li S, Shi J. Odontoblast-like cell differentiation and dentin formation induced with TGF-beta1. Arch Oral Biol. 2011;56(11):1221–9. https://doi.org/10.1016/j.archoralbio.2011.05.002.
6. Niwa T, Yamakoshi Y, Yamazaki H, Karakida T, Chiba R, Hu JC, et al. The dynamics of TGF-beta in dental pulp, odontoblasts and dentin. Sci Rep. 2018;8(1):4450. https://doi.org/10.1038/s41598-018-22823-7.
7. Mitsiadis TA, Caton J, Pagella P, Orsini G, Jimenez-Rojo L. Monitoring notch signaling-associated activation of stem cell niches within injured dental pulp. Front Physiol. 2017;8:372. https://doi.org/10.3389/fphys.2017.00372.
8. Ferracane JL, Cooper PR, Smith AJ. Can interaction of materials with the dentin-pulp complex contribute to dentin regeneration? Odontology. 2010;98(1):2–14. https://doi.org/10.1007/s10266-009-0116-5.
9. Goldberg M, Smith AJ. Cells and extracellular matrices of dentin and pulp: a biological basis for repair and tissue engineering. Crit Rev Oral Biol Med. 2004;15(1):13–27. https://doi.org/10.1177/154411130401500103.
10. Fuks AB. Pulp therapy for the primary and young permanent dentitions. Dent Clin N Am. 2000;44(3):571–96, vii.
11. Lewis B. The obsolescence of formocresol. Br Dent J. 2009;207(11):525–8. https://doi.org/10.1038/sj.bdj.2009.1103.
12. Sultana A, Karim FA, Sheikh MH. Better outcome in pulpotomy on primary molar with Biodentine. Update Dent Coll J. 2016;5(2):57–62. https://doi.org/10.3329/updcj.v5i2.27277.
13. Sheikh MAH, Khanum S, Shaikh AK, Nisa SS. Pulpotomy of primary molar teeth with bio-dentine—a case report. BIRDEM Med J. 2017;7(3):238–41.
14. Poornima P, Shagun S, Roopa K, Neena I. Clinical and radiographic evaluation of primary molars treated with Biodentine pulpotomy: a series of eight case reports. Niger J Exp Clin Biosci. 2017;5:48–52. https://doi.org/10.4103/njecp.njecp_15_16.
15. Akhtar M, Rana SAA, Rana MJA, Parveen N, Kashif M. Clinical and radiological success rates of Biodentine for pulpotomy in children. Int J Contemp Med Res. 2016;3(8):2300–2.

16. Nasseh HN, El Noueiri B, Pilipili C, Ayoub F. Evaluation of Biodentine pulpotomies in deciduous molars with physiological root resorption (stage 3). Int J Clin Pediatr Dent. 2018;11(5):393–4. https://doi.org/10.5005/jp-journals-10005-1546.

17. Nasrallah H, El Noueiri B, Pilipili C, Ayoub F. Clinical and radiographic evaluations of Biodentine pulpotomies in mature primary molars (stage 2). Int J Clin Pediatr Dent. 2018;11(6):496–504. https://doi.org/10.5005/jp-journals-10005-1564.

18. Waterhouse PJ, Nunn JH, Whitworth JM. An investigation of the relative efficacy of Buckley's Formocresol and calcium hydroxide in primary molar vital pulp therapy. Br Dent J. 2000;188(1):32–6.

19. Willard RM. Radiographic changes following formocresol pulpotomy in primary molars. ASDC J Dent Child. 1976;43(6):414–5.

20. Tziafas D, Smith AJ, Lesot H. Designing new treatment strategies in vital pulp therapy. J Dent. 2000;28(2):77–92.

21. Subramaniam P, Konde S, Mathew S, Sugnani S. Mineral trioxide aggregate as pulp capping agent for primary teeth pulpotomy: 2 year follow up study. J Clin Pediatr Dent. 2009;33(4):311–4. https://doi.org/10.17796/jcpd.33.4.r83r38423x58h38w.

22. International Agency for Research on Cancer, World Health Organization, Press Release No. 153, 15 Jun 2004. http://www.iarc.fr/ENG/Press_Releases/archives/pr153a.html.

23. Ahuja S, Surabhi K, Gandhi K, Kapoor R, Malhotra R, Kumar D. Comparative evaluation of success of Biodentine and mineral trioxide aggregate with formocresol as pulpotomy medicaments in primary molars: an in vivo study. Int J Clin Pediatr Dent. 2020;13(2):167–73. https://doi.org/10.5005/jp-journals-10005-1740.

24. Chotitnmapong T, Asvanund Y, Mitrakul K. A one-year treatment outcome comparison of pulpotomies in primary molars using Biodentine and formocresol in Thai children: a randomised control trial. J Clin Diagn Res. 2019;13(10):17–21. https://doi.org/10.7860/JCDR/2019/41960.13223.

25. El Aziem Elbardissy AA, El Sayed MA. Clinical and radiographic evaluation of Biodentine versus formocresol in vital pulpotomy of primary molars (a randomized control clinical trial). Egypt Dent J. 2019;65(1):9–20. https://doi.org/10.21608/EDJ.2019.71241.

26. Juneja P, Kulkarni S. Clinical and radiographic comparison of Biodentine, mineral trioxide aggregate and formocresol as pulpotomy agents in primary molars. Eur Arch Paediatr Dent. 2017;18(4):271–8. https://doi.org/10.1007/s40368-017-0299-3.

27. El Meligy O, Alamoudi NM, Allazzam SM, El-Housseiny AAM. Biodentine(TM) versus formocresol pulpotomy technique in primary molars: a 12-month randomized controlled clinical trial. BMC Oral Health. 2019;19(1):3. https://doi.org/10.1186/s12903-018-0702-4.

28. El Meligy OA, Allazzam S, Alamoudi NM. Comparison between Biodentine and formocresol for pulpotomy of primary teeth: a randomized clinical trial. Quintessence Int. 2016;47(7):571–80. https://doi.org/10.3290/j.qi.a36095.

29. Khatab A, Deraz E. Clinical, radiographical and histopathological evaluation of Biodentine versus formocresol in primary teeth pulpotomy. Egypt Dent J. 2019;65(4):3199–212. https://doi.org/10.21608/edj.2019.73996.

30. Musale PK, Kulkarni N, Kothare SS. An in vivo evaluation of Biodentine™ as a pulpotomy agent in primary teeth. J South Asian Assoc Pediatr Dent. 2018;1(2):39–46. https://doi.org/10.5005/jp-journals-10077-3011.

31. Rubanenko M, Petel R, Tickotsky N, Fayer I, Fuks AB, Moskovitz M. A randomized controlled clinical trial comparing tricalcium silicate and formocresol pulpotomies followed for two to four years. Pediatr Dent. 2019;41(6):446–50.

32. Verma S, Choudhari S, Goyal S, Vispute GK, Bharti KD, Choudhari S. Comparative evaluation of success of pulpotomy in primary molars treated with Formocresol, Pulpotec and Biodentine—6 month follow up study. Int J Appl Dent Sci. 2019;5:77–82.

33. Peng L, Ye L, Tan H, Zhou X. Evaluation of the formocresol versus mineral trioxide aggregate primary molar pulpotomy: a meta-analysis. Oral Surg Oral Med Oral Pathol Oral Radiol Endod. 2006;102(6):e40–4. https://doi.org/10.1016/j.tripleo.2006.05.017.

34. Rocha M, Baroni R, Santos L, Girardi K. Ca(OH)2 and MTA pulpotomies in primary teeth: one year results. Int J Paediatr Dent. 1999;9:102.
35. Ng FK, Messer LB. Mineral trioxide aggregate as a pulpotomy medicament: an evidence-based assessment. Eur Arch Paediatr Dent. 2008;9(2):58–73.
36. Ng FK, Messer LB. Mineral trioxide aggregate as a pulpotomy medicament: a narrative review. Eur Arch Paediatr Dent. 2008;9(1):4–11.
37. Fouad WA, Youssef R. Clinical and radiographic assessment of vital pulpotomy in primary molars using mineral trioxide aggregate and a novel bioactive cement. Egypt Dent J. 2013;59(3):3007–13.
38. Togaru H, Muppa R, Srinivas N, Naveen K, Reddy VK, Rebecca VC. Clinical and radiographic evaluation of success of two commercially available pulpotomy agents in primary teeth: an in vivo study. J Contemp Dent Pract. 2016;17(7):557–63.
39. Ramanandvignesh P, Gyanendra K, Mridula DJKG. Clinical and radiographic evaluation of pulpotomy using MTA, Biodentine and Er,Cr:YSGG laser in primary teeth—a clinical study. Laser Ther. 2020;29(1):29–34. https://doi.org/10.5978/islsm.20-OR-03.
40. Rajasekharan S, Martens LC, Vandenbulcke J, Jacquet W, Bottenberg P, Cauwels RG. Efficacy of three different pulpotomy agents in primary molars: a randomized control trial. Int Endod J. 2017;50(3):215–28. https://doi.org/10.1111/iej.12619.
41. Afroz S, Sultana S, Saki N, Wahiduzzaman M, Sheikh MAH, Karim FA, et al. A comparative study of Biodentine and calcium hydroxide as pulpotomy material in primary teeth. Update Dent Coll J. 2019;9(1):37–41. https://doi.org/10.3329/updcj.v9i1.41205.
42. Grewal N, Salhan R, Kaur N, Patel HB. Comparative evaluation of calcium silicate-based dentin substitute (Biodentine) and calcium hydroxide (Pulpdent) in the formation of reactive dentin bridge in regenerative pulpotomy of vital primary teeth: triple blind, randomized clinical trial. Contemp Clin Dent. 2016;7(4):457–63. https://doi.org/10.4103/0976-237X.194116.
43. Kusum B, Rakesh K, Richa K. Clinical and radiographical evaluation of mineral trioxide aggregate, Biodentine and propolis as pulpotomy medicaments in primary teeth. Restor Dent Endod. 2015;40(4):276–85. https://doi.org/10.5395/rde.2015.40.4.276.
44. Sirohi K, Marwaha M, Gupta A, Bansal K, Srivastava A. Comparison of clinical and radiographic success rates of pulpotomy in primary molars using ferric sulfate and bioactive tricalcium silicate cement: an in vivo study. Int J Clin Pediatr Dent. 2017;10(2):147–51. https://doi.org/10.5005/jp-journals-10005-1425.
45. Guven Y, Aksakal SD, Avcu N, Unsal G, Tuna EB, Aktoren O. Success rates of pulpotomies in primary molars using calcium silicate-based materials: a randomized control trial. Biomed Res Int. 2017;2017:4059703. https://doi.org/10.1155/2017/4059703.
46. Niranjani K, Prasad MG, Vasa AA, Divya G, Thakur MS, Saujanya K. Clinical evaluation of success of primary teeth pulpotomy using mineral trioxide aggregate((R)), laser and Biodentine(™)—an in vivo study. J Clin Diagn Res. 2015;9(4):ZC35–7. https://doi.org/10.7860/JCDR/2015/13153.5823.
47. Mythraiye R, Rao VV, Minor Babu MS, Satyam M, Punithavathy R, Paravada C. Evaluation of the clinical and radiological outcomes of pulpotomized primary molars treated with three different materials: mineral trioxide aggregate, Biodentine, and pulpotec. An in-vivo study. Cureus. 2019;11(6):e4803. https://doi.org/10.7759/cureus.4803.
48. Cuadros-Fernandez C, Lorente Rodriguez AI, Saez-Martinez S, Garcia-Binimelis J, About I, Mercade M. Short-term treatment outcome of pulpotomies in primary molars using mineral trioxide aggregate and Biodentine: a randomized clinical trial. Clin Oral Investig. 2016;20(7):1639–45. https://doi.org/10.1007/s00784-015-1656-4.
49. Carti O, Oznurhan F. Evaluation and comparison of mineral trioxide aggregate and Biodentine in primary tooth pulpotomy: clinical and radiographic study. Niger J Clin Pract. 2017;20(12):1604–9. https://doi.org/10.4103/1119-3077.196074.
50. Fouad W, Abd Al Gawad R. Is Biodentine, as successful as, mineral trioxide aggregate for pulpotomy of primary molars? A split-mouth clinical trial. Tanta Dent J. 2019;16(2):115–9. https://doi.org/10.4103/tdj.tdj_35_18.

51. Kamboj V, Gupta M, Pandit IK, Gugnani N. Comparative evaluation of mineral trioxide aggregate and Biodentine as pulpotomy agents in primary molars—an in vivo study. Int J Sci Healthc Res. 2019;4(4):160–7.
52. Celik BN, Mutluay MS, Arikan V, Sari S. The evaluation of MTA and Biodentine as a pulpotomy materials for carious exposures in primary teeth. Clin Oral Investig. 2019;23(2):661–6. https://doi.org/10.1007/s00784-018-2472-4.
53. El Habashy LM. Biodentine versus MTA as pulpotomy agents in primary molars: clinical and radiographic study. Egypt Dent J. 2020;66(3):1423–34. https://doi.org/10.21608/EDJ.2020.26182.1079.
54. Caruso S, Dinoi T, Marzo G, Campanella V, Giuca MR, Gatto R, et al. Clinical and radiographic evaluation of Biodentine versus calcium hydroxide in primary teeth pulpotomies: a retrospective study. BMC Oral Health. 2018;18(1):54. https://doi.org/10.1186/s12903-018-0522-6.
55. Koubi G, Colon P, Franquin JC, Hartmann A, Richard G, Faure MO, et al. Clinical evaluation of the performance and safety of a new dentine substitute, Biodentine, in the restoration of posterior teeth—a prospective study. Clin Oral Investig. 2013;17(1):243–9. https://doi.org/10.1007/s00784-012-0701-9.
56. Dawood AE, Manton DJ, Parashos P, Wong RH. The effect of working time on the displacement of Biodentine() beneath prefabricated stainless steel crown: a laboratory study. J Investig Clin Dent. 2016;7(4):391–5. https://doi.org/10.1111/jicd.12162.
57. Palma PJ, Marques JA, Falacho RI, Vinagre A, Santos JM, Ramos JC. Does delayed restoration improve shear bond strength of different restorative protocols to calcium silicate-based cements? Materials (Basel). 2018;11(11) https://doi.org/10.3390/ma11112216.
58. Palma PJ, Marques JA, Antunes M, Falacho RI, Sequeira D, Roseiro L, et al. Effect of restorative timing on shear bond strength of composite resin/calcium silicate-based cements adhesive interfaces. Clin Oral Investig. 2020; https://doi.org/10.1007/s00784-020-03640-7.
59. Bolhari B, Ashofteh Yazdi K, Abbasi M, Sanjari S, Meraji N, Ozcan M. Calcium silicate cement interface with restorative materials through layering after different time intervals. Odontology. 2020; https://doi.org/10.1007/s10266-020-00521-z.

Biodentine™ Applications in Traumatology and Fractures

7

Luc Martens and Rita Cauwels

7.1 Introduction

Crown fractures with pulp exposure represent 18–20% of traumatic dental injuries, the majority being in young permanent central incisors [1]. These injuries produce changes in the exposed pulp tissues, and a biological and functional restoration of immature young permanent teeth with immature root formation represents a high clinical challenge [2]. The treatment of pulpal injury during this period provides a significant challenge for the clinician as a conventional endodontic treatment protocol for these immature teeth is demanding because of the open apex [3, 4].

The goal of this treatment is to maintain pulp vitality via apexogenesis, which allows continued root development along the entire root length [5]. Apexogenesis after traumatic pulp exposure in vital young permanent teeth can be accomplished by implementing the appropriate vital pulp therapy such as pulp capping or pulpotomy depending on the time elapsed after the injury, the degree of root development and the size of the pulp exposure and as a consequence the degree of pulp vitality [6]. Histologic examination of traumatised pulp shows that the depth of infection does not exceed 2 mm from the exposed surface within 48 h [7]. Therefore, if treated within 48 h, 2 mm of the injured pulp can be successfully removed, leaving the non-inflamed healthy radicular pulp to reorganise.

In this era of regenerative endodontics, it is of utmost importance to define the real meaning of regenerative endodontics. As long as vital pulp is present, repair of the dentine-pulp complex using tricalcium silicate-based cements (TCSCs) is the treatment of choice. When no vital pulp is left, revitalisation by allowing a fresh blood clot in an empty canal being covered with tricalcium silicate-based cements in combination with/without scaffolds makes regeneration of new (dental) tissue

L. Martens (✉) · R. Cauwels
Department of Paediatric Dentistry, Ghent University, Ghent, Belgium
e-mail: luc.martens@ugent.be; rita.cauwels@ugent.be

possible [8]. According to the above, the goal of treating dental trauma in immature incisors is mainly to perform a therapy to repair the dentine-pulp complex.

7.1.1 Paradigm Shift

For decades calcium hydroxide was the material of choice for (in)direct capping and pulpotomies to achieve apexogenesis. A significant progress in the prevention and treatment of pulpal and periradicular pathology took place thanks to advances in research on the dentine-pulp complex with special attention to pulp repair and regeneration of mineralised tissue. Also as a consequence of the better knowledge of the interaction between stem cells and bioactive cements, new techniques have been developed with the aim of avoiding pulpectomy of the contaminated pulp and preventing extraction in case of a severe infection.

Bioactive materials such as TCSCs became the golden standard for all the aforementioned indications owing to its increased desirable interaction with biological tissues. They represent a paradigm shift in the treatment of dental trauma of immature permanent incisors with pulpal involvement.

It has been demonstrated that many proteins and growth factors are present within the dentine structure during odontogenesis. These molecules have been shown to have a particular role in dentine remineralisation [9]. The solubilisation of proteins from dentine, exposed to certain materials, i.e. tricalcium silicate-based cements, has been demonstrated. The ability to extract these potentially bioactive molecules to facilitate their interaction with pulpal cells creates the potential to enhance the process of repair of the dentine-pulp complex [10]. Regarding the endodontic treatment of immature teeth, continued root formation to its maturity and an increased thickness of root dentine are anticipated. Ideally, this occurs when pulp tissue and apical papilla tissue are still present. The dental papilla at the apex contains stem cells (SCAP) [11]. In case of infection (see illustration in Sect. 7.1.2) the SCAP may survive the infection and keep the ability to give rise to new odontoblasts influenced by HERS (Hertwig's epithelial root sheet), allowing root dentine to form and, additionally, together with the existing primary odontoblasts from the residual pulp tissue, to proceed to root maturation [11, 12].

Due to an open apex, providing a good communication from the pulp space to the periapical tissues, it has been shown that, even with the presence of periapical disease, pulp tissue is only partially necrotic and infected. Stem cells may also have survived the infection allowing regeneration of pulp and root maturation. It is suggested that the infection has spread through the survived pulp tissue reaching the periapex, leaving vital pulp and vital SCAP [13].

7.1.2 Casuistics

A 10-year-old boy presented with a painful mucosal infection of tooth 11 (Fig. 7.1a, b). He suffered from a dental trauma 2 years earlier but never went to his dentist for a

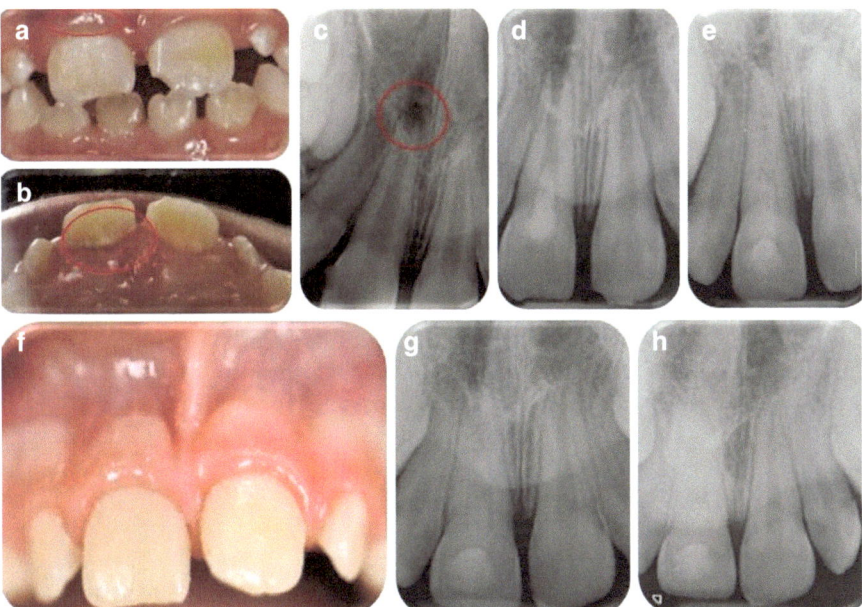

Fig. 7.1 A 10-year-old boy with mucosal infection (**a**, **b**) 2 years after trauma. The X-ray showed arrested maturation and a periapical lesion (**c**). Biodentine in close contact with vital pulpal tissue (**d**); periapical healing was found (**e**); mucosal healing (**f**) and full maturation of the tooth after 2- (**g**) and 3-year (**h**) follow-up

follow-up. The periapical radiograph revealed a periapical reaction and arrested root maturation of tooth 11 (Fig. 7.1c). The affected tooth did not respond to sensitivity tests. After local anaesthesia, rubber dam isolation, opening the pulp chamber and superficial irrigation with NaOCl (2.5%) a sensation was felt by the patient while exploring the working length with blunt paper points. At that level, existing vital pulp remnants were located. Further irrigation was done at the same level minus 1 mm in order not to harm vital tissue. Saline was used for the final irrigation. The canal was dried by blunt paper points on working length. Biodentine was then placed in contact with the vital tissue and finished by a coronal seal (Fig. 7.1d). Figure 7.1e, f shows the healing of the periapical area, a healthy mucosa and further maturation of the root. Figure 7.1g, h shows further post-operative maturation after 2- and 3-year follow-up, respectively.

7.1.3 Choice for Biodentine

Calcium silicate-based materials have gained enormous attention and use in traumatic injuries. Biodentine is a hydraulic self-setting cement which has frequently been acknowledged in the literature as a promising material and serves as an important representative of tricalcium silicate-based cements used in dentistry. Biodentine has earned positive reviews in the literature owing to its superior physical properties, setting time, biocompatibility and wide range of clinical applications including dental traumatic injuries [14, 15].

Progressive discolouration of the tooth crown is a potential aesthetic complication after endodontic treatment of anterior teeth. Discolouration is a result of either material ingress into dentinal tubules or material remnants in the pulp chamber, which get darker over time and are transmitted through the hard tissues [16]. Biodentine seems to exhibit colour stability independent of oxygen and light irradiation unlike other tricalcium silicate cements such as mineral trioxide aggregate [17]. Biodentine maintained colour stability up to 6 months and exhibited significantly less discolouration compared with ProRoot MTA [18, 19], OrthoMTA [20], grey MTA and white MTA [21], and bioaggregate and MTA Angelus [22]. The presence of bismuth oxide and uptake of blood components in the porosities of various Portland cement-based products were considered to be causal factors of discolouration [16]. Clinically perceptible discolouration was observed with Biodentine in the presence of sodium hypochlorite [23, 24], chlorhexidine gluconate [23] and blood [20]. Delayed tooth discolouration was detected in both ProRoot MTA and Biodentine at the 1-year evaluation, but it was more evident for ProRoot MTA than Biodentine [25].

Traumatic injuries are very frequent and it has been reported that 20% of children entering the emergency care unit suffer from dental trauma [26]. The performance of an adequate pulp treatment is of utmost importance. In this respect it is most advantageous that Biodentine can be used as pulp dressing and as temporary filling. From a 6-month report, it became clear that Biodentine remains in the oral cavity for at least 6 months as an enamel replacement material [27].

7.2   Direct Pulp Capping in Traumatised Immature Incisors

When a complicated crown fracture occurs, the treatment choice is often a matter of time elapsed after the fracture, the grade of possible infection of the pulp and the size of pulp exposure. Direct pulp capping can be the choice of treatment in case of pinpoint exposure; however when a TCSC is used, it is advised to change to a 'small' pulpotomy to allow the material to be secured [28].

7.2.1   Casuistics

A 9-year-old boy came to the emergency unit due to a dental trauma that occurred a few hours earlier (Fig. 7.2). Clinical and radiographic diagnosis revealed a pinpoint exposure of the pulp of incisor 21 (Fig. 7.2a, d). After local anaesthesia and proper isolation, a 'small' cavity of 2 mm was prepared to have better access to the pulp. No infection was suspected, and bleeding stopped spontaneously as expected (Fig. 7.2b). The cavity was filled with Biodentine, making sure that the cement came in close contact with the pulp without pressure. According to the mechanical properties of the cement, Biodentine was used as a temporary filling (Fig. 7.2c, e).

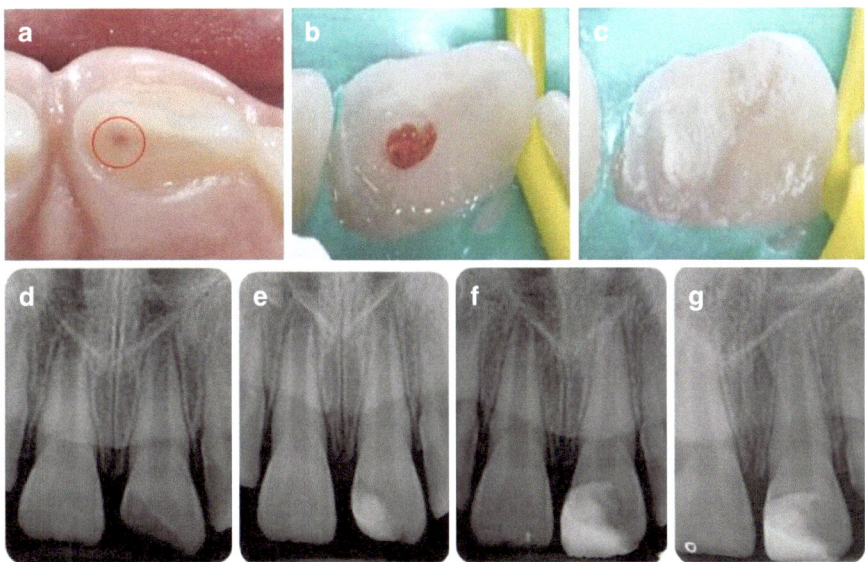

Fig. 7.2 Clinical (**a–c**) and radiographic (**d–g**) follow-up of a pinpoint pulp exposure (**a**) and treatment (**b, c**) with subsequent further root maturation of incisor 21

In a second appointment, the superficial layer of Biodentine was replaced by composite as permanent restoration (Fig. 7.2f). Follow-up sessions show a further maturation of 21 without complications (Fig. 7.2g).

7.3   Pulpotomy in Traumatised Immature Incisors

Vital pulp therapy is a well-known and widely practiced therapy after traumatic complicated crown fractures in young immature teeth with pulp exposure. Partial pulpotomy with calcium hydroxide has shown a high success rate in previous reports [29]. The outcome criteria for successful vital pulp therapy treatment after dental trauma include asymptomatic teeth (clinically and radiographically), new hard-tissue formation (dentine-like bridge), apexogenesis (indicates tooth vitality) and absence of tooth discolouration (for aesthetic reasons). In Fig. 7.3 the formation of a hard-tissue barrier is illustrated 3 months (Fig. 7.3c) after partial pulpotomy with Biodentine (Fig. 7.3b) in a central incisor with a complicated crown fracture (Fig. 7.3a) and pinpoint pulp exposure. Long-term follow-up of case series with TCSs is necessary to establish the success rate.

7.3.1   Casuistics

In a 7-year-old Caucasian female, who visited the emergency service after an accident in the playground, an enamel dentine fracture with pulp exposure on tooth 11

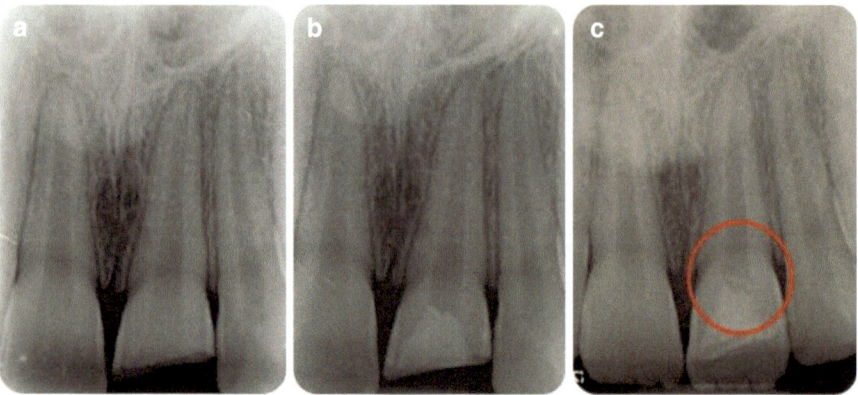

Fig. 7.3 A complicated crown fracture (**a**); partial pulpotomy with Biodentine (**b**); hard-tissue formation after 3 months (**c**)

was diagnosed (Fig. 7.4a). Due to severe anxiety, it was impossible to treat her under local analgesia. The treatment was performed the following day under general anaesthesia [30]. The pulp exposure was further opened with a sterile high-speed diamond bur with sufficient water cooling. The pulp tissue to the cement-enamel junction level was removed (cervical pulpotomy). Haemostasis was achieved with a cotton pellet, and the pulp exposure was capped with Biodentine which was used as a temporary filling (Fig. 7.4b–e). A radiograph at this appointment showed an immature open apex and the Biodentine pulpotomy could be noted at the cingulum level (Fig. 7.4f). Three weeks later, a permanent composite restoration was made. Pulp sensibility and digital radiographical evaluation were performed after 12, 24 and 48 months (Fig. 7.4g–i). No subjective discomfort was reported during the entire follow-up period. Clinically, the tooth remained vital, and no discolouration was observed. Radiographically, starting from 18 months, complete apexogenesis was evident, and this was further confirmed at the 24- and 48-month follow-up.

7.4   Full Obturation in Traumatised Incisors

Endodontic treatment of immature traumatised teeth with pulp necrosis is a challenge for the clinicians because of the widely open apices and the thin dentinal walls which are strong predictors for teeth fractures especially in the cervical area [31, 32]. Besides, canal debridement is challenging and working length determination and obturation are difficult [33]. For decades $Ca(OH)_2$ (calcium hydroxide) had been used for the apexification technique forming an apical calcified barrier. The duration for this varied from 5 to 19 months [34]. This technique allowed an improvement in root canal treatment using gutta-percha and sealing material [35]. On the other hand, it has been reported that after long-term application of $Ca(OH)_2$ tooth strength is reduced up to 50% in 1 year [36] due to its proteolytic action [35].

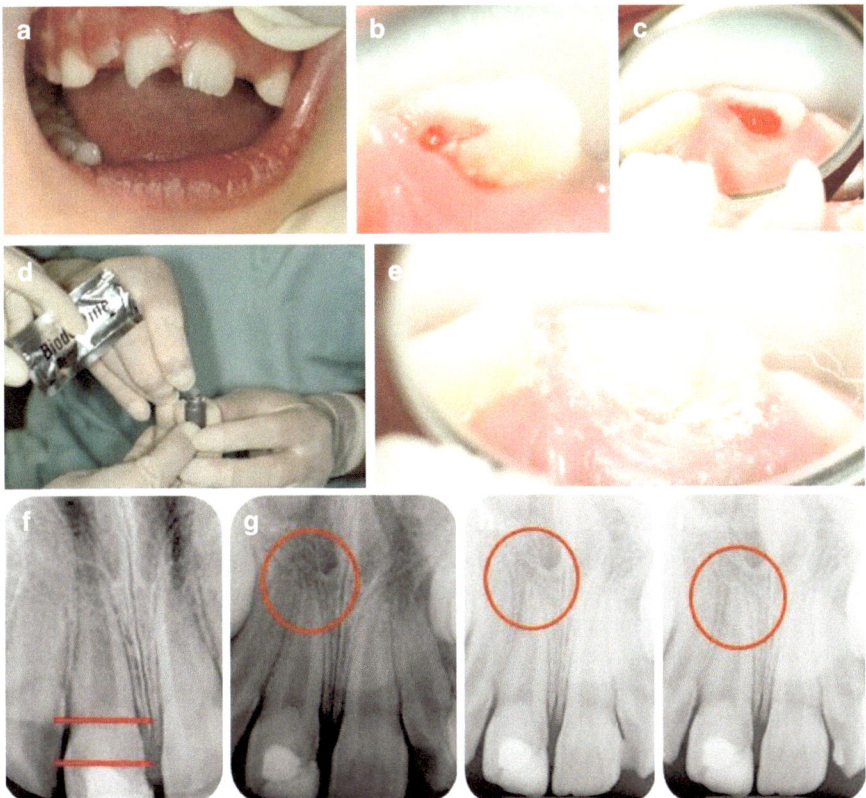

Fig. 7.4 A 7-year-old girl presented with a complex crown fracture with pulp exposure (**a**, **c**). After further opening (**d**) a Biodentine pulpotomy was performed (**b**, **e**). This bioceramic material was also used as a temporary filling. Radiographical follow-up after Biodentine pulpotomy at baseline (**f**) up to 12–24–48 months with full apexogenesis (**g–i**)

It has been reported that cervical root fracture incidence is high (>60%) caused by minor impacts, or else subsequent to root canal treatment in weakened immature teeth [37].

Although Biodentine was reported as being successful as a plug material in the apical area with favourable prognosis [38–41], the gutta-percha endodontic filling on top gives no strength to the cervical area. Minimising the incidence of root fracture in immature teeth can be done by enhancing the resistance of these teeth to fracture [42].

In this respect, full obturation of an immature root is a possible alternative endodontic therapy that could provide equally satisfying clinical results in cases where revitalisation/regenerative endodontic treatment is not a viable option. Calcium silicate-based cements adhere to root dentine, forming a crystalline bond in a biochemical process termed biomineralisation [43]. The biomineralisation ability of Biodentine initiates calcium and silicate uptake by the dentine, which in turn can lead to chemical and structural modification of the dentine that may result in higher acid resistance and physical strength [44]. Hence, the use of Biodentine in the present cases as an obturation material may eventually improve the resistance of the endodontically treated immature teeth against fracture. In order to strengthen the weakened roots, one should seal the cervical area up to the enamel-dentin junction. From an earlier in vitro study, it could be concluded that mineral trioxide aggregate significantly strengthened immature root canals [35]. Moreover, Biodentine exhibits higher compressive strength in comparison to other tricalcium silicate cements, which is attributed to the low water/cement ratio thanks to the addition of a water-soluble polymer in the liquid. The physical properties of Biodentine such as flexural strength, elastic modulus and Vickers hardness are comparable to those of dentine [45, 46].

7.4.1 Casuistics

7.4.1.1 Case 1: 9-Year-Old Girl with Infection of 22

A 9-year-old girl presented at the emergency service with an infection of the lateral incisor 22 of unknown origin. She complained of a mucosal painful swelling. Clinical and radiographical examination revealed a periapical reaction of the immature 22. The cusp of the erupting 23 was seen at the level of the source of infection (Fig. 7.5a). Following local anaesthesia, proper isolation and access opening to the pulp, the canal was irrigated with NaOCl (2.5%), followed by final rinsing with saline and canal drying with blunt paper points. A complete empty pulp canal was found and therefore it was temporarily filled with $Ca(OH)_2$ paste for further disinfection (Fig. 7.5b). Two weeks later, the $Ca(OH)_2$ paste was replaced by Biodentine since the patient had no complaints within a few days after the former treatment. Two months later, the infection source was healed and a further eruption of 23 was seen (Fig. 7.5c). Figure 7.5d, e shows the mature 22 and fully erupted 23 after 4 years of initial treatment.

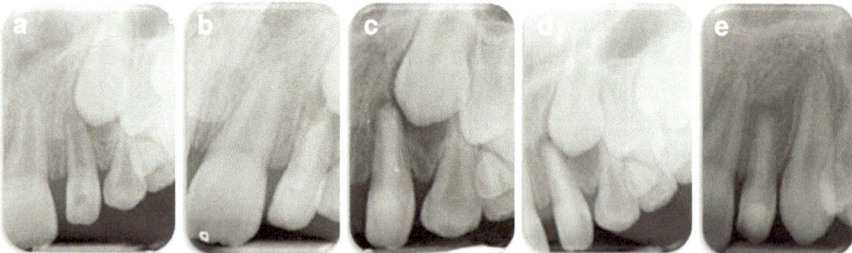

Fig. 7.5 Infection of immature 22 (**a**); calcium hydroxide dressing (**b**); Biodentine obturation (**c**, **d**); 4-year follow-up with complete healing and eruption of 23 (**e**)

7.4.1.2 Case 2: 8-Year-Old Girl with Recurrent Infection After Trauma of 11

An 8-year-old girl came to the department 2.5 months after a trauma with an abscess in tooth 11. Uncomplicated crown fractures of 11 and 21 were diagnosed and glass ionomer cement dressing was placed. Percussion and palpation tests were positive and cold test was negative. There was no mobility. Radiographic diagnosis revealed apical radiolucency on 11 (Fig. 7.6a). After proper opening of the cavity (Fig. 7.6b) necrotic pulp tissue (Fig. 7.6c) was removed. The root canal was irrigated with NaOCl (2.5%), dried with paper points and filled with a $Ca(OH)_2$ dressing for 2 weeks (Fig. 7.6d).

During follow-up after 2 weeks the abscess clinically disappeared, and there was no percussion sensitivity. Decision was made to replace the $Ca(OH)_2$ dressing with Biodentine. Figure 7.6e shows the radiographical situation after 1 month. Although the patient had no complaints, recurrent infection could be seen at tooth 11 after 12-month (Fig. 7.6f) and 18-month interval (Fig. 7.6g). After consulting an endodontist, decision was made to perform an apicoectomy on 11. During surgery, apical infection became obvious and could be properly removed. Moreover, it was seen that the Biodentine was well sealed in the canal which showed very thin dentinal walls (Fig. 7.6h). Follow-up at 1 month (Fig. 7.6i) and 1 year (Fig. 7.6j) showed a healing process. After 1 year, complete bone healing and an intact periodontal ligament were found. The complete maturation of 21 without any symptom was also observed.

7.5 Root Fractures

Root fractures involving dentine, cementum and pulp are relatively uncommon among dental traumas, comprising 0.5–7% and affecting permanent dentition. Several potential healing events are described depending on the integrity of the pulp at the fracture site. Callus formation and connective tissue healing are possible when no ingress of bacteria occurs [47]. If bacteria gain access to the coronal pulp, pulp necrosis occurs with potential accumulation of inflamed tissue between the two root fragments or with pus formation within the canal. Especially in this particular case where pulp did not survive, Biodentine treatment in the coronal part may be the treatment of choice.

7.5.1 Casuistics

A 10-year-old boy presented with a trauma which had occurred 7 days earlier (Fig. 7.7). Clinically, the mucosa around 11 and 21 was blueish. He suffered from pain and 21 showed a slightly increased mobility (Fig. 7.7a). The radiograph revealed a horizontal root fracture in the apical third (Fig. 7.7b). Tooth 21 was put

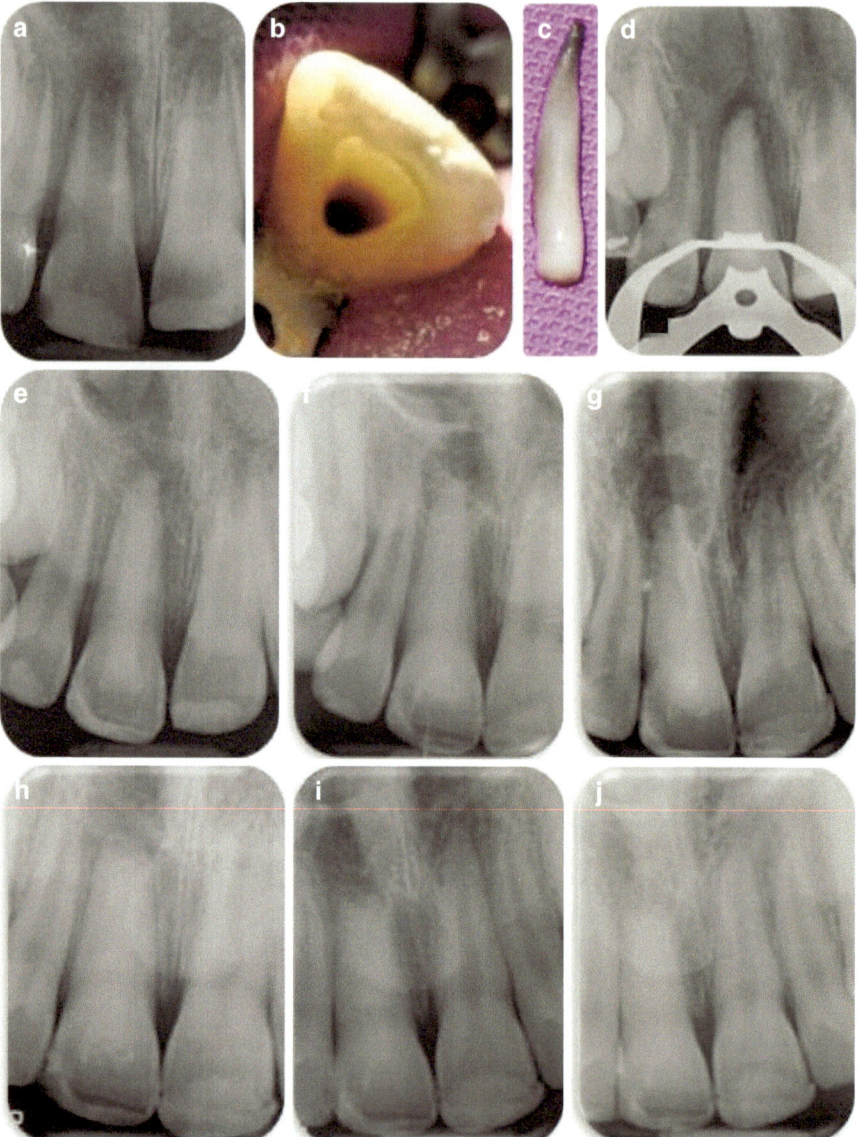

Fig. 7.6 Uncomplicated crown fractures at 11 and 21 with infection on 11 (**a**); access to the pulp chamber (**b**); necrotic pulp tissue (**c**); canal of tooth 11 filled up with calcium hydroxide (**d**). Biodentine follow-up after 1 month (**e**); 12 (**f**) and 18 months (**g**); apicectomy of 11 (**h**); follow-up at 6 (**i**) and 12 months (**j**) with complete bone healing and an intact periodontal ligament

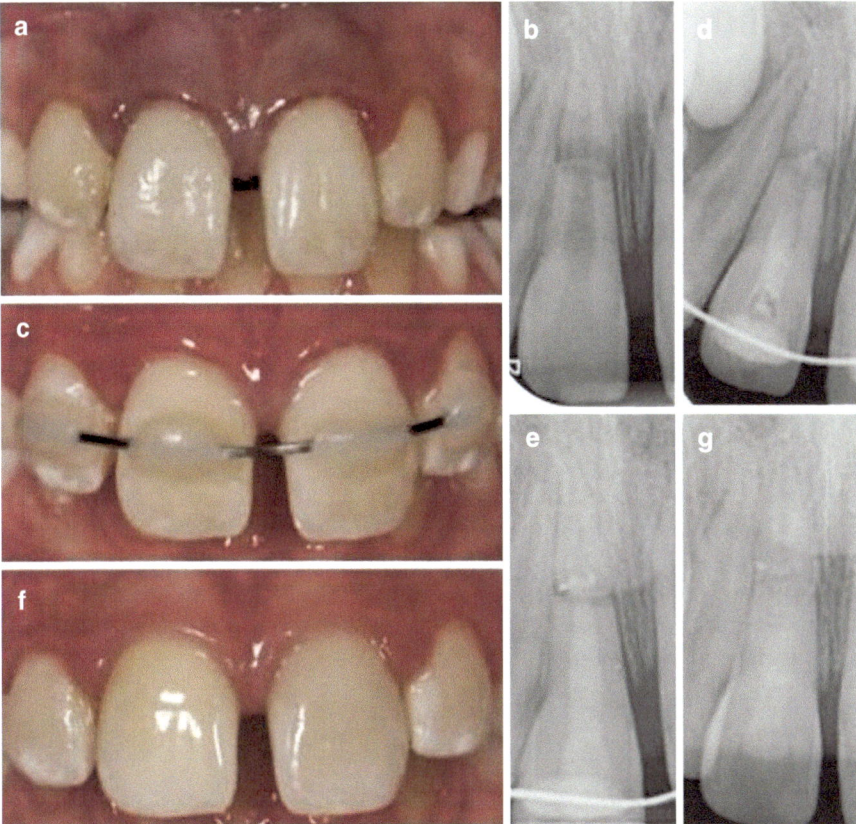

Fig. 7.7 A 10-year-old boy presented with tooth 11 and 21 one week after trauma (**a**) with a middle third root fracture on 11 (**b**); splinting of 11 (**c**); calcium hydroxide dressing (**d**); Biodentine obturation (**e**); clinical picture after 22 months (**f**); complete healing and hard-tissue formation after 22 months (**g**)

in its original place as far as possible, and splinted with a flexible wire and composite for 4 weeks (Fig. 7.7c). A few days later the patient presented with a discoloured 21 and access to the canal was opened after proper isolation. An empty coronal pulp canal confirmed the suspected pulp necrosis. In order to control the infection Ca(OH)$_2$ was applied until the level of the fracture line (Fig. 7.7d). The crown was sealed with a temporary filling. Within the 4 weeks of splinting, the Ca(OH)$_2$ was replaced by Biodentine (Fig. 7.7e). The splint was removed after 4 weeks (Fig. 7.7f) and canal treatment was followed up to 22 months (Fig. 7.7g). A complete healing with normal periodontal ligament and new hard-tissue formation at the fracture area were observed.

7.6   Save the Unsaved

Due to a lack of expertise, general dentists do not feel familiar with complex dental injuries. These cases, also when presented at emergency services in local hospitals, often do not receive an adequate immediate treatment and follow-up. However international guidelines are available [48].

As a result, necrotic immature teeth with fistula, abscesses and pus formation are referred to dental hospitals. Taking into account the current guidelines to avoid systemic and intra-canal antibiotics, Biodentine offers a perfect choice to save these compromised teeth. The same applies when trauma occurs in freshly erupted incisors with partial root formation.

7.6.1   Necrotic Immature Teeth After Trauma

Pulp necrosis is the second most common complication after traumatic dental injuries and occurs mostly within the first 6–24 months of the follow-up period, depending on the type of dental trauma and the maturity of the tooth [49]. Apexification by induction of a calcified barrier and revitalisation treatment aiming at regeneration of pulp tissue are the choice of treatments currently available for retaining an immature necrotic permanent tooth [5, 50, 51].

7.6.1.1 Casuistics
An 8-year-old boy was referred to the dental hospital by his general dental practitioner for further endodontic treatment of an immature maxillary central incisor (tooth 21) under general anaesthesia [52]. Medical history of the patient did not give any relevant information and dental history revealed that the tooth had suffered a luxation injury of tooth 21 about 6 months earlier. The general dentist had administered $Ca(OH)_2$ after pulpectomy.

Percussion and palpation revealed negative results and the tooth was asymptomatic. Besides a clear dentinal bridge formation that was seen in the apical third (Fig. 7.8a), digital radiographic examination disclosed a radiolucency along the periapical region. The tooth was diagnosed as necrotic and the absolute non-cooperation of the patient required the endodontic treatment to be performed under general anaesthesia. Access to tooth 21 was obtained using a high-speed bur. Black pulp tissue indicative of complete necrosis was noted. Working length was manually determined (Fig. 7.8a), followed by irrigation with 2.5% sodium hypochlorite. Subsequently, complete drying of the canal using paper points was obtained and the root canal was filled with $Ca(OH)_2$ (Fig. 7.8b). The access cavity was sealed with a glass-ionomer cement. Six weeks later, $Ca(OH)_2$ from the root canal was removed by irrigation with saline and 2.5% sodium hypochlorite. The root canal was dried with paper points and completely obturated with Biodentine (Fig. 7.8c). Two days

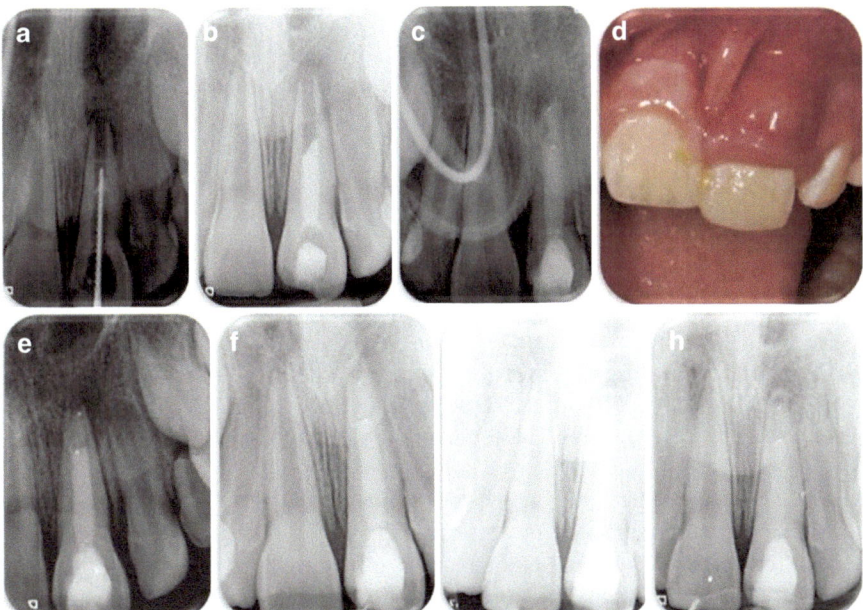

Fig. 7.8 An 8-year-old boy with recurrent infection on 21 after a first calcium hydroxide therapy in private practice (**a**); renewed calcium hydroxide dressing (**b**); length determination (**c**); full obturation with Biodentine (**d**); 2 weeks post-op (**e**); 3-month follow-up (**f**); 15- and 27-month follow-up (**g, h**)

thereafter, the patient reported labial swelling and pus discharge from the labial sulcus of 21 (Fig. 7.8d). Antibiotic therapy (amoxicillin 1500 mg/day) was prescribed alongside chlorhexidine mouthwash for 1 week. In the next visit, the glass-ionomer restoration was replaced by composite resin (A2 shade, Clearfil, Kuraray, New York, USA) (Fig. 7.8e). Subsequently, the swelling and pus discharge disappeared, and the patient remained symptomless for the rest of the observation period. The patient was initially followed up at 3-month interval (Fig. 7.8f) and then at 6-month interval. Radiographically, normal periodontal ligament and apexification indicative of healing were noted at the follow-up appointments at 15 and 27 months (Fig. 7.8g, h). In further follow-ups apical areas remained unchanged.

7.6.2 Saving the Unsaved

Besides necrosis severe atypical traumatic injury can happen at a very young age (root fracture in a recently erupted tooth, necrosis after a severe blow, etc.). In the past these cases could not be saved. The regenerative potential of Biodentine gives an opportunity to save these lost cases.

7.6.2.1 Casuistics

Case 1: 5-Year-Old Boy with a Unilateral Root Fracture on the Immature Tooth 21

A 5-year-old boy presented several weeks after a severe blow on tooth 21. Baseline radiograph showed a severe fracture of the immature root and apparently an infection (Fig. 7.9a). Opening of the tooth revealed a necrotic tissue with a bad smell. After irrigation with NaOCl (2.5%) and gently drying, AB-paste (Ledermix) was placed for 5 days (Fig. 7.9b). Five days later, the tooth was opened, rinsed again and gently dried. Biodentine was placed in the best possible way using a carrier and endo plug-gers (Fig. 7.9c). Follow-ups after 3 (Fig. 7.9d) and 6 months (Fig. 7.9e) showed complete healing and hard-tissue formation. Also, a periodontal ligament became visible around the root structure. These healthy processes were confirmed at 12–24 and 36 months (Fig. 7.9f–h). This tooth was functional without any mobility.

Case 2: 6-Year-Old Boy with a Severe Trauma on a Freshly Erupted Incisor

A 6-year-old boy was referred by his dentist, 2 weeks after a dental injury. He suf-fered from a painful swelling of the mucosa around tooth 21. Clinical investigation showed increased mobility of 21, no sensitivity to cold stimulus and no pulp expo-sure but pus was released from the sulcus by palpation. His dentist prescribed sys-temic antibiotics. The diagnostic radiograph revealed a periapical reaction (Fig. 7.10a). After local anaesthesia, proper isolation of the tooth and palatal access

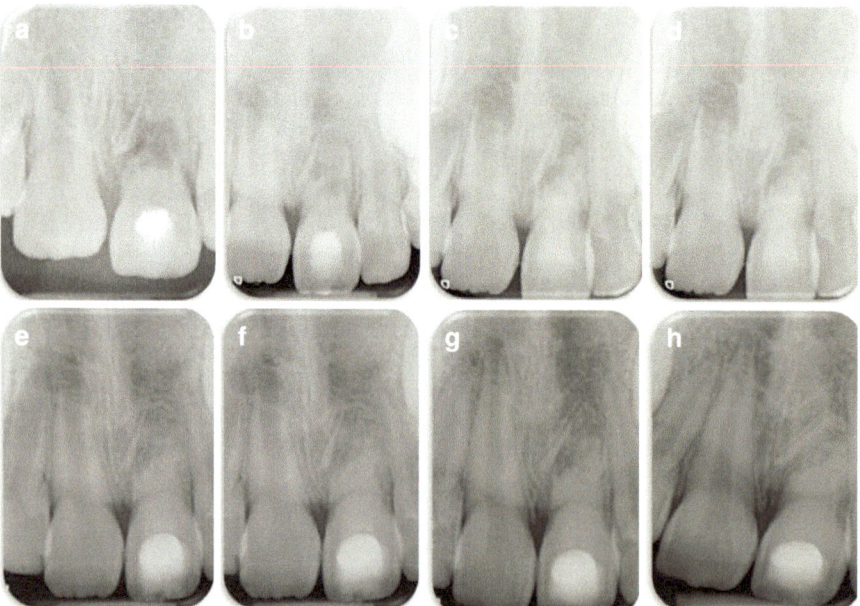

Fig. 7.9 A 5-year-old boy with severe infection on immature 21 (**a**); application of AB-paste (**b**); application of Biodentine (**c**); 3-month follow-up (**d**); follow-up at 6 (**e**); 12 (**f**), 24 (**g**) and 36 months (**h**)

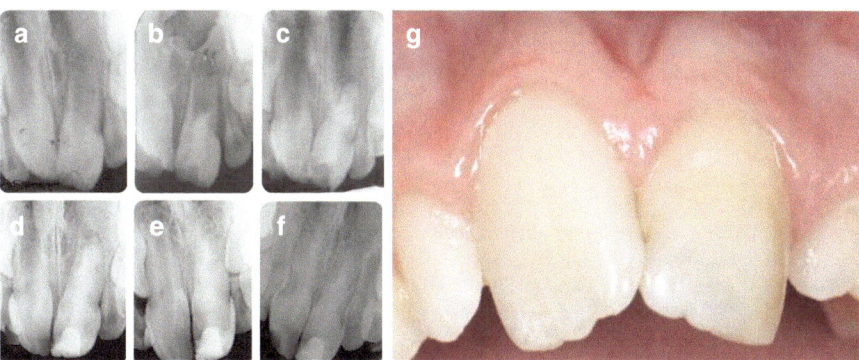

Fig. 7.10 Severe trauma on immature tooth 21 (**a**); calcium hydroxide dressing (**b**); Biodentine obturation (**c**); follow-up at 6 (**d**), 18 (**e**) and 54 months (**f**); clinical picture after 54 months (**g**)

to the pulp chamber, an important flow of pus was released from the canal. After thorough irrigation with NaOCl (2.5%) followed by saline rinsing, Ca(OH)$_2$ was left in the canal for 2 weeks (Fig. 7.10b). At the next appointment the patient did not complain anymore, and within 1 week the swelling disappeared. Access was again made to the pulp chamber and medication was removed by irrigation as in the first appointment. The pulp chamber was dried with blunt paper points to a depth of contact with tissue, feeling its resistance, after which the endodontic open space was filled with Biodentine in contact with the remaining tissue (Fig. 7.10c). A continuing maturation of the root is shown in the follow-up radiographs at 6 and 18 months (Fig. 7.10d, e). Figure 7.10f, g shows the radiographical and clinical result after 4 years and 6 months. X-ray showed a perfect PDL, allowing safe orthodontic treatment in the future.

7.7 Conclusion

Thanks to a better understanding of the dentine-pulp complex and its molecular biology in combination with the development of newer bioceramic materials especially based on tricalcium silicate cements, a total paradigm shift became possible regarding the management of traumatic injuries. Although high evidence is difficult to obtain, it may be accepted that due to worldwide reported clinical success, the use of Biodentine is the best clinical practice for treating dental injuries including (root) fractures and recurrent infection, with a most favourable outcome.

References

1. de Blanco LP. Treatment of crown fractures with pulp exposure. Oral Surg Oral Med Oral Pathol Oral Radiol Endod. 1996;82(5):564–8.
2. Ojeda-Gutierrez F, Martinez-Marquez B, Arteaga-Larios S, Ruiz-Rodriguez MS, Pozos-Guillen A. Management and follow-up of complicated crown fractures in young patients treated with partial pulpotomy. Case Rep Dent. 2013;2013:597563.

3. Rafter M. Apexification: a review. Dent Traumatol. 2005;21:1–8.
4. Shabahang S. Treatment options: apexogenesis and apexification. J Endod. 2013;39(3 Suppl):S26–9. https://doi.org/10.1016/j.joen.2012.11.046.
5. Shabahang S. Treatment options: apexogenesis and apexification. Pediatr Dent. 2013;35(2):125–8.
6. Guideline on pulp therapy for primary and immature permanent teeth. Pediatr Dent. 2016;38(6):280–8.
7. Cvek M, Cleaton-Jones PE, Austin JC, Andreasen JO. Pulp reactions to exposure after experimental crown fractures or grinding in adult monkeys. J Endod. 1982;8:391–7.
8. Tziafas D, Kodonas K. Differentiation potential of dental papilla, dental pulp, and apical papilla progenitor cells. J Endod. 2010;36(5):781–9.
9. Smithe AJ, Murray PE, Sloan AJ, Matthews JB, Zhao S. Transdentinal stimulation of tertiary dentinogenesis. Adv Dent Res. 2001;15:51–4.
10. Ferracane JL, Cooper PR, Smith AJ. Can interaction of materials with the dentin-pulp complex contribute to dentin regeneration. Odontology. 2010;98:2–14.
11. Huang GTJ. Apexification: the beginning of its end. Int Endod J. 2009;42:855–66.
12. Sonoyama W, Liu Y, Yamaza T, et al. Characterization of the apical papilla and its resiing stem cells from human immature permanent teeth: a pilot study. J Endod. 2008;34:166–71.
13. Huang GTJ, Sonoyama W, Liu H, Wang S, Shi S. The hidden treasure in apical papilla: the potential role in pulp/dentin regeneration and bioroot engineering. J Endod. 2008;34:645–51.
14. Rajasekharan S, Martens LC, Cauwels R, Anthonappa RP, Verbeeck RMH. Biodentine material characteristics and clinical applications: a 3 year literature review and update. Eur Arch Paediatr Dent. 2018;19(1):1–22.
15. Malkondu Ö, Kazandağ MK, Kazazoğlu E. A review on biodentine, a contemporary dentine replacement and repair material. Biomed Res Int. 2014;2014:160951.
16. Lenherr P, Allgayer N, Weiger R, Filippi A, Attin T, Krastl G. Tooth discoloration induced by endodontic materials: a laboratory study. Int Endod J. 2012;45:942–9.
17. Valles M, Mercade M, Duran-Sindreu F, Bourdelande JL, Roig M. Influence of light and oxygen on the color stability of five calcium silicate-based materials. J Endod. 2013;39(4):525–8. https://doi.org/10.1016/j.joen.2012.12.021.
18. Valles M, Roig M, Duran-Sindreu F, Martinez S, Mercade M. Color stability of teeth restored with Biodentine: a 6-month in vitro study. J Endod. 2015;41:1157–60.
19. Marconyak LJ Jr, Kirkpatrick TC, Roberts HW, et al. A comparison of coronal tooth discoloration elicited by various endodontic reparative materials. J Endod. 2016;42:470–3.
20. Shokouhinejad N, Nekoofar MH, Pirmoazen S, Shamshiri AR, Dummer PM. Evaluation and comparison of occurrence of tooth discoloration after the application of various calcium silicate-based cements: an ex vivo study. J Endod. 2016;42:140–4.
21. Kohli MR, Yamaguchi M, Setzer FC, Karabucak B. Spectrophotometric analysis of coronal tooth discoloration induced by various bioceramic cements and other endodontic materials. J Endod. 2015;41:1862–6.
22. Yoldas SE, Bani M, Atabek D, Bodur H. Comparison of the potential discoloration effect of bioaggregate, Biodentine, and white mineral trioxide aggregate on bovine teeth in vitro research. J Endod. 2016;42:1815–8.
23. Camilleri J. Staining potential of Neo MTA plus, MTA plus, and Biodentine used for pulpotomy procedures. J Endod. 2015;41:1139–45.
24. Keskin C, Demiryurek EO, Ozyurek T. Color stabilities of calcium silicate-based materials in contact with different irrigation solutions. J Endod. 2015;41:409–11.
25. Ramos JC, Palma PJ, Nascimento R, et al. 1-year in vitro evaluation of tooth discoloration induced by 2 calcium silicate-based cements. J Endod. 2016;42:1403–7.
26. Martens LC, Rajasekharan S, Jacquet W, Vandenbulcke JD, Van Acker JWG, Cauwels RGEC. Paediatric dental emergencies: a retrospective study and a proposal for definition and guidelines including pain management. Eur Arch Paediatric Dent. 2018;19(4):245–253.

27. Koubi G, Colon P, Franquin JC, et al. Clinical evaluation of the performance and safety of a new dentine substitute, Biodentine, in the restoration of posterior teeth—a prospective study. Clin Oral Investig. 2013;17(1):243–9.
28. Andreasen F, Andreasen J, Tsilingardis G. Chapter 25: Management of trauma-related pulp disease and tooth reposition. In: Traumatic injuries of the teeth. 5th ed. Copenhagen: Wiley Blackwell; 2019. ISBN: 9781119167051.
29. Fong CD, Davis MJ. Partial pulpotomy for immature permanent teeth, its present and future. Pediatr Dent. 2002;24(1):29–32.
30. Martens L, Rajasekharan S, Cauwels R. Pulp management after traumatic injuries with a tricalcium silicate-based cement (Biodentine): a report of two cases, up to 48 months follow-up. Eur Arch Paediatr Dent. 2015;16:491–6.
31. Guven Y, Tuna EB, Dincol ME, Ozel E, Yilmaz B, Aktoren O. Long-term fracture resistance of simulated immature teeth filled with various calcium silicate-based materials. Biomed Res Int. 2016;2016:2863817.
32. Carvalho CA, Valera MC, Oliveira LD, Camargo CH. Structural resistance in immature teeth using root reinforcements in vitro. Dent Traumatol. 2005;21(3):155–9.
33. Peroz I, Blankenstein F, Lange KP, Naumann M. Restoring endodontically treated teeth with posts and cores—a review. Quintessence Int. 2005;36(9):737–46.
34. Ghose LJ, Baghdady VS, Hikmat YM. Apexification of immature apices of pulpless permanent anterior teeth with calcium hydroxide. J Endod. 1987;13(6):285–90.
35. Cauwels RG, Pieters IY, Martens LC, Verbeeck RM. Fracture resistance and reinforcement of immature roots with gutta percha, mineral trioxide aggregate and calcium phosphate bone cement: a standardized in vitro model. Dent Traumatol. 2010;26(2):137–42.
36. Andreasen JO, Farik B, Munksgaard EC. Long-term calcium hydroxide as a root canal dressing may increase risk of root fracture. Dent Traumatol. 2002;18(3):134–7.
37. Elnaghy AM, Elsaka SE. Fracture resistance of simulated immature teeth filled with Biodentine and white mineral trioxide aggregate—an in vitro study. Dent Traumatol. 2016;32(2):116–20.
38. Vidal K, Martin G, Lozano O, Salas M, Trigueros J, Aguilar G. Apical closure in apexification: a review and case report of apexification treatment of an immature permanent tooth with biodentine. J Endod. 2016;42(5):730–4.
39. Bajwa NK, Jingarwar MM, Pathak A. Single visit apexification procedure of a traumatically injured tooth with a novel bioinductive material (Biodentine). Int J Clin Pediatr Dent. 2015;8(1):58–61.
40. Sinha N, Singh B, Patil S. Cone beam-computed topographic evaluation of a central incisor with an open apex and a failed root canal treatment using one-step apexification with Biodentine: a case report. J Conserv Dent. 2014;17(3):285–9.
41. Nayak G, Hasan MF. Biodentine—a novel dentinal substitute for single visit apexification. Restor Dent Endod. 2014;39(2):120–5.
42. Cvek M. Prognosis of luxated non-vital maxillary incisors treated with calcium hydroxide and filled with gutta-percha. A retrospective clinical study. Endod Dent Traumatol. 1992;8(2):45–55.
43. Reyes-Carmona JF, Felippe MS, Felippe WT. The biomineralization ability of mineral trioxide aggregate and portland cement on dentin enhances the push-out strength. J Endod. 2010;36:286–91.
44. Han L, Okiji T. Uptake of calcium and silicon released from calcium silicate-based endodontic materials into root canal dentine. Int Endod J. 2011;44:1081–7.
45. Grech L, Mallia B, Camilleri J. Characterization of set intermediate restorative material, biodentine, bioaggregate and a prototype calcium silicate cement for use as root-end filling materials. Int Endod J. 2013;46:632–41.
46. Grech L, Mallia B, Camilleri J. Investigation of the physical properties of tricalcium silicate cement-based root-end filling materials. Dent Mater. 2013;29:E20–8.
47. Andreasen F, Andreasen J, Tsilingardis G. Chapter 15: Root fractures. In: Traumatic injuries of the teeth. 5th ed. Copenhagen: Wiley Blackwell; 2019. ISBN: 9781119167051.

48. Cauwels R, Martens L, Verbeeck R. Educational background and perceptions of emergency treatment in dental traumatology of Flemish dental practitioners. Dent Traumatol. 2014;30(2):133–9.
49. Nosrat A, Homayounfar N, Oloomi K. Drawbacks and unfavorable outcomes of regenerative endodontic treatments of necrotic immature teeth: a literature review and report of a case. J Endod. 2012;38:1428–34.
50. Bucher K, Neumann C, Thiering E, Hickel R, Kuhnisch J. Complications and survival rates of teeth after dental trauma over a 5-year period. Clin Oral Investig. 2013;17:1311–8.
51. Nosrat A, Li KL, Vir K, Hicks ML, Fouad AF. Is pulp regeneration necessary for root maturation? J Endod. 2013;39:1291–5.
52. Martens L, Rajasekharan S, Cauwels R. Endodontic treatment of trauma-induced necrotic immature teeth using a tricalcium silicate-based bioactive cement. A report of 3 cases with 24-month follow-up. Eur J Paediatr Dent. 2016;17:24–8.

Biodentine™ Applications in Irreversible Pulpitis Management in Children and Adults

Nessrin Taha and Papimon Chompu-inwai

8.1 Pulpal Status Beneath Carious Exposures and the Classification of Pulpitis

Dental caries is induced by biofilms and maintained by fermentable carbohydrates; the acidogenic by-products produced by biofilms induce demineralization of enamel and initiate inflammatory and defensive mechanisms in both dentine and pulp. If demineralization continues, invasion of dentine occurs with subsequent cavitation, and if the lesion is left untreated, it will progress toward the pulp where inflammation will intensify, causing abscess and areas of pulp necrosis leading eventually to death of the dental pulp. On the other hand, if the stimulus is removed and the tooth is adequately restored, the pulp is capable of healing [1]. However, the cutoff point where the pulp is no longer capable of repair is not clear and it is impossible to determine this point by the available sensibility tests, including thermal and electrical ones.

The terms reversible and irreversible pulpitis have long been used as part of the endodontic diagnostic scheme to guide the clinical decision-making process. Reversible pulpitis refers to mild pulpal inflammation and that the pulp is capable of healing, and it is characterized by a mild-to-severe pain response to stimuli, usually from thermal changes but not biting pressure. The pain resolves within seconds. On the other hand, irreversible pulpitis refers to a pulpal status that implies the presence of a more severe degenerative process that will not heal, and it is characterized by mild-to-severe pain that lingers after removal of the stimulus or might be

N. Taha (✉)
Department of Conservative Dentistry, Jordan University of Science and Technology, Irbid, Jordan
e-mail: n.taha@just.edu.jo

P. Chompu-inwai
Division of Pediatric Dentistry, Department of Orthodontics and Pediatric Dentistry, Faculty of Dentistry, Chiang Mai University, Chiang Mai, Thailand

spontaneous. It might be sharp or dull depending on the nerve fibers that respond to the inflammatory mediators [2].

The validity of these diagnostic terms, reversible and irreversible pulpitis, has been questioned previously by Dummer et al. [3], who showed poor correlation between clinical symptoms and actual histological status of the pulp, and subsequently the healing potential of the inflamed pulp tissue. In teeth with savable pulps, i.e., pulps without necrosis, pain was present in 40% and loss of sleep occurred in 36% of these teeth, whereas in teeth with chronic partial pulpitis and partial necrosis, the percentage of pain increased to 94% and teeth with total necrosis had 79% incidence of pain, while the rest were asymptomatic.

Therefore, many of the signs and symptoms traditionally associated with progressive disease do occur more frequently but not exclusively with inflamed pulps. Currently, clinicians can only indicate the probable state of the pulp based on signs and symptoms and findings of clinical tests.

Histologically in teeth with reversible pulpitis, bacteria are confined to the deepest dentine, while teeth with irreversible pulpitis have a necrotic area of varying dimension, colonized by bacteria in the pulp chamber [4]. In this study, 84% of cases with clinical symptoms of irreversible pulpitis had a matching histological picture, although it was common to find healthy architecture in the pulp away from the site of carious exposure. Despite the fact that the authors contradict the conclusion of Dummer et al. [3] by reporting good correlation between clinical and histologic diagnosis, they both agree on the main point that it is not possible to clinically diagnose the extent of pulp degeneration based on clinical symptoms. Taking this into consideration will affect the choice between vital pulp therapy (VPT) and root canal treatment and how much tissue should be removed if VPT is attempted.

In conclusion, the use of diagnostic terminology that is based on the predicted outcome of treatment rather than the actual pulp status before intervention is unusual: "reversible" or "irreversible" inflammation can be decided only after the carious insult is actually removed, the lesion is appropriately restored, and the outcome is assessed.

8.2   Diagnosis of Irreversible Pulpitis and Its Limitations in Children and Adults

Clinicians are unable to directly examine the dental pulp tissue preoperatively because of its location within a relatively hard tissue. Histological examination is currently the only method that can exactly determine the pulpal condition; unfortunately, it is impractical in the clinical situation. Therefore, clinicians currently make an educated guess about the histological status of the pulp from preoperative clinical (signs and symptoms and sensibility tests) and radiographic examination. Moreover, intraoperative clinical examination from direct evaluation of the pulp is also important for the diagnosis of the pulp status. While the obtained data are supported by scientific evidence, all of them have some limitations. These limitations, with particular attention to children, will be further described.

8.2.1 Preoperative Clinical and Radiographic Examination

Despite the premise that the preoperative diagnosis in pulpitis cases is a tentative diagnosis, it is still essential for developing a treatment plan. However, reliance on the preoperative diagnosis alone can lead to misdiagnosis and mistreatment; for example, overtaking root canal therapy in all teeth with symptoms of irreversible pulpitis, without directly evaluating the pulp tissue, can be considered overtreatment. Only through intraoperative assessment or after follow-up periods that clinicians could determine the accuracy of a tentative preoperative diagnosis [5].

8.2.1.1 Signs and Symptoms

Signs and symptoms are usually considered important parts of the preoperative clinical diagnosis; however, confusion exists between different diagnostic systems. Irreversible pulpitis, defined by the American Association of Endodontists (AAE), consists of spontaneous pain together with sharp and lingering pain on cold testing and it is contraindicated for VPT [6]. However, if a recent classification by Wolters et al. [7] is followed, the symptoms matched with irreversible pulpitis can be categorized as mild-to-moderate pulpitis, which on the other hand, the application of VPT can be recommended. However, as the extent of pulp degeneration cannot be actually ascertained on the primary basis of clinical symptoms, the classification of mild, moderate, and severe pulpitis is actually impractical, and it is not possible to recommend treatments based primarily on symptoms. Moreover, the term irreversible pulpitis is misleading because the clinical diagnosis cannot be equated with the ability of the tissue to heal after therapeutic intervention.

Characteristics of pain are usually used as a criterion for the diagnosis of pulp disease; however, pain is a subjective experience and variation in pain intensity between individuals exists. According to Ricucci et al. [4], teeth with a clinical diagnosis of irreversible pulpitis are commonly associated with severe pain that urges the patient to seek professional help. Moreover, pain reported by patients is often defined as throbbing, dull, or sharp, and often graded as severe. However, there were differences in pain intensity level reported in studies for patients with a tooth diagnosed with irreversible pulpits. The patients in one study reported a mean initial visual analog scale (VAS) reading of 124 mm which is equal to the level of severe pain [8], whereas in another study, patients' initial VAS reading was 98 mm which is equal to the level of a moderate pain [9]. The range of pain duration in teeth with irreversible pulpitis also varied greatly from few minutes to several hours [10]. Moreover, teeth histologically determined as irreversible pulpitis were reported to be completely asymptomatic in 14–60% of cases [11, 12].

Pain caused by pulpitis was reported to be one of the most common reasons for emergency dental visits in children [13, 14]. Therefore, there is a high chance that dentists will have to face with the management of irreversible pulpitis in children on a daily basis. In children, pain is even more difficult to measure because young patients may not be able to adequately describe their pain history [15]. Several pain scale indicators have been recommended for pain assessment in children and they should routinely be used to aid in the diagnosis of the pulp condition. The evidence indicates a relatively high reliability of Wong-Baker Faces Pain Scale in children from 3 to 18 years old [16].

While symptoms alone do not reflect the true inflammatory stage of the entire pulp, gathering information on the pain level is still important. Ricucci et al. [4] found high correlation of clinical and histological status in teeth with normal pulp or symptoms of reversible pulpitis (96.6%), which infers that these teeth could be conservatively managed by direct pulp capping. The relatively high correlation in teeth with symptoms of irreversible pulpitis (84.4%) and the fact that variations do exist in the extent of pulpal inflammation within the same clinical diagnostic category, as the histological definition of irreversible pulpitis can be either partial or total necrosis of the coronal pulp, suggest that these teeth could be managed by pulp tissue removal that can start with partial to full pulpotomy or even pulpectomy depending on the intraoperative assessment of the pulp status under magnification.

Although there is no good correlation between clinical symptoms and actual histological findings of the pulp, there is a good correlation between the depth of carious bacterial penetration in the dentine and the histologic response of the pulp to caries [17].

The clinical classification of the symptoms provides slight information about the regenerative capacity of the tissue. It merely facilitates the treatment decision for the practitioner, since a schematic approach can be taken. Treatment of pulpitis depends on the extent of the bacterial infection, which unfortunately cannot be accurately determined clinically. Vitality-preserving measures can only be successful if infection of the pulp can be ruled out during and after therapy.

8.2.1.2 Sensibility Tests

Vitality of the pulp is the main criterion commonly used to determine the choice between vital and non-vital pulp treatment. By its definition, pulp vitality testing should actually assess the pulp's blood supply; however, most of the current tests, referred to as vitality tests, do not directly assess the pulp's vascularity.

Pulp sensibility tests rely on the distribution, diameter size, conduction speed, and myelin sheath of the A-delta fibers. The A fibers appear relatively late in pulpal development explaining why the EPT is not reliable, often resulting in false-negative response in young teeth [18]. Therefore, cold testing is more reliable for immature permanent teeth and should be performed routinely [18, 19]. Both false-positive and false-negative responses were also reported in adults using cold and electrical pulp tests [20].

Besides the limitations in the immature tooth itself, controversies also exist regarding the reliability of children toward pulp testing. The unreliability and inconsistent results on repeated attempts in children could be due to the child's apprehension associated with the test itself, or due to the tests being uncomfortable for the child [21].

8.2.1.3 Radiographic Examination

Another essential part for pulp diagnosis is radiographic examination. Radiographic examination is one of the essential diagnostic tools to determine caries extension into the dental tissues and the status of root-supporting structures. The interpretation of radiographs of young immature permanent teeth can be challenging due to their normally large open apex and radiolucent apical papilla. Less experienced dentists treating these teeth should avoid confusing pathologic changes with normal apical anatomy.

Traditionally, it has been taught that any tooth with a suspected radiographic lesion is likely to be non-vital. However, it has been shown through biopsies of pulps that necrosis can be limited to only specific portions of the pulp [22] and total inflammation or necrosis of the pulp is not a prerequisite to the appearance of a periapical lesion [23]. Periapical inflammatory infiltrates, increased osteoclast numbers, and bone destruction can appear in advance of total pulp necrosis [24, 25].

Radiographically, a young permanent tooth with advanced stage of carious lesions often presents with early periapical changes such as widened periodontal ligament space or condensing osteitis [26–29]. In one study conducted in children under 18 years old [30], vitality was assessed in teeth with radiolucencies and the results showed that 45% of teeth with periapical lesions were vital upon visual inspection of the pulp.

Thus, the previous assumption that periapical radiolucency of pulpal origin is only associated with non-vital teeth is no longer valid. The presence of periapical lesion in an inflamed vital pulp is not a contraindication for VPT, and several clinical studies reported successful outcomes of VPT in teeth with clinical symptoms of irreversible pulpitis and periapical lesions in both children and adults [26–29, 31].

8.2.2 Intraoperative Assessment

When there is a pulp exposure during an operative procedure, the appearance of pulp tissue, color of bleeding, and time used to control bleeding have mainly been used as indicators of pulp status in previous studies [26, 28, 29, 31–33]. Direct observation of the pulp wound under magnification is recommended; the ideal characteristics of a healthy pulp wound include a resilient, continuous blood-filled tissue surrounded by clean sound dentine. If there is necrotic tissue, dentine debris, or light-yellow areas within the pulp, then the pulp is not a candidate for direct pulp capping and more tissue should be removed as in partial pulpotomy, and then the color and bleeding of pulp tissue should be reassessed for the need of full pulpotomy. A healthy-appearing architecture of pulp tissue must be encountered; otherwise total pulpectomy should be initiated [34].

The correlation between bleeding and inflammation of the pulp is still unclear. Several authors suggested that pulpal bleeding can be used as a clinical indicator of pulpal inflammation [35–37]. However, these suggestions are empirical and despite the fact that Matsuo et al.'s [37] is a highly quoted article, it was on direct pulp capping in teeth with symptoms of reversible pulpitis. In their study, they classified the degree of bleeding into four categories: oozing, slight but apparent from the pulp exposure site, overflowing from the pulp exposure site but arrested within 30 s, and overflowing from the pulp exposure site but not arrested within 30 s. The success rate of the first two groups was higher than the last two groups; however, the success rate of group 4 was higher than group 3, which actually makes it very difficult to explain. Moreover, their findings cannot actually be applied in partial pulpotomy or full pulpotomy since if there is minimal bleeding, one would suspect that the tooth is undergoing necrosis. Furthermore, the degree of bleeding on pulp exposure is not sufficient as a clinical index of the prognosis of treatment of pulp capping because of its low specificity by virtue that 55% of the cases with conspicuous bleeding included in Matsuo et al.'s [37] study were successful.

What actually matters for decision-making in VPT is the fact that the amount of bleeding flowing from the pulp exposure site should be easily controlled in order to be able to place the bioactive material on top of the exposed pulp tissue. However, the exact time needed to control pulpal bleeding and beyond which point the pulp can be considered unsuitable for VPT is still inconclusive, and several studies reported variable times from 1 to 25 min with successful outcomes [38–40]. In 84% of teeth with clinical signs and symptoms suggestive of irreversible pulpitis, vital pulp tissue was present clinically and hemostasis could be achieved within 6 min after partial or full pulpotomy [32, 33].

Obviously, the current methods used for diagnosis of the pulp have some limitations. The chairside application of rapid molecular tests that target the level of biomarkers of pulpal inflammation has been suggested as a potential tool of diagnosis of the pulp condition [41].

8.3   Case Selection for Vital Pulp Therapy in Teeth with Irreversible Pulpitis in Children

Prior to the decision to perform any treatment for teeth with irreversible pulpitis in children, clinicians should always take into consideration some unique characteristics of young permanent teeth in young patients.

8.3.1   Restorability of the Affected Tooth and Stage of Developing Dentition

The young permanent molar (especially the first permanent molar) is one of the teeth most commonly affected from massive destruction by carious lesion and/or developmental defect (i.e., hypomineralization). Although the young pulp may have high ability to repair, the remaining tooth structure can be thin, thus leading to a high risk of fracture and compromised longevity of the treated tooth [42, 43]. Restorability of the affected tooth, restoration complexity, financial burden, and its long-term outcome should always be weighted prior to a decision to either save (VPT or root canal treatment) or extract a young permanent tooth with irreversible pulpitis. Orthodontic consultation and comprehensive evaluation prior to extraction are required.

8.3.2   Incomplete Root Formation and Thin Dentine Wall

In young vital permanent teeth with incomplete root formation, it is unavoidable that vitality of the treated tooth is preserved so the tooth can continue its dentine apposition and root formation. Apexogenesis, performed with some forms of VPT, has long been recommended in this group [44].

In addition, VPT, a biologically based minimally invasive pulp treatment, is preferred in young permanent teeth of children regardless of its root development stage. It could not be overemphasized that VPT promotes the apposition of dentine and root development, and hence, it decreases the risk of cervical crown-root fracture due to poor crown-root ratio [45, 46]. Moreover, the prognosis and survival of a root canal-treated tooth were shown to be inferior to those of a vital tooth [47].

8.4   Is Vital Pulp Therapy a Viable and Even Preferred Alternative to Pulpectomy for Teeth with Clinical Diagnosis of Irreversible Pulpitis in Children and Adults?

Vital pulp therapy has long been indicated for young permanent teeth in children, however, with quite a narrow indication. Traditionally, VPT has been indicated mainly, but not limited to the young permanent teeth with immature root formation. Additionally, the causes of pulp exposure were restricted to traumatic, mechanical, or carious exposure with small pulp exposure size [44]. Moreover, VPT was indicated for teeth with diagnosis that is not severe than normal pulp or reversible pulpitis, and definitely with normal periapical tissue. Based on the AAE guide to clinical endodontics and the American Academy of Pediatric Dentistry (AAPD) guidelines on pulp therapy for primary and immature permanent teeth, mature permanent teeth with irreversible pulpitis should be treated with root canal treatment [6, 44].

In the past few decades, better understanding of pulp biology and advances in bioactive endodontic cement (i.e., calcium silicate cements) have played a major role in making VPT, a procedure once considered an unreliable treatment with limited indications, become a more reliable option with extended indications. Considering calcium silicate cements, a recent systematic review and meta-analysis [48] showed that mineral trioxide aggregate (MTA) has a higher success rate, with a lower inflammatory response and a more predictable hard-tissue barrier formation than calcium hydroxide (CH) cements. However, there were no differences, in these parameters, when MTA was compared with other calcium silicate cements (i.e., Biodentine, Endocem, and MTA Angelus). Dental adhesive systems showed the lowest success rates.

Calcium silicate cements increased the success of VPT and played an essential part for it in becoming a proposed definitive alternative for root canal treatment for both immature and mature teeth in both children and adults [26–29, 31, 49–51]. Based on the success reported in these previous studies, carious exposure is no longer considered a contraindication for VPT. Moreover, the traditionally limited indications for VPT have recently been extended to the older age group as well as to the more challenging indications such as teeth with symptoms of irreversible pulpitis or even teeth with periapical lesions.

8.4.1 Does Age Matter in Decision-Making in Vital Pulp Therapy?

There is currently no clear definition of young and old pulp. Traditionally, VPT has long been recommended mainly for the young teeth because of their characteristics that favor the VPT treatment [44]. Pulpal circulation is an important factor in the repair process. An adequate blood supply is important for transporting immune cells to the pulpal injury site and removing irritants from that area. Thus a young pulp, especially one with an open apex, with plentiful blood and nerve supply, has a much better healing potential than an aged pulp [52].

During the aging process, there is a decrease in blood vessels and nerves that supply the pulp [53]. At the level of pulpal microcirculation, aging was associated with altered blood flow levels, contributing to a decreased adaptability of aged dental pulp to pathological stimuli [54].

From the differences in structure between the young and aged pulp described above, it may be assumed that the ability of pulpal healing between these age groups may also be different. However, this conventional assumption has recently been challenged by the recent evidence on VPT using bioactive calcium silicate cements; several studies reported that the age of the patient has no significant effect on the success of VPT [33, 55, 56]. Therefore, age should not be the sole criterion that discriminates the VPT from mature teeth in adults.

8.4.2 Cost-Effectiveness of Vital Pulp Therapy

Compared to root canal treatment, VPT is a much simpler and less expensive treatment, making it more affordable and acceptable, especially for children. Because root canal treatment is very challenging and technically demanding, malpractice claims are most commonly associated with technical complications and mishaps [57]. After 10 years, molars treated by endodontists were reported to have significantly higher survival rates than those treated by non-endodontists [58].

Based on the German healthcare system, direct pulp capping was more cost effective in younger patients and for occlusal exposure sites, whereas root canal treatment was more effective in older patients or teeth with proximal exposures. However, these findings might change depending on the healthcare system and underlying literature-based probabilities [59]. Cost-effectiveness by means of a Markov simulation model was studied in a Scandinavian setting and pulp capping was considered to be a cost-effective alternative to root canal treatment in young patients [60].

When compared to CH, the traditional pulp dressing material, the cost of the calcium silicate cement, the currently recommended pulp dressing material, may raise a concern in some countries. However, VPT with calcium silicate cements has been shown to be cost effective when compared to root canal treatment [59, 60].

8.5 Outcome of Vital Pulp Therapy in Teeth with Irreversible Pulpitis in Children and Adults

Several clinical studies reported on the use of calcium silicate materials in VPT procedures in teeth with clinical diagnosis of irreversible pulpitis. It is important to note that inclusion criteria (patient age, caries extension, severity of preoperative symptoms) and clinical procedures (isolation, disinfection, time to hemostasis, capping material) vary among studies which makes direct comparisons of success rates difficult to establish. Below is a summary of these studies supplemented by Tables 8.1 and 8.2.

8.5.1 Coronal Pulpotomy

In a tooth diagnosed with irreversible pulpitis, coronal pulpotomy is probably the most common type of VPT performed. The histological outcome of MTA pulpotomy for treatment of irreversible pulpitis in human teeth from patients 16–28 years old was investigated in one study [66]. Histological observation revealed that all samples had complete hard-tissue barrier formation and the pulps were vital and free of inflammation. In another case report, a second premolar with irreversible pulpitis and symptomatic apical periodontitis in a 19-year-old female patient was treated with MTA pulpotomy. Ten months after the initial treatment, the tooth was extracted for orthodontic reasons and processed for histological examination. Microscopically, the pulpal wound treated with MTA was free from inflammation and covered with a thin layer of reparative dentine [67].

Subsequently, several clinical studies have shown success of coronal pulpotomy with bioactive endodontic cements across a wide range of patient ages (Table 8.1). Taha et al. [31] reported success rates of 100% at 1 year and 92.7% at 3 years in their study with regard to outcome MTA pulpotomy in mature permanent teeth. The pulp was exposed due to caries in patients aged between 11 and 51 years, more than 84% of the included cases had a diagnosis of irreversible pulpitis, and 27% had preoperative periapical lesions. Asgary et al. [50] reported a comparable success for coronal pulpotomy using CEM and root canal treatment performed by general dentists in teeth with irreversible pulpitis in patients with age range from 9 to 65 years and 60-month follow-up.

In a systematic review evaluating the clinical success rate of coronal pulpotomy in permanent teeth presented with symptomatic irreversible pulpitis, the success rate of coronal pulpotomy was 97.4% clinically and 95.4% radiographically

Table 8.1 Outcome of full pulpotomy in teeth with carious pulp exposure and symptoms of irreversible pulpitis using calcium silicate cements

Author	Age (years)	Type of study	Root maturity	Diagnosis	Material	Number of treated teeth	Follow-up	Overall success (%)
Nosrat et al. (2013) [61]	6–10	Randomized clinical trial	Immature	Reversible and irreversible pulpitis	MTA	24	1 year	100
					CEM	25		100
Asgary and Eghbal (2013) [62]	27 ± 8	Randomized clinical trial	Mature	Irreversible pulpitis	CEM	205	1 year	92
	26 ± 9				MTA	208		95
Asgary et al. (2015) [50]	9–65	Randomized clinical trial	Mature	Irreversible pulpitis	CEM	137	5 years	78.1
					RCT	134		75.3
Taha et al. (2017) [31]	11–51	Prospective study	Mature	Reversible and irreversible pulpitis	MTA	50	3 years	92.7
Linsuwanont et al. (2017) [63]	7–68	Retrospective study	Mature	Reversible and irreversible pulpitis	MTA	55	Up to 62 months	87
Asgary et al. (2018) [64]	26.5 ± 7.4	Randomized clinical trial	Mature	Normal, reversible, irreversible pulpitis, and the presence of apical periodontitis	CEM	69	1 year	95.5
Taha and Abdelkhader (2018) [32]	19–69	Prospective study	Mature	Irreversible pulpitis	Biodentine	64	1 year	98.4
Taha and Abdulkhader (2018) [29]	9–17	Prospective study	Mature Immature	Irreversible pulpitis	Biodentine	20	1 year	95

MTA mineral trioxide aggregate, *CEM* calcium-enriched mixture, *RCT* root canal treatment

Table 8.2 Outcome of partial pulpotomy in teeth with carious pulp exposure and symptoms of irreversible pulpitis using calcium silicate cements

Authors	Age (years)	Type of study	Root maturity	Diagnosis	Material	Number of treated teeth	Follow-up	Overall success rate (%)
Peng et al. (2015) [65]	6.1–15.4	Prospective study	Immature	Irreversible	MTA	20	1 year	91
Taha and Khazali (2017) [33]	20–52	Randomized clinical trial	Mature	Irreversible	MTA CH	26 23	2 years	85 43
Asgary et al. (2018) [64]	26.8 ± 7.6	Randomized clinical trial	Mature	Normal, reversible, and irreversible pulpitis	CEM	76	1 year	91.4
Uesrichai et al. (2019) [26]	6–18	Randomized clinical trial	Mature 27 Immature 40	Irreversible	MTA Biodentine	37 32	32.2 ± 17.9 months	92 87

MTA mineral trioxide aggregate, *CEM* calcium-enriched mixture, *CH* calcium hydroxide

at 12-month follow-up, reduced to 93.7% clinical and 88.3% radiographic success at 3 years [68].

The findings of Cushley et al. [68] showed an overall encouraging outcome for full pulpotomy in teeth with signs and symptoms indicative of irreversible pulpitis which is comparable to the success reported by a systematic review for teeth diagnosed with reversible pulpitis [69], in which they reported an overall success rate of 94% at 1 year and 92% at 2 years. They proposed that full pulpotomy treatment can be considered as a treatment option in managing carious pulp exposures in teeth with closed root apices; furthermore, this success rate was comparable to that reported for root canal treatment over 2 years [70].

Full pulpotomy to the canal orifices is technically less challenging than partial pulpotomy and may provide better restorative options, and total removal of coronal pulp tissue in full pulpotomy definitely benefits the certainty of infected pulp tissue removal. However, it may at the same time overly unnecessarily remove healthy, noninfected pulp tissue. The preservation of the coronal portion is of significance because it may yield in advantageous repairing process. The coronal pulp has higher odontoblast density and nearly twice the capillary blood flow as the root portion [71]. Moreover, the degree of age-related decrease of the density of odontoblasts and sub-odontoblasts in the root is greater than that in the crown [72]. Total removal of the pulp tissue may cease dentine apposition on the coronal thin dentine wall in young permanent teeth, thus resulting in the risk of cervical fracture of the treated tooth [45].

Additionally, total removal of pulp tissue in coronal pulpotomy often prohibits its response to the sensibility test while partial removal of the pulp in partial pulpotomy still allows for the confirmation of pulp status with sensibility tests. Therefore, to preserve coronal pulp tissue as much as possible, other more conservative forms of VPT (i.e., partial pulpotomy, direct pulp capping) have also been proposed in teeth with irreversible pulpitis.

8.5.2   Partial Pulpotomy and Miniature Pulpotomy

Partial pulpotomy and miniature pulpotomy are the forms of VPT that aim to remove only partial, but not the entire, coronal pulp tissue. Partial pulpotomy provides the advantage of preserving the healthy coronal pulp tissue, thus reducing the risk of cervical root fracture, especially in young permanent tooth.

The outcome of partial pulpotomy using CH in teeth with carious pulp exposure was reported in the early 1990s [63]. Five teeth included in that study had temporary pain, widened periodontal space peri-apically, and/or condensing osteitis. After a mean observation time of 56 months, healing had occurred in four out of five teeth.

The first prospective study to report on MTA partial pulpotomy in young teeth with irreversible pulpitis and open apices (age 6–15) was written in Chinese; it included only ten teeth and the success rate was 90% at 12-month follow-up [65] (Table 8.2).

A randomized clinical trial on partial pulpotomy for teeth with irreversible pulpitis in adults above 20 years reported a significantly higher success rate for MTA over CH at 1- and 2-year follow-up. Calcium hydroxide was considered unsuitable material for partial pulpotomy in teeth with irreversible pulpitis [33]. When MTA was used, the success rate was 85% over 2-year follow-up, which appears to be lower than that reported for full pulpotomy (92.7% at 3 years) in teeth with irreversible pulpitis [31].

A systematic review concluded that partial pulpotomy could be effective in both mature and immature teeth; neither the patient's age nor the root apex closure affected the prognosis of partial pulpotomy. Only the preoperative status held significance; teeth with preoperative symptoms of irreversible pulpitis had lower success rates compared to teeth with reversible pulpitis symptoms. However the success rate for partial pulpotomy was equal to that of full pulpotomy in teeth with reversible pulpitis symptoms [73].

8.5.3 Direct and Indirect Pulp Capping

Based on histobacteriologic findings of pulp status beneath a carious exposure in teeth with symptoms of irreversible pulpitis, current recommendations consider direct and indirect pulp capping unacceptable treatment in such teeth, as inflammation and bacterial invasion have extended within a distance from the caries front. Removal of the irritant, i.e., caries, will not be sufficient to promote healing and partial or complete removal of the infected pulp tissue via partial or full pulpotomy is recommended [4, 34, 74].

In a randomized clinical trial, Asgary et al. [64] reported on the outcome of VPT procedures including indirect pulp capping, direct pulp capping, and partial and full pulpotomy in mature teeth with variable clinical symptoms using CEM. The four VPTs were associated with favorable/comparable clinical and radiographic outcomes at 1 year and the pulpal and periapical status had no effect on treatment outcomes. Considering the different pulp status of cases included in this study (normal, reversible, irreversible pulpitis), and hence their different histologic and microbiologic baseline condition, the results of this study might be taken with caution.

8.6   Biodentine Applications in Irreversible Pulpitis Management

Recent developments in bioactive materials have been found to be extremely advantageous in the treatment of irreversibly inflamed pulpal tissues. MTA is one of the most evidenced bioactive cements studied; a systematic review reported that pulpotomy with MTA has higher clinical and radiographic success rate at 12 months as compared to that of CH pulpotomy [75]. By virtue of its high biocompatibility, sealing ability, antibacterial effect, and induction of hard-tissue barrier formation, MTA has been the recommended material for VPT procedures [76].

However, to address the limitations of MTA which include technique sensitivity of manual mixing, long initial setting time (4 h), and high discoloration potential, several new formulations of calcium silicate-based materials with more favorable properties that overcome MTA limitations have been introduced.

Biodentine (Septodont, Saint-Maur-des-Fossés, France) is a bioactive dentine substitute which consists of a powder and liquid; the powder contains calcium silicate, calcium carbonate, and zirconium oxide as the radiopacifier. Biodentine has several advantages including good sealing ability, adequate compressive strength, a relatively short initial setting time (12 min), promotion of hard-tissue barrier formation with a positive effect on vital pulp cells, higher level of calcium ion release, and better color stability [77, 78].

Biodentine and ProRoot MTA have equal interim results of inflammatory response and hard-tissue barrier formation [79]. A systematic review reported that MTA has a higher success rate, with a lower inflammatory response and a more predictable hard-tissue barrier formation than CH. However, there were no differences, in these parameters, between MTA and Biodentine [48].

In terms of tooth discoloration, Biodentine was shown to produce less tooth discoloration. From a study of direct pulp capping procedure in children, grey discoloration was observed only with ProRoot MTA (55%) and none in the Biodentine group [28]. Also in a partial pulpotomy study in children, Uesrichai et al. [26] reported that while perceptible grey discoloration was observed in both MTA and Biodentine group, there was a significant difference between the two materials (80% for teeth treated with ProRoot MTA and 27% for teeth treated with Biodentine). The main reason for MTA-induced discoloration is the oxidative reaction of the radiopacifier bismuth oxide. In Biodentine, bismuth oxide is replaced with zirconium oxide, thus resulting in less discoloration [80].

Randomized clinical trials compared Biodentine with MTA in pulp capping of carious exposures and reported a high success rate approaching 100% at 1-year follow-up in asymptomatic teeth of young patients [81, 82] and in mature teeth with a clinical diagnosis of reversible pulpitis [83].

Taha and Abdulkhader [29] reported on the use of Biodentine as a pulpotomy agent in young permanent teeth with carious pulp exposure and symptoms of irreversible pulpitis. Patient age ranged from 9 to 17 years (mean 12.3 years). Symptomatic apical periodontitis was present in 14/20 cases; hemostasis was achieved within 6 min using a cotton pellet moistened with 2.5% NaOCl. Three mm of Biodentine was placed over the canal orifices and the teeth were subsequently restored with resin composite over a Vitrebond layer, amalgam, or stainless steel crowns, depending on the remaining tooth structure. The treatment was highly successful; 2 days after the treatment the patients reported complete relief of pain. At 6-month and 1-year follow-up, they found a high clinical success rate of 100% and radiographic success of 95%. Teeth with immature apex showed continued root development; hard-tissue barrier formation was detected in 5/20 teeth, with no evidence of canal narrowing or obliteration. All teeth with periapical lesions showed signs of healing with one tooth exhibiting internal root resorption. Biodentine offered the advantage of dentine substitute, and either a resin restoration or a stainless steel crown could be placed on top. No perceptible discoloration was noted in any of the cases.

Similar findings were reported for Biodentine full pulpotomy in adult teeth with symptoms of irreversible pulpitis [32]. Sixty-four teeth in 52 patients aged 19–69 years were included, and periapical rarefaction was present in 9 teeth. The study included teeth with spontaneous pain (40.6%), lingering pain (59.4%), and percussion sensitivity (44%). After 2 days, 93.8% reported complete relief of pain. At 1-year follow-up, the teeth had 100% clinical and 98.4% radiographic success. Seven out of eight cases with periapical radiolucency who attended recall had improvement in the periapical index score, and none of the preoperative variables (pain level, caries extent, periapical status, bleeding time, final restoration) acted as a potential negative factor. No evidence of internal resorption, canal narrowing, or crown discoloration was noted in any of the reviewed cases, and hard-tissue barrier was detected radiographically in four cases.

A hard-tissue barrier is a deposit of reparative dentine or other calcific substances that forms across and reseals the exposed pulp. This barrier can be detected clinically after re-intervention by removal of the filling, but this is discouraged to avoid contamination. Pulp capping materials such as Biodentine, besides their excellent sealing properties, are placed in sufficient bulk (3 mm) to provide a physical barrier even in the absence of a physiological calcific barrier.

Biodentine has also been successfully used in partial pulpotomy for young permanent teeth with symptoms of irreversible pulpitis in children. Villat et al. [84] reported success of Biodentine partial pulpotomy in a mandibular premolar with incomplete root formation and diagnosis of irreversible pulpitis. The patient reported complete relief of pain within 12 h after the treatment. At 6-month recall, normal pulp sensibility, continued root formation, and hard-tissue barrier formation were reported.

Another case report also showed a 5-year success of Biodentine partial pulpotomy in a young permanent molar, with signs and symptoms indicative of irreversible pulpitis and periapical lesion, in a 9-year-old patient. After partial pulpotomy hemorrhage was controlled within 4 min with 2.5% NaOCl-moistened cotton pellets. Biodentine was placed as both a pulp dressing and a temporary restoration. At the following visit, composite resin was placed over Biodentine as a final restoration. At 5-year follow-up, the tooth was asymptomatic, had positive responses to sensibility tests, showed no discoloration, and showed a hard-tissue barrier formation and periapical healing [27].

In a randomized controlled trial, Uesrichai et al. [26] compared the outcome of partial pulpotomy using MTA and Biodentine in permanent teeth of children (mean age 10 years) with signs and symptoms indicative of irreversible pulpitis. Early periapical changes presented in 46% of the included teeth. Partial pulpotomy of 2–3 mm or more of pulp tissue removal was performed, and hemostasis was achieved within 10 min using cotton pellet moistened with 2.5% NaOCl. Sixty-seven teeth were followed up every 6 months; the follow-up time ranged from 7 to 69 months with a mean of 32 ± 17.9 months. The success rate of Biodentine pulpotomy was 87% compared to 92% for MTA; however, the difference was not statistically significant.

The success rate of Biodentine full pulpotomy in teeth with irreversible pulpitis appears higher than that for partial pulpotomy, which is explained by the fact that full pulpotomy has higher chances for removal of the infected tissue than partial pulpotomy. However, studies with direct comparisons of the two procedures are required before definite conclusions can be made.

For direct pulp capping, a randomized clinical trial compared Biodentine with MTA in children (6–18 years) [28]. Fifty-nine young permanent teeth with small carious exposures (≤2.5 mm) were included; the diagnosis included teeth with normal pulp (32.7%), reversible pulpitis (27.3%), and irreversible pulpitis (40%), with early apical changes in 30.9% of the included teeth; hemostasis was achieved within 4 min. At a mean follow-up of 18 months, the Biodentine group had higher success rate than MTA group (96.4% vs. 92.6%); however, the difference was not statistically significant. Moreover, failures were distributed equally in all categories of pulpal diagnosis and occurred in teeth with no periapical involvement and small exposures. Since small sample size was included in the three different diagnostic categories, one should be cautious in withdrawing conclusions regarding the effect of preoperative status on the outcome of direct pulp capping.

In general, Biodentine demonstrated higher success rate or at least equal success rates to MTA in all VPT procedures; added to this are the advantages of easy handling, fast set, low discoloration potential, and ability to be used as a bulk fill temporary restoration up to 6 months [85]. However, it is recommended that the VPT-treated tooth should be restored with a bacteria-proof, definitive restoration in the same session or as soon as possible.

8.7   Which Irreversible Pulpitis Tooth Can Be a Candidate for Vital Pulp Therapy in Children and Adults?

Case selection in VPT is of utmost importance for predicting and maximizing the outcome. In this section, a summary of some of the key steps in the clinical management of the vital pulp derived from clinical studies using newer materials will be presented. According to ESE position statement, direct pulp capping is contraindicated for teeth with symptoms of irreversible pulpitis [74]. Tooth candidates for partial or full pulpotomy may include the following:

1. A tooth with deep caries extending ≥2/3 of dentine or exposing the pulp radiographically.
2. Patient age is not a limiting factor, both children and adults' teeth can be treated successfully.
3. Clinical diagnosis of irreversible pulpitis, judged from patient's symptoms (spontaneous pain, exaggerated pain, or lingering pain after stimulus that may disturb sleep and quality of life) and which can be reproduced by sensibility test (thermal tests).

4. Absence of clinical swelling, fistula, or abnormal tooth mobility.
5. Absence of internal or external root resorption, calcification, or pulp canal obliteration.
6. Presence of periapical lesion in an inflamed vital pulp is not a contraindication for VPT if the provided diagnostic tests confirmed tooth vitality/sensibility.
7. A tooth that is restorable with intracoronal restoration or stainless steel crown in children and does not require intra-radicular retention via post and core restoration in adults.
8. Under magnification the pulp tissue should appear vital, as judged from the appearance of sound surrounding dentine, bright red in color with no light-yellow greyish areas indicating abscess or necrosis, and should bleed normally.
9. Size of pulp exposure: for partial or full pulpotomy there is no contraindication based on the size of pulp exposure. It is more of modification of the amount or direction of tissue removal. In case of partial pulpotomy with single pulp exposure, 2 mm can be removed toward the base of the exposure. While in the presence of two small exposures, partial pulpotomy can be performed horizontally to connect the two exposures and remove 2 mm of underlying tissues.
10. Bleeding from the exposure site should be controlled within 10 min following subsequent application of cotton pellet moistened with low concentration of NaOCl (1–2.5%) repeated on 2-min interval. Studies reported control of bleeding within 6 min in 84% of teeth with irreversible pulpitis after partial or full pulpotomy [29, 31, 32].

8.8 Vital Pulp Therapy Using Biodentine in Teeth with Irreversible Pulpitis: Procedure

Examples of different cases treated successfully with Biodentine full and partial pulpotomy are presented in Figs. 8.1 and 8.2.

The step-by-step procedure is shown in Figs. 8.3 and 8.4.

1. Topical anesthesia is applied at the injection site.
2. Local anesthesia is administered.
3. Rubber dam isolation is placed.
4. Disinfection of the tooth surface with full-strength NaOCl or 0.2% chlorhexidine for microbial control.
5. Caries is removed until resistance is felt when spoon excavator is used to detect the hard dentine.
6. When there is a pulp exposure, the cavity is rinsed with 1–2.5% NaOCl and the pulp status is evaluated. Vitality of the pulp is judged by its appearance along with color and amount of bleeding. The pulp tissue is removed until the healthy vital pulp is met and either direct pulp capping, partial pulpotomy, or coronal pulpotomy can be performed depending on the vitality of the pulp. Clinicians progress in tissue removal from partial to full pulpotomy and try to achieve hemostasis within 10 min. If not successful, then root canal therapy is indicated.

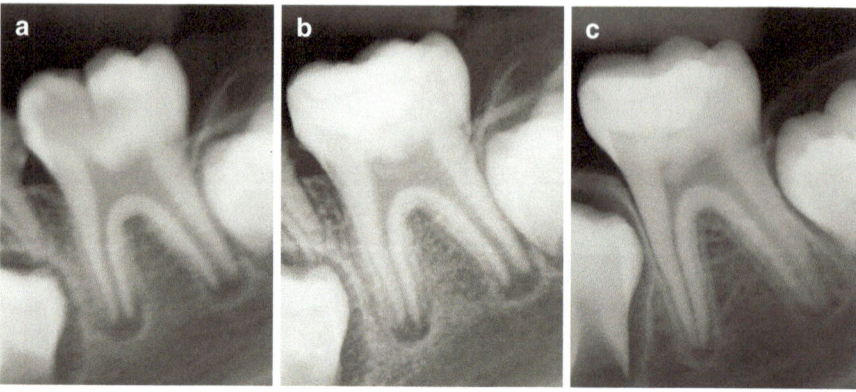

Fig. 8.1 Apexogenesis after Biodentine partial pulpotomy in an irreversible pulpitis tooth in a 7-year-old boy, (**a**) preoperative periapical radiograph revealing tooth 36 with open apex and carious pulp exposure, (**b**) immediate postoperative radiograph after partial pulpotomy with Biodentine and resin composite restoration, (**c**) 19-month postoperative radiograph showing hard-tissue formation and complete root formation. The tooth is normally responsive to cold test

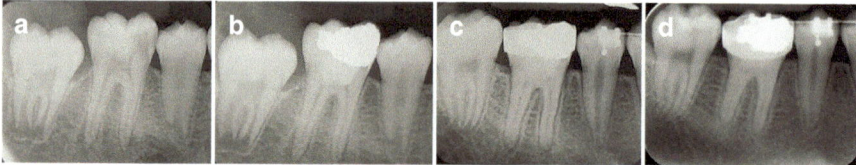

Fig. 8.2 Full pulpotomy using Biodentine in tooth 46 with clinical diagnosis of irreversible pulpitis and symptomatic apical periodontitis in a 12-year-old boy, (**a**) preoperative periapical radiograph showing deep caries exposing the pulp and periapical lesion, (**b**) immediate postoperative radiograph after Biodentine full pulpotomy and amalgam restoration, (**c**) 1-year follow-up radiograph with complete healing of the periapical lesion, (**d**) 4-year follow-up radiograph with normal periapical area

7. The pulpal tissue is irrigated with 1–2.5% NaOCl and bleeding is controlled with gentle pressure using cotton pellet moistened with low-concentration (1–2.5%) NaOCl.

8. Pulp amputation should preferably be performed with a high-speed handpiece and a diamond bur under ample water cooling or continuous rinsing with physiological saline solution [86, 87]. For reasons of practicability, however, pulpal amputation is frequently performed under water cooling directly from the high-speed handpiece. It has not been proven whether the use of cooling water from the high-speed handpieces can be expected to have disadvantages in terms of lower reliability of success.

9. If bleeding is not evident from the exposure site or from any of the pulp canals, necrosis is expected, and the tooth cannot be treated with VPT.

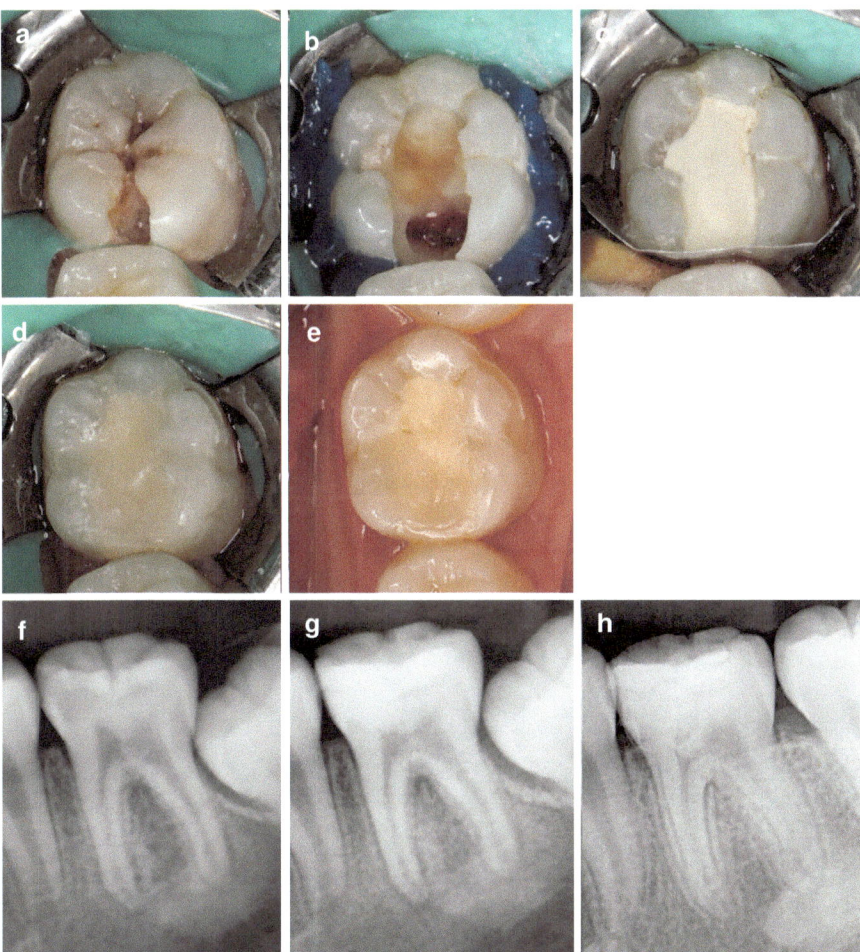

Fig. 8.3 Partial pulpotomy with Biodentine, (**a**) mesio-occlusal deep carious lesion on tooth 36, (**b**) after pulp tissue removal and hemorrhage was controlled using cotton pellet soaked with 2.5% NaOCl, (**c**) Biodentine was placed as a pulp dressing material and base material, (**d**) tooth was finally restored with composite resin, (**e**) no discoloration of Biodentine partial pulpotomy-treated tooth after 15 months, (**f**) preoperative radiograph of tooth 36 showing deep caries and periapical changes, (**g**) 8-month postoperative radiograph, (**h**) 17-month postoperative radiograph showing hard-tissue barrier formation and normal periapical tissue

10. Biodentine is mixed according to the manufacturer's instructions, by adding five drops of the liquid to the powder and activating the capsule for 30 s. The material is then carried by a plastic instrument and/or an amalgam carrier and placed to serve as both a pulp dressing material and a protective base, leaving 2 mm of space for restorative material. Biodentine is allowed to set for 12 min from the start of mixing time.

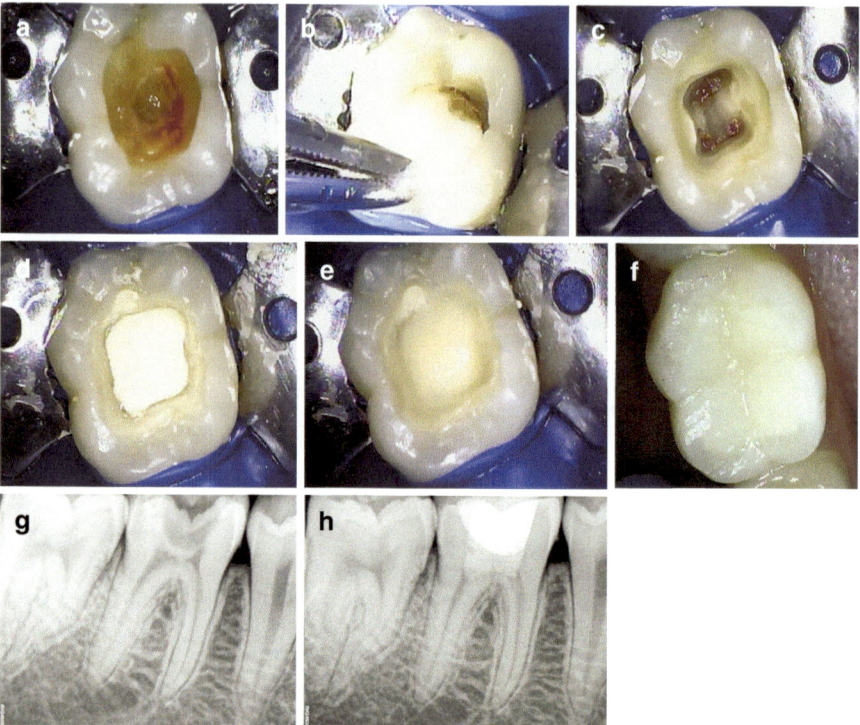

Fig. 8.4 Full pulpotomy with Biodentine, (**a**) deep occlusal caries exposing the pulp in tooth 46, (**b**) application of cotton pellet soaked with 2.5% NaOCl to achieve hemostasis after full pulpotomy, (**c**) hemostasis after full pulpotomy to canal orifices, (**d**) Biodentine placed over pulp tissue and as base material, (**e**) resin-modified glass-ionomer liner placed on top of Biodentine, (**f**) resin composite restoration on top of Biodentine, (**g**) preoperative periapical radiograph of tooth 46, (**h**) immediate postoperative radiograph of tooth 46

11. Teeth can be restored with resin composite or stainless steel crown depending on the amount of tooth structure left.
12. In cases that a tooth is planned for stainless steel crown, Biodentine is placed as a bulk in the cavity and left until set, and then tooth preparation for the stainless steel crown can be performed at the same visit.
13. If composite restoration is planned, a resin-modified glass-ionomer liner can be placed over Biodentine, and then conventional etching and bonding are performed with subsequent resin composite placement.
14. For young permanent teeth, stainless steel crown can be used as a semipermanent restoration.
15. Postoperative periapical radiograph with parallel technique is recommended immediately after procedure to serve as baseline for future follow-up.

8.9   Outcome Measures for Successful Vital Pulp Therapy

Teeth that received VPT should be followed up both clinically and radiographically, 6 months after the procedure and yearly up to 5 years [31, 74, 88]. The treated tooth is considered to have successful outcome if it has

1. Positive to cold testing, corresponding to normal pulp (however, the test may not be possible in a tooth with coronal pulpotomy or a tooth restored with stainless steel crown)
2. Absence of signs and symptoms of reversible or irreversible pulpitis
3. Absence of swelling or sinus tract
4. Absence of abnormal tooth mobility
5. Continued root formation of the previously incomplete root formation
6. Radiographically no signs of internal and/or external root resorption
7. No new periapical pathosis and healing of periapical pathosis if it was present preoperatively

8.10   Possible Complications Following Vital Pulp Therapy with Biodentine in Teeth with Irreversible Pulpitis

The major complications following VPT in teeth with irreversible pulpitis are pulp necrosis and apical periodontitis, cervical root fracture, and pulp canal obliteration.

8.10.1 Pulp Necrosis and Apical Periodontitis

Pulp necrosis and apical periodontitis can be the sequela of pulpal infection, which can be the results of incomplete pulp disinfection, inaccurate diagnosis of the pulp status, or micro-leakage of coronal restoration in VPT-treated teeth. While early failures reflect inaccurate assessment of the inflammatory status of the pulp, late failures usually reflect reinfection of the pulp space via a leaky restoration [89].

There is currently no agreement on the appropriate recommended follow-up period; 2-year follow-up has been considered adequate for direct pulp capping and for pulpotomy using MTA [56, 88], as failures tended to occur within this time frame. Longer term studies of 5–10 years would be helpful to confirm the recommendation of 2 years as sufficient follow-up.

8.10.2 Cervical Root Fracture

In young permanent tooth with thin dentine wall, cervical root fracture is frequently observed as a postoperative complication [42, 43]. Therefore, the evaluation of the remaining tooth structure prior to the decision to save or to extract the tooth is essential for long-term survival of the tooth. Moreover, the necessity of the full coverage (i.e., stainless steel crown in permanent teeth in children) should be considered to protect the tooth from cervical root fracture in cases with thin dentine wall.

8.10.3 Pulp Canal Obliteration

Evaluation of canal narrowing or obliteration from overlapping two dimensional radiographs is not very accurate. Several studies suggest that a high risk of obliteration of the root canal is not to be expected after partial pulpotomy [90–93].

While a retrospective study reported canal narrowing in 17/55 teeth that received pulpotomy [55] and only 1 of these 17 teeth had periapical lesion, it is noteworthy here that this study did not have immediate postoperative radiographs for accurate comparisons. Others reported no canal obliteration at 1–2-year follow-up [32, 88]. Furthermore, the actual concern is if canal obliteration is concurrent with apical periodontitis, then intervention needs to be done. Otherwise, obliteration by itself is not a problem, and in the majority of teeth that may appear obliterated on radiographs, there is actually a canal space and a pulp tissue clinically.

8.11 Conclusions

- From pulp biology perspective, VPT of permanent teeth with irreversible pulpitis can be an alternative to root canal therapy.
- Partial and full pulpotomy using calcium silicate materials is a successful treatment option for cariously exposed pulps in mature and immature permanent molar teeth with clinical signs and symptoms of irreversible pulpitis.
- Biodentine is a suitable alternative to MTA in VPT procedures.
- Parallel with the need for an update of the diagnostic terminology of the state of the pulp, there is an urgent need for more representative pulpal diagnostic methods.

References

1. Bjørndal L, Simon S, Tomson PL, Duncan HF. Management of deep caries and the exposed pulp. Int Endod J. 2019;52(7):949–73.
2. Levin LG, Law AS, Holland GR, Abbott PV, Roda RS. Identify and define all diagnostic terms for pulpal health and disease states. J Endod. 2009;35(12):1645–57.
3. Dummer PM, Hicks R, Huws D. Clinical signs and symptoms in pulp disease. Int Endod J. 1980;13(1):27–35.
4. Ricucci D, Loghin S, Siqueira JF Jr. Correlation between clinical and histologic pulp diagnoses. J Endod. 2014;40(12):1932–9.
5. Rosenberg PA, Schindler WG, Krell KV, Hicks ML, Davis SB. Identify the endodontic treatment modalities. J Endod. 2009;35(12):1675–94.

6. The American Association of Endodontists. Endodontic Diagnosis. Endodontics. Colleagues for Excellence. American Association of Endodontists. Clinical considerations for a regenerative procedure, 2013. Available from: https://www.aae.org/uploadedfiles/publications_and_research/research/currentregenerativeendodonticconsiderations.pdf.

7. Wolters WJ, Duncan HF, Tomson PL, Karim IE, McKenna G, Dorri M, et al. Minimally invasive endodontics: a new diagnostic system for assessing pulpitis and subsequent treatment needs. Int Endod J. 2017;50(9):825–9.

8. Webster S Jr, Drum M, Reader A, Fowler S, Nusstein J, Beck M. How effective is supplemental intraseptal anesthesia in patients with symptomatic irreversible pulpitis? J Endod. 2016;42(10):1453–7.

9. Dianat O, Mozayeni MA, Layeghnejad MK, Shojaeian S. The efficacy of supplemental intraseptal and buccal infiltration anesthesia in mandibular molars of patients with symptomatic irreversible pulpitis. Clin Oral Investig. 2020;24(3):1281–6.

10. Goldberg M, Farges JC, Lacerda-Pinheiro S, Six N, Jegat N, Decup F, et al. Inflammatory and immunological aspects of dental pulp repair. Pharmacol Res. 2008;58(2):137–47.

11. Seltzer S, Bender IB, Ziontz M. The dynamics of pulp inflammation: correlations between diagnostic data and actual histologic findings in the pulp. Oral Surg Oral Med Oral Pathol. 1963;16:846–71.

12. Michaelson PL, Holland GR. Is pulpitis painful? Int Endod J. 2002;35(10):829–32.

13. Lygidakis NA, Marinou D, Katsaris N. Analysis of dental emergencies presenting to a community paediatric dentistry centre. Int J Paediatr Dent. 1998;8(3):181–90.

14. Shqair AQ, Gomes GB, Oliveira A, Goettems ML, Romano AR, Schardozim LR, et al. Dental emergencies in a university pediatric dentistry clinic: a retrospective study. Braz Oral Res. 2012;26(1):50–6.

15. Barrêtto Ede P, Ferreira e Ferreira E, Pordeus IA. Evaluation of toothache severity in children using a visual analogue scale of faces. Pediatr Dent. 2004;26(6):485–91.

16. Gharaibeh M, Abu-Saad H. Cultural validation of pediatric pain assessment tools: Jordanian perspective. J Transcult Nurs. 2002;13(1):12–8.

17. Lin LM, Ricucci D, Saoud TM, Sigurdsson A, Kahler B. Vital pulp therapy of mature permanent teeth with irreversible pulpitis from the perspective of pulp biology. Aust Endod J. 2020;46(1):154–66.

18. Fuss Z, Trowbridge H, Bender IB, Rickoff B, Sorin S. Assessment of reliability of electrical and thermal pulp testing agents. J Endod. 1986;12(7):301–5.

19. Fulling HJ, Andreasen JO. Influence of maturation status and tooth type of permanent teeth upon electrometric and thermal pulp testing. Scand J Dent Res. 1976;84(5):286–90.

20. Peters DD, Baumgartner JC, Lorton L. Adult pulpal diagnosis. I. Evaluation of the positive and negative responses to cold and electrical pulp tests. J Endod. 1994;20(10):506–11.

21. McDonald R, Avery D, Dean J. McDonald and Avery's dentistry for the child and adolescent. 9th ed. St. Louis, MO: Mosby Elsevier; 2011.

22. Lin L, Shovlin F, Skribner J, Langeland K. Pulp biopsies from the teeth associated with periapical radiolucency. J Endod. 1984;10(9):436–48.

23. Lin L, Langeland K. Light and electron microscopic study of teeth with carious pulp exposures. Oral Surg Oral Med Oral Pathol. 1981;51(3):292–316.

24. Yamasaki M, Kumazawa M, Kohsaka T, Nakamura H, Kameyama Y. Pulpal and periapical tissue reactions after experimental pulpal exposure in rats. J Endod. 1994;20(1):13–7.

25. Stashenko P, Teles R, D'Souza R. Periapical inflammatory responses and their modulation. Crit Rev Oral Biol Med. 1998;9(4):498–521.

26. Uesrichai N, Nirunsittirat A, Chuveera P, Srisuwan T, Sastraruji T, Chompu-Inwai P. Partial pulpotomy with two bioactive cements in permanent teeth of 6- to 18-year-old patients with signs and symptoms indicative of irreversible pulpitis: a noninferiority randomized controlled trial. Int Endod J. 2019;52(6):749–59.

27. Chinadet W, Sutharaphan T, Chompu-Inwai P. Biodentine™ partial pulpotomy of a young permanent molar with signs and symptoms indicative of irreversible pulpitis and periapical lesion: a case report of a five-year follow-up. Case Rep Dent. 2019;2019:8153250.

28. Parinyaprom N, Nirunsittirat A, Chuveera P, Na Lampang S, Srisuwan T, Sastraruji T, et al. Outcomes of direct pulp capping by using either ProRoot mineral trioxide aggregate or Biodentine in permanent teeth with carious pulp exposure in 6- to 18-year-old patients: a randomized controlled trial. J Endod. 2018;44(3):341–8.
29. Taha NA, Abdulkhader SZ. Full pulpotomy with Biodentine in symptomatic young permanent teeth with carious exposure. J Endod. 2018;44(6):932–7.
30. Lentini E. Endodontic radiolucency on a mature permanent tooth in the pediatric population: can the tooth be vital? Richmond, VA: Virginia Commonwealth University; 2014.
31. Taha NA, Ahmad MB, Ghanim A. Assessment of mineral trioxide aggregate pulpotomy in mature permanent teeth with carious exposures. Int Endod J. 2017;50(2):117–25.
32. Taha NA, Abdelkhader SZ. Outcome of full pulpotomy using Biodentine in adult patients with symptoms indicative of irreversible pulpitis. Int Endod J. 2018;51(8):819–28.
33. Taha NA, Khazali MA. Partial pulpotomy in mature permanent teeth with clinical signs indicative of irreversible pulpitis: a randomized clinical trial. J Endod. 2017;43(9):1417–21.
34. Ricucci D, Siqueira JF Jr, Li Y, Tay FR. Vital pulp therapy: histopathology and histobacteriology-based guidelines to treat teeth with deep caries and pulp exposure. J Dent. 2019;86:41–52.
35. Aminabadi NA, Parto M, Emamverdizadeh P, Jamali Z, Shirazi S. Pulp bleeding color is an indicator of clinical and histohematologic status of primary teeth. Clin Oral Investig. 2017;21(5):1831–41.
36. Bogen G, Chandler NP. Pulp preservation in immature permanent teeth. Endod Top. 2010;23(1):131–52.
37. Matsuo T, Nakanishi T, Shimizu H, Ebisu S. A clinical study of direct pulp capping applied to carious-exposed pulps. J Endod. 1996;22(10):551–6.
38. Bogen G, Kim JS, Bakland LK. Direct pulp capping with mineral trioxide aggregate: an observational study. J Am Dent Assoc. 2008;139(3):305–15; quiz 15.
39. Qudeimat MA, Alyahya A, Hasan AA. Mineral trioxide aggregate pulpotomy for permanent molars with clinical signs indicative of irreversible pulpitis: a preliminary study. Int Endod J. 2017;50(2):126–34.
40. Cao Y, Bogen G, Lim J, Shon WJ, Kang MK. Bioceramic materials and the changing concepts in vital pulp therapy. J Calif Dent Assoc. 2016;44(5):278–90.
41. Brizuela C, Meza G, Mercadé M, Inostroza C, Chaparro A, Bravo I, et al. Inflammatory biomarkers in dentinal fluid as an approach to molecular diagnostics in pulpitis. Int Endod J. 2020; https://doi.org/10.1111/iej.13343.
42. Schröder U. Pedodontic endodontics. In: Koch G, Poulsen S, editors. Pediatric dentistry: a clinical approach. 2nd ed. Chichester: Wiley-Blackwell Publishing Ltd.; 2009. p. 161.
43. Baba N, White SN, Bogen G. Restoration of endodontically treated teeth. In: Chugal N, Lin LM, editors. Endodontic prognosis. Cham: Springer International Publishing; 2017. p. 171.
44. The American Academy of Pediatric Dentistry. Pulp therapy for primary and immature permanent teeth. Pediatr Dent. 2018;40(6):343–51.
45. Camp JH. Diagnosis dilemmas in vital pulp therapy: treatment for the toothache is changing, especially in young, immature teeth. Pediatr Dent. 2008;30(3):197–205.
46. Gudkina J, Mindere A, Locane G, Brinkmane A. Review of the success of pulp exposure treatment of cariously and traumatically exposed pulps in immature permanent incisors and molars. Stomatologija. 2012;14(3):71–80.
47. Caplan DJ, Cai J, Yin G, White BA. Root canal filled versus non-root canal filled teeth: a retrospective comparison of survival times. J Public Health Dent. 2005;65(2):90–6.
48. Paula AB, Laranjo M, Marto CM, Paulo S, Abrantes AM, Casalta-Lopes J, et al. Direct pulp capping: what is the most effective therapy?—systematic review and meta-analysis. J Evid Based Dent Pract. 2018;18(4):298–314.
49. Asgary S, Eghbal MJ, Bagheban AA. Long-term outcomes of pulpotomy in permanent teeth with irreversible pulpitis: a multi-center randomized controlled trial. Am J Dent. 2017;30(3):151–5.

50. Asgary S, Eghbal MJ, Fazlyab M, Baghban AA, Ghoddusi J. Five-year results of vital pulp therapy in permanent molars with irreversible pulpitis: a non-inferiority multicenter randomized clinical trial. Clin Oral Investig. 2015;19(2):335–41.
51. Aguilar P, Linsuwanont P. Vital pulp therapy in vital permanent teeth with cariously exposed pulp: a systematic review. J Endod. 2011;37(5):581–7.
52. Eşian D, Monea A. Management of the young permanent teeth with pulp diseases—a therapeutic guide of teeth with open apex. Acta Medica Transilvanica. 2011;16(3):446–9.
53. Bernick S, Nedelman C. Effect of aging on the human pulp. J Endod. 1975;1(3):88–94.
54. Dzeletovic B, Stratimirovic DJ, Stojic D, Djukic LJ. Linear and nonlinear analysis of dental pulp blood flow oscillations in ageing. Int Endod J. 2020;53:1033–9.
55. Linsuwanont P, Wimonsutthikul K, Pothimoke U, Santiwong B. Treatment outcomes of mineral trioxide aggregate pulpotomy in vital permanent teeth with carious pulp exposure: the retrospective study. J Endod. 2017;43(2):225–30.
56. Çalışkan MK, Güneri P. Prognostic factors in direct pulp capping with mineral trioxide aggregate or calcium hydroxide: 2- to 6-year follow-up. Clin Oral Investig. 2017;21(1):357–67.
57. Bjørndal L, Reit C. Endodontic malpractice claims in Denmark 1995-2004. Int Endod J. 2008;41(12):1059–65.
58. Burry JC, Stover S, Eichmiller F, Bhagavatula P. Outcomes of primary endodontic therapy provided by endodontic specialists compared with other providers. J Endod. 2016;42(5):702–5.
59. Schwendicke F, Stolpe M. Direct pulp capping after a carious exposure versus root canal treatment: a cost-effectiveness analysis. J Endod. 2014;40(11):1764–70.
60. Brodén J, Davidson T, Fransson H. Cost-effectiveness of pulp capping and root canal treatment of young permanent teeth. Acta Odontol Scand. 2019;77(4):275–81.
61. Nosrat A, Seifi A, Asgary S. Pulpotomy in caries-exposed immature permanent molars using calcium-enriched mixture cement or mineral trioxide aggregate: a randomized clinical trial. Int J Paediatr Dent. 2013;23(1):56–63.
62. Asgary S, Eghbal MJ. Treatment outcomes of pulpotomy in permanent molars with irreversible pulpitis using biomaterials: a multi-center randomized controlled trial. Acta Odontol Scand. 2013;71(1):130–6.
63. Mejàre I, Cvek M. Partial pulpotomy in young permanent teeth with deep carious lesions. Endod Dent Traumatol. 1993;9(6):238–42.
64. Asgary S, Hassanizadeh R, Torabzadeh H, Eghbal MJ. Treatment outcomes of 4 vital pulp therapies in mature molars. J Endod. 2018;44(4):529–35.
65. Peng C, Zhao Y, Yang Y, Qin M. [Mineral trioxide aggregate pulpotomy for the treatment of immature permanent teeth with irreversible pulpitis: a preliminary clinical study]. Zhonghua Kou Qiang Yi Xue Za Zhi. 2015;50(12):715–9.
66. Eghbal MJ, Asgary S, Baglue RA, Parirokh M, Ghoddusi J. MTA pulpotomy of human permanent molars with irreversible pulpitis. Aust Endod J. 2009;35(1):4–8.
67. Chueh LH, Chiang CP. Histology of irreversible pulpitis premolars treated with mineral trioxide aggregate pulpotomy. Oper Dent. 2010;35(3):370–4.
68. Cushley S, Duncan HF, Lappin MJ, Tomson PL, Lundy FT, Cooper P, et al. Pulpotomy for mature carious teeth with symptoms of irreversible pulpitis: a systematic review. J Dent. 2019;88:103158.
69. Alqaderi H, Lee CT, Borzangy S, Pagonis TC. Coronal pulpotomy for cariously exposed permanent posterior teeth with closed apices: a systematic review and meta-analysis. J Dent. 2016;44:1–7.
70. Ng YL, Mann V, Rahbaran S, Lewsey J, Gulabivala K. Outcome of primary root canal treatment: systematic review of the literature—part 2. Influence of clinical factors. Int Endod J. 2008;41(1):6–31.
71. Kim S, Schuessler G, Chien S. Measurement of blood flow in the dental pulp of dogs with the 133xenon washout method. Arch Oral Biol. 1983;28(6):501–5.
72. Murray PE, Stanley HR, Matthews JB, Sloan AJ, Smith AJ. Age-related odontometric changes of human teeth. Oral Surg Oral Med Oral Pathol Oral Radiol Endod. 2002;93(4):474–82.

73. Elmsmari F, Ruiz XF, Miró Q, Feijoo-Pato N, Durán-Sindreu F, Olivieri JG. Outcome of partial pulpotomy in cariously exposed posterior permanent teeth: a systematic review and meta-analysis. J Endod. 2019;45(11):1296–1306.e3.
74. Duncan HF, Galler KM, Tomson PL, Simon S, El-Karim I, Kundzina R, et al. European Society of Endodontology position statement: management of deep caries and the exposed pulp. Int Endod J. 2019;52(7):923–34.
75. Li Y, Sui B, Dahl C, Bergeron B, Shipman P, Niu L, et al. Pulpotomy for carious pulp exposures in permanent teeth: a systematic review and meta-analysis. J Dent. 2019;84:1–8.
76. Parirokh M, Torabinejad M, Dummer PMH. Mineral trioxide aggregate and other bioactive endodontic cements: an updated overview—part I: vital pulp therapy. Int Endod J. 2018;51(2):177–205.
77. Vallés M, Roig M, Duran-Sindreu F, Martínez S, Mercadé M. Color stability of teeth restored with Biodentine: a 6-month in vitro study. J Endod. 2015;41(7):1157–60.
78. Rajasekharan S, Martens LC, Cauwels R, Anthonappa RP, Verbeeck RMH. Biodentine™ material characteristics and clinical applications: a 3 year literature review and update. Eur Arch Paediatr Dent. 2018;19(1):1–22.
79. Nowicka A, Wilk G, Lipski M, Kołecki J, Buczkowska-Radlińska J. Tomographic evaluation of reparative dentin formation after direct pulp capping with Ca(OH)2, MTA, Biodentine, and dentin bonding system in human teeth. J Endod. 2015;41(8):1234–40.
80. Camilleri J. Staining potential of Neo MTA Plus, MTA Plus, and Biodentine used for pulpotomy procedures. J Endod. 2015;41(7):1139–45.
81. Katge FA, Patil DP. Comparative analysis of 2 calcium silicate-based cements (Biodentine and mineral trioxide aggregate) as direct pulp-capping agent in young permanent molars: a split mouth study. J Endod. 2017;43(4):507–13.
82. Brizuela C, Ormeño A, Cabrera C, Cabezas R, Silva CI, Ramírez V, et al. Direct pulp capping with calcium hydroxide, mineral trioxide aggregate, and Biodentine in permanent young teeth with caries: a randomized clinical trial. J Endod. 2017;43(11):1776–80.
83. Linu S, Lekshmi MS, Varunkumar VS, Sam Joseph VG. Treatment outcome following direct pulp capping using bioceramic materials in mature permanent teeth with carious exposure: a pilot retrospective study. J Endod. 2017;43(10):1635–9.
84. Villat C, Grosgogeat B, Seux D, Farge P. Conservative approach of a symptomatic carious immature permanent tooth using a tricalcium silicate cement (Biodentine): a case report. Restor Dent Endod. 2013;38(4):258–62.
85. Koubi G, Colon P, Franquin JC, Hartmann A, Richard G, Faure MO, et al. Clinical evaluation of the performance and safety of a new dentine substitute, Biodentine, in the restoration of posterior teeth—a prospective study. Clin Oral Investig. 2013;17(1):243–9.
86. Granath LE, Hagman G. Experimental pulpotomy in human bicuspids with reference to cutting technique. Acta Odontol Scand. 1971;29(2):155–63.
87. Sluka H, Lehmann H, Elgün Z. [Comparative experiments on treatment technics in vital amputation in view of the preservation of the remaining pulp]. Quintessenz. 1981;32(9):1571–7.
88. Simon S, Perard M, Zanini M, Smith AJ, Charpentier E, Djole SX, et al. Should pulp chamber pulpotomy be seen as a permanent treatment? Some preliminary thoughts. Int Endod J. 2013;46(1):79–87.
89. Tan SY, Yu VSH, Lim KC, Tan BCK, Neo CLJ, Shen L, et al. Long-term pulpal and restorative outcomes of pulpotomy in mature permanent teeth. J Endod. 2020;46(3):383–90.
90. Kang CM, Sun Y, Song JS, Pang NS, Roh BD, Lee CY, et al. A randomized controlled trial of various MTA materials for partial pulpotomy in permanent teeth. J Dent. 2017;60:8–13.
91. Barrieshi-Nusair KM, Qudeimat MA. A prospective clinical study of mineral trioxide aggregate for partial pulpotomy in cariously exposed permanent teeth. J Endod. 2006;32(8):731–5.
92. Qudeimat MA, Barrieshi-Nusair KM, Owais AI. Calcium hydroxide vs mineral trioxide aggregates for partial pulpotomy of permanent molars with deep caries. Eur Arch Paediatr Dent. 2007;8(2):99–104.
93. Mass E, Zilberman U. Long-term radiologic pulp evaluation after partial pulpotomy in young permanent molars. Quintessence Int. 2011;42(7):547–54.

Calcium Silicate-Based Cement (Biodentine™) as a Bioactive Material for the Long-Term Preservation of Pulp Vitality in Restorative Dentistry and Prosthodontics

9

Athina Bakopoulou, Anna Koutrouli, and Imad About

9.1 Introduction

Preservation of pulp vitality in cases of deep carious lesions or pulp exposure after mechanical trauma is one of the critical factors determining the prognosis of teeth after restorative treatment. This is of higher importance when these teeth serve as abutments of fixed or removable partial dentures. Previous studies have shown that loss of pulp vitality is one of the major biological complications leading to failure of different types of prosthetic restorations [1]. On the other hand, use of endodontically treated teeth as abutments for such restorations is associated with a significantly higher number of mechanical (e.g., tooth facture) or biological (e.g., recurrent periapical pathology) complications, overall compromising their long-term prognosis [2].

Current treatment modalities of deep carious lesion restoration include direct (DPC) or indirect pulp capping (IPC) by means of calcium hydroxide (CH) covered by a glass-ionomer (GICs), resin-modified glass-ionomer cement (RMGICs), or calcium silicate-based cement, applied as cavity liners. This is then followed by the application of the definitive restoration, which can be either direct composite fillings or composite/ceramic inlays and onlays [3]. In the case of teeth serving as abutments of fixed/removable partial dentures, core buildups using metal-reinforced

A. Bakopoulou (✉)
Department of Prosthodontics, School of Dentistry, Faculty of Health Sciences, Aristotle University of Thessaloniki (AUTh), Thessaloniki, Greece
e-mail: abakopoulou@dent.auth.gr

A. Koutrouli
Department of Paediatric Dentistry, School of Dentistry, Faculty of Health Sciences, Aristotle University of Thessaloniki, Thessaloniki, Greece

I. About
Aix Marseille University, CNRS, ISM, Institute of Movement Science, Marseille, France
e-mail: imad.about@univ-amu.fr

© Springer Nature Switzerland AG 2022
I. About (ed.), *Biodentine™*, https://doi.org/10.1007/978-3-030-80932-4_9

GICs or resin composites are frequently used to restore the full shape of these abutment teeth. This is done in order to ensure the greatest possible retention and stability in the prosthetic reconstruction, while facilitating the individual stages of the clinical process, such as making the impression and fabricating the provisional restorations [4]. This process has been shown to give acceptable clinical outcomes, as it provides fracture-resistant abutments, which can support long-span prosthetic restorations [5].

Ideally, core buildup materials should protect the underlying healthy pulpal tissues by promoting healing and repair. This healing process is mainly assessed by the absence of pain and/or radiographical signs of periapical pathology. The assessment should precede the fabrication of an extracoronal restoration, as pulp sensitivity tests or radiographical evidence of a dentin-bridge formation cannot be performed in teeth covered with full crowns. It is also requested that core buildup materials possess enhanced mechanical properties, to preserve the structural integrity of abutment teeth, especially those serving in long-span fixed or removable partial dentures receiving multidirectional forces for many years [5]. It is also desirable for core buildup materials to form a long-lasting and strong bond with the remaining tooth structure. Moreover, the core material should possess dentin-like properties in terms of hardness and modulus of elasticity. The strength and the bonding of core materials on dental tissues are crucial for the prognosis of prosthetic restorations. Indeed, this will determine whether or not additional retaining elements, or even prophylactic endodontic treatment and placement of a post and core, will be required. Other ideal properties of core buildup materials include toothlike color properties, fast setting rates, and ease of handling [6].

Calcium hydroxide (CH) was first introduced in dentistry in the 1920s and was considered as the "gold standard" in pulp capping [7], with a success rate of 80–90%, calculated by over 2000 cases of DPC. Success was mostly determined by lack of symptoms and/or radiographic lesions and not by pulp vitality tests. According to the literature the success rates drop between approximately 65% and 80% in 2 years, and to 55–70% in 10 years [8]. Studies have shown that the failure of calcium hydroxide is attributed to several drawbacks, such as poor bonding to dentin, reduced mechanical strength, and chemical instability, leading to its gradual dissolution under composite fillings, and subsequent pulp complications, usually within the first 2 years after its application [9]. Although CH allows a dentin bridge formation, the resulting bridge contains a relatively porous structure, favoring pulp infection and/or necrosis [10].

On the other hand, GICs present chemical and mechanical stability, adhesive bonding to the dentin, and acceptable biocompatibility, which are considered as significant advantages. However, they lack the required and essential dentin-forming effect, which is desirable [11]. The mechanical properties of composites and GICs have been tested both in vitro [12] and in clinical studies [13] to determine their suitability as core buildup materials. Their mechanical properties, such as compressive strength, diametrical tensile strength, fracture toughness, and elasticity, have also been tested. Besides, with the development of modern—up to the eighth generation—adhesive systems, composite resins have an acceptable clinical behavior in terms of chemical bonding to enamel. However, their bonding to organic, humid, and carries-affected dentin is of a lesser quality [14, 15]. Another issue related to GICs and resin-modified GICs is their volumetric expansion, which makes them unsuitable under all-ceramic crowns, as there is an increased risk of fracture of these restorations [16]. Of note, resin composite materials present a questionable biological behavior in deep caries, as several studies have shown that, when these materials are used for DPC or IPC even in combination with CH, they lead to pulp inflammation and subsequent irreversible pulp damage [17]. This adverse effect is quite common after the application of resin-based materials, and it is directly related to the proximity of the material to the pulp [13]. The polymerization shrinkage of these materials combined with the monomer release upon incomplete polymerization leads to marginal leakage and cell toxicity, which are responsible for the observed postoperative sensitivity [18]. All these critical issues raise the need to develop more biocompatible and/or bioactive materials in DPC or IPC of vital abutment teeth while maintaining the superior mechanical properties of resin composites.

The tremendous evolution of bioactive materials in the past decade has significantly changed the world of restorative dentistry and endodontics. Mineral trioxide aggregate (MTA) was the first calcium silicate-based cement introduced in the 1990s, and very rapidly it became the ideal replacement of CH in pulp capping procedures. This was mainly due to its ability to produce a hard-tissue barrier, along with its radiopacity and antibacterial properties [19]. Another advantage was the absence of tunnel defects observed in 89% of dentin bridges formed in CH-treated cases [20]. In 2010, a synthetic tricalcium silicate-based cement (Biodentine™, Septodont, Saint Maur des Fossés) became commercially available. Clinical and experimental results have clearly demonstrated a successful outcome with respect to its application in vital pulp therapy, i.e., IPC, DPC, and pulpotomy [21]. The main advantages of this material include its ability to create a firm anchorage to dentin, its bioactivity leading to reparative dentin formation, its antibacterial effects, and its improved mechanical properties. The latter are similar to those of dentin, which presents an elastic modulus of 22 GPa, a compressive strength of 220 MPa, and a microhardness of 60 VHN [22]. Biodentine acts through the formation of CH, through the chemical setting reaction of its two principal components (tricalcium silicate = Ca_3SiO_5 and dicalcium silicate = Ca_3SiO_4). It should be noted however that dentin bridge formation is more homogenous compared to the CH-based materials [23]. The material can exert its bioactive action within a period of 6 weeks, allowing then for the placement of the permanent restoration. However, in cases of a questionable pulp status, the material can be kept in situ as a provisional filling material for up to 6 months, preserving acceptable surface properties regarding anatomic form, marginal adaptation, and interproximal contact [24]. Moreover, its mechanical properties are not affected by restorative procedures, such as acid etching, so that the material can be used in combination with resin-based luting cements [25, 26]. Biodentine has been shown to have better handling properties, while showing similar clinical properties to MTA, and for this reason, it has been proposed as a viable substitute to MTA in vital pulp treatment [27]. Despite the appealing mechanical and biological properties of Biodentine, data regarding its potential application as a core buildup material underneath a prosthetic restoration are entirely lacking.

This chapter focuses on the critical review of current clinical evidence on the efficacy of Biodentine, in terms of long-term preservation of pulp vitality after IPC or DPC. This chapter also examines the material properties that provide exemplary justification for the application of Biodentine as a promising material for the core buildup of prosthetic abutment teeth bearing lesions in proximity to the dental pulp. Furthermore, this review presents a case series of successful application of Biodentine in deep carious lesions in abutment teeth restored with indirect restorations, i.e., inlays or onlays, as well as with full-coverage crowns.

9.2 Clinical Evidence on the Efficacy of Biodentine as an IDP or DPC Material in Vital Pulp Therapy

A literature survey of the electronic database (PubMed, Cochrane Library, Scopus, Google Scholar) was conducted, including studies published between 2015 and 2020. Randomized controlled and non-randomized clinical trials; retrospective, comparative, and longitudinal studies; as well as case series were evaluated. A total of 13 studies were included, and a summary is depicted in Table 9.1.

In order to determine the successful outcome, the selected studies included clinical and radiographic outcome measures. At each recall, the clinical success was determined by positive response to cold/electric pulp testing, absence of spontaneous pain or sensitivity to percussion, absence of sinus/fistula/swelling, or pathological tooth mobility. In three studies, the integrity of the coronal restoration was also evaluated [28–30]. Radiographic success was determined by the presence of an intact lamina dura, absence of excessive periodontal ligament widening, absence of periapical radiolucency and/or internal/external root resorption, and continued root formation in immature permanent teeth. In one study, the absence of pulpal calcification or root canal obliteration was considered as a factor for success, in conjunction with other signs and symptoms indicating pulp necrosis [31]. Dentin bridge formation was assessed in many studies as a significant criterion indicating success [30, 32–34]. Overall, success was confirmed when the treated tooth maintained its vitality and did not present any signs/symptoms of irreversible pulpitis or necrosis.

9.3 Studies Evaluating IPC with Biodentine

Regarding the use of Biodentine in the IPC procedure, only a few studies were identified in the literature. Besides, the majority included a small sample size and limited follow-up periods.

A randomized controlled trial (RCT) evaluated the efficacy of Biodentine as an IPC material in adult patients [35]. Sixty-six teeth with reversible pulpitis were analyzed, and 12 months after treatment, the clinical success rate for both Biodentine™

Table 9.1 Studies published between 2015 and 2020 (PubMed, Cochrane Library, Scopus, Google Scholar) providing clinical evidence on the efficacy of Biodentine as an indirect (IDP) or direct (DPC) pulp capping material in vital pulp therapy

Author, year	Title	Study design	Materials and methods	Restoration	Outcomes analyzed	Results	Follow-up
Hashem et al., 2015 [35]	Clinical and radiographic assessment of the efficacy of calcium silicate indirect pulp capping: a randomized controlled clinical trial	Random-ized controlled clinical trial	IPC—66[a] restorations (31 **Biodentine™**, 35 **Fuji IX™ GIC**) Teeth with clinical symptoms of reversible pulpitis, positive pulp response to electric pulp test/thermal stimulation, no periapical changes viewed on PA radiographs were included Age group: 18–76 years	The permanent **resin composite veneer restoration** (N'Durance; Septodont, Louisville, KY, USA) was placed 1 month after treatment	Clinical: Response to cold/electric pulp testing, presence of spontaneous pain, sensitivity to percussion, presence of sinus/fistula/swelling and mobility Radiographic: CBCT/PA radiographs were taken to evaluate the presence of PA radiolucencies	Clinical success rate for both Biodentine™ and Fuji IX™ GIC after 12 months was 83.3% A significant correlation was found between pulp vitality and symptom intensity at the baseline A significant difference was observed between teeth with healing/healed lesions identified using CBCT receiving BD (71%) and those with new/progressed lesions receiving Fuji IX™ (88%)	Clinical controls were performed at 1, 6, and 12 months (±2 weeks). Radiographic controls at 12 months after treatment
Hashem et al., 2019 [28]	Evaluation of the efficacy of calcium silicate vs. glass-ionomer cement indirect pulp capping and restoration assessment criteria: a randomized controlled clinical trial—2-year results	Random-ized controlled clinical trial	IPC—66[a] restorations (31 **Biodentine™**, 35 **Fuji IX™**) At the 2-year follow-up 42 teeth were analyzed (21 BD, 21 Fuji IX™) Teeth with clinical symptoms of reversible pulpitis, positive pulp response to electric pulp test/thermal stimulation, no periapical changes viewed on PA radiographs were included Age group: 18–76 years	The permanent **resin composite veneer restoration** (N'Durance®, Septodont, Louisville, KY, USA) was placed 1 month after treatment	Clinical: Response to cold test, electric pulp testing, presence of spontaneous pain, sensitivity to percussion, sinus/fistula/swelling and abnormal mobility, assessment of the restoration Radiographic: Presence of PA radiolucencies	Clinical success rate for Biodentine™ was 77.8% and for Fuji IX™ 66.7% after 24 months (not statistically significant) No difference was found between 12-month and 24-month recall in the periapical radiographs and in the integrity of the resin composite restorations overlying BD compared to Fuji IX™	Clinical controls were performed at 1, 6, 12, and 24 months (±2-week). Radiographic controls at 12 and 24 months after treatment

(continued)

Table 9.1 (continued)

Author, year	Title	Study design	Materials and methods	Restoration	Outcomes analyzed	Results	Follow-up
Arshad et al., 2019 [36]	Comparative evaluation of clinical outcome of indirect pulp treatment with calcium hydroxide, calcium silicate, and Er;Cr:YSGG laser in permanent molars	Longitudinal experimental study	IPC—30 restorations (10 **Dycal™**, 10 **Biodentine™**, 10 with cavity decontamination using **Er;Cr:YSGG laser**) Permanent molars with normal appearance of gingiva, absence of spontaneous pain, tenderness, swelling, fistula, abscess formation, abnormal tooth mobility, absence of radiographic thickening of periodontal spaces, interradicular or periapical radiolucencies, internal or external root resorption Age group: 6–14 years	The permanent **composite resin restoration** (Z 100, 3M) was placed immediately after treatment	Clinical: Presence of spontaneous pain and/or sensitivity to pressure, presence of sinus, fistula, edema, and/or abnormal mobility Radiographic: Presence of radiolucencies at the interradicular and/or periapical regions, internal/external root resorption	Overall success rate for CH was 90%, and for both Biodentine™ and laser decontaminated cavities 80% after 9 months (not statistically significant)	Clinical and radiographic controls were performed at 3, 6, and 9 months after treatment

Kusum-valli et al., 2019 [37]	Clinical evaluation of Biodentine™: its efficacy in the management of deep dental caries	Clinical trial	DPC/IPC—12 restorations (7 DPC, 5 IPC) with **Biodentine™** Posterior teeth with a positive cold test, absence of spontaneous/lingering pain/pain on percussion, no sinus tract or swelling, and absence of periapical changes or open apex were included Age group: 15–40 years	The permanent **resin composite restoration** (Tetric EvoCeram, Ivoclar Vivadent) was placed immediately after treatment	Clinical: Presence of signs/symptoms of irreversible pulpitis/necrosis, response to vitality tests, presence of tooth discoloration Radiographic: Presence of periapical changes	Overall success rate was 83.4% after 12 months	Clinical and radiographic controls were performed at 1, 3, 6, and 12 months after treatment
Katge and Patil, 2017 [33]	Comparative analysis of 2 calcium silicate-based cements (Biodentine™ and mineral trioxide aggregate) as direct pulp capping agent in young permanent molars: a split-mouth study	Random-ized clinical trial/split mouth	DPC—42ᵃ restorations in bilateral first permanent molars (21 **Biodentine™**, 21 **gray MTA Angelus™**) Teeth with pinpoint inadvertent pulp exposure (≤ 1 mm) during caries excavation, bleeding controlled under pressure at exposure site, vital pulp, and absence of periapical pathology radiographically were included Age group: 7–9 years	The permanent **composite resin restorative material** (Filtek Z350 XT Universal Restorative; 3M ESPE) was placed 3 months after treatment	Clinical: Presence of pain, swelling, abscess and sinus tract formation, response to electrical pulp vitality test Radiographic: Presence of dentin bridge over the lesion, presence of PA radiolucency, periodontal ligament space widening, calcification, internal/external resorption	Clinical and radiographical success rate for both Biodentine™ and MTA Angelus™ was 100% after 12 months Radiographically: Dentin bridge formation was evident for 95.24% of teeth treated with Biodentine™ and 85.71% of teeth treated with MTA Angelus™ after 12 months (not statistically significant)	Clinical and radiographic controls were performed at 6 and 12 months after treatment

(continued)

Table 9.1 (continued)

Author, year	Title	Study design	Materials and methods	Restoration	Outcomes analyzed	Results	Follow-up
Brizuela et al., 2017 [38]	Direct pulp capping with calcium hydroxide, mineral trioxide aggregate, and Biodentine™ in permanent young teeth with caries: a randomized clinical trial	Randomized clinical trial	DPC—69ᵃ restorations in carious permanent molars (22 **CH**, 25 **Biodentine™**, 22 **white ProRoot® MTA**) Teeth with carious exposure (<2 mm) and complete/incomplete radicular growth, with normal pulp or reversible pulpitis, compatible with normal pulpal testing that was included Age group: 7–16 years	The permanent **direct resin restoration** (Filtek Z350 XT Universal Restorative; 3M ESPE) was placed immediately after treatment	Clinical: Presence of pain, facial edema, fistula, response to sensitivity tests (thermal and electrical) and percussion test Radiographic: Presence of internal/external resorption, periradicular disease, assessment of periodontal ligament width	The overall success rate for Biodentine™ was 100% and for both ProRoot MTA™ and CH 86.4% after 12 months (not statistically significant)	Clinical controls were performed at 1 week, and 3, 6, and 12 months Radiographic controls at 6 and 12 months after treatment

	Treatment	Study type	Materials/groups	Restoration	Outcome measures	Results	Follow-up
Linu et al., 2017 [34]	Treatment outcome following direct pulp capping using bioceramic materials in mature permanent teeth with carious exposure: a pilot retrospective study	Retrospective study/comparative	DPC—Clinical records of 26 restorations (13 ProRoot® MTA, 13 Biodentine™) in molars treated from January 2015 to June 2015 were retrieved Mandibular molars with caries restricted to occlusal surface, no history of night/spontaneous pain, positive response to pulp sensibility tests, no signs of periapical pathology were included Age group: 15–30 years	The permanent **composite resin restoration** (3M ESPE, St. Paul, MN) for the Biodentine™ group was placed 2 weeks after treatment	Clinical: Presence of pain (on percussion/spontaneous/at night) after treatment, response to sensitivity tests Radiographic: Signs of periapical pathology and dentin bridge formation	Overall success rate for ProRoot® MTA was 84.6% and for Biodentine™ 92.3% after 18 months (not statistically significant) Coronal discoloration was observed only in MTA cases (69.2%). Radiographically: Dentin bridge formation was evident in 69.2% of MTA cases and in 61.5% of BD-treated teeth (not statistically significant)	Clinical and radiographic controls were performed at 1, 3, 6, 12, and 18 months after treatment
Hegde et al., 2017 [32]	Clinical evaluation of mineral trioxide aggregate and Biodentine™ as direct pulp capping agents in carious teeth	Clinical trial/comparative	DPC—24 restorations in molars (12 **white ProRoot® MTA**, 12 **Biodentine™**) Teeth with class I or class II cavities, no symptoms, positive response to thermal and electrical tests, no tenderness on percussion, and no pathologic changes on periapical radiographs were included Age group: 18–40 years	The permanent **composite restoration** was placed 3 weeks after treatment	Clinical: Presence of postoperative sensitivity and pain, response to cold/electric pulp testing Radiographic: Presence of PA radiolucencies and formation of dentin bridge on postoperative radiographs	Overall success rate for ProRoot® MTA was 91.7% and for Biodentine™ 83.3% after 6 months (not statistically significant). There was a significant association between tooth vitality and presence of dentin bridge	Clinical and radiographic controls were performed at 3 weeks and 3 and 6 months after treatment

(continued)

Table 9.1 (continued)

Author, year	Title	Study design	Materials and methods	Restoration	Outcomes analyzed	Results	Follow-up
Awawdeh et al., 2018 [29]	Outcomes of vital pulp therapy using mineral trioxide aggregate or Biodentine™: a prospective randomized clinical trial	Randomized clinical trial	DPC/PP—68 restorations (34 **Biodentine™**, 34 white **MTA angelus™**) in vital permanent teeth with deep caries At the 3-year follow-up 49 teeth were analyzed (24 BD, 25 MTA) Teeth with carious lesion involving 2 surfaces, severe symptoms but diagnosis indicating reversible pulpitis based on the cold test, complaints of tooth pain, and radiographic findings were included Age group: 16–59 years	The permanent **amalgam** (15)/**resin composite** (Z250, 3M ESPE) (53) restoration was placed 1 week after treatment	Clinical: Presence of soft-tissue swelling, integrity of coronal restoration, crown discoloration, response to cold sensitivity test Radiographic: Evaluation of periapical status, formation of a dentine bridge, pulpal calcifications, and canal obliteration	Overall success rate for Biodentine™ was 91.7% and for MTA Angelus™ 96.0% after 3 years (not statistically significant) The success rates for the DPC and PP procedures at each time interval exhibited no significant differences	Clinical and radiographic controls were performed at 6 months and 1, 2, and 3 years after treatment
Parin-yaprom et al., 2018 [39]	Outcomes of direct pulp capping by using either ProRoot mineral trioxide aggregate or Biodentine™ in permanent teeth with carious pulp exposure in 6–18-year-old patients: a randomized controlled trial	Randomized controlled clinical trial	DPC—55ª restorations (27 **ProRoot® MTA**, 28 **Biodentine™**) in cariously exposed permanent teeth Teeth with diagnosis of normal pulp, reversible pulpitis, or irreversible pulpitis, early periapical involvement, and exposure size of up to 2.5 mm were included Age group: 6–18 years	The permanent **resin composite** (39)/**amalgam** (1)/**SSC** (15) restoration was placed depending on the amount of tooth structure left immediately after treatment	Clinical: Response to cold test, presence of pain on percussion, swelling, pus exudates/fistulae in soft/periodontal tissues, tooth mobility, crown discoloration Radiographic: Loss of lamina dura, discontinued root formation, more advanced periapical lesion	Overall success rate for ProRoot® MTA was 92.6% and for Biodentine™ 96.4% after a mean follow-up of 18.9+/−12.9 months (not statistically significant) Gray discoloration was observed only with ProRoot® MTA (55%)	Clinical and radiographic controls were performed every 6 months, with mean follow-up: 18.9+/−12.9 months

| Lipski et al., 2018 [31] | Factors affecting the outcomes of direct pulp capping using Biodentine™ | Clinical trial | DPC—86 restorations with Biodentine™ Teeth with signs and/or symptoms of reversible pulpitis, no sinus tract, swelling, percussion pain, periodontal inflammation, radiographic evidence of calcification of the pulp chamber/canals, internal/external resorption, or furcal/periapical radiolucency were included The following factors were tested: (1) sex, (2) age of <40 years or ≥40 years, (3) anterior or posterior tooth, (4) maxilla or mandible, (5) initial or secondary caries treatment, (6) occlusal or proximal/cervical caries localization, and (7) immediate restoration (>1 day) or delayed placement of a permanent filling (2–3 months) Age group: 11–79 years | The permanent resin composite restoration was placed immediately (49 teeth) or 2–3 months after treatment (37 teeth) | Clinical: Assessment of pulpal vitality and tooth crown discoloration Radiographic: Presence of periodontal ligament widening, loss of lamina dura, apical periodontitis, calcific alterations in pulpal space | Overall success rate was 82.6% at 1–1.5 years after treatment 8.5% of vital teeth seemed to be yellower than the adjacent after 1–1.5 years (no gray discoloration) Only age had a significant effect on the pulpal survival rate: the success rate was 90.9% in patients younger than 40 years and 73.8% in patients 40 years or older | Clinical controls were performed at 2–3 months and 1–1.5 years. Radiographic controls were performed at 1–1.5 years after treatment |

(continued)

Table 9.1 (continued)

Author, year	Title	Study design	Materials and methods	Restoration	Outcomes analyzed	Results	Follow-up
Pesker-soy et al., 2020 [30]	Efficacy of different calcium silicate materials as pulp capping agents: randomized clinical trial	Random-ized clinical trial	DPC—525 restorations (105 **Dycal™**, 105 **LC Calcihyd™**, 105 **TheraCal LC™**, 105 **Biodentine™**, 105 **MTA+™**) Molars with class II profound caries, negative to percussion and palpation tests, mobility within normal limits, positive response to pulp vitality tests (electric, cold), clinical and radiographic diagnosis of reversible pulpitis were included Age group: 18–42 years	The permanent **nanohybrid composite resin restoration** (Beautifil II, Shofu Corp) was placed immediately after treatment	Clinical: Presence of abnormal signs/symptoms, function assessment, response to vitality tests and percussion, mobility and restoration assessment Radiographic: Assessment of periodontal ligament space, periapical region, root and alveolar bone status, presence of dentin bridge formation	Clinical and radiographic success of MTA+™ (86.3%, 85.4%) and Biodentine™ (79.4%, 80.1%) after 36 months was found the highest (statistically significant) Dentin bridge thickness: Statistically significant difference between calcium silicate groups (MTA+, TLC, BD) and calcium hydroxide groups (CCH, LCC), after 36 months	Clinical and radiographic controls were performed at 1, 6, 12, and 36 months after treatment

| Dube et al., 2018 [40] | Preventive endodontics by direct pulp capping with restorative dentin substitute-Biodentine™: a series of 15 cases | Case series | DPC—with Biodentine™ First and second molars with deep class I caries, positive to vitality tests (electric and cold), negative on percussion, with no evidence of periodontal ligament widening/periradicular changes were included Age group: 15–30 years | The permanent restoration was performed using **RMGIC** as base and **composite resin** (Filtek Z350-3M) immediately after treatment | Clinical: Response to vitality tests, presence of sensitivity, pain, swelling, mobility, tenderness on percussion, presence of sinus tract Radiographic: Presence of root obliteration, root resorption, or periapical changes | In the follow-up period that ranged from 12 to 24 months, all teeth were asymptomatic (100% success) | Clinical and radiographic controls were performed at 1, 2, 6, and 12 months after treatment |

IPC indirect pulp capping, *DPC* direct pulp capping, *PP* pulpotomy, *CBCT* cone beam computed tomography, *PA* periapical, *BD* Biodentine, *MTA* mineral trioxide aggregate, *CH* calcium hydroxide, *SSC* stainless steel crown, *GIC* glass-ionomer cement, *RMGIC* resin-modified glass-ionomer cement, *TLC* light-cured calcium silicate, *CCH* conventional calcium hydroxide, *LCC* light-cured calcium hydroxide

aExcluded dropouts

and Fuji IX™ GIC was 83.3%. Radiographic evaluation through conical beam computed tomography (CBCT) performed at baseline and the 12-month follow-up period identified cases where preexisting periapical lesions which were not discernible in periapical radiographs were healed, but—in contrast—some cases showed new/deteriorated lesions. It was further demonstrated that 71% of the healed cases were treated with Biodentine, whereas 88% of the new/deteriorated lesions were treated with GIC, thus implying a healing advantage of Biodentine towards the periapical tissues [35]. A subsequent RCT published in 2019, by the same authors, followed the same group of patients for another 12 months [28]. The results of that study demonstrated that the success rate for Biodentine dropped to 77.8%, although no teeth from the Biodentine group failed within the second year. This drop is attributed to the lower recall rate during the second year of follow-up. The success rate for Fuji IX™ at 24 months was 66.7%, and three teeth restored with this GIC lost vitality during this period. This difference between the two materials was not statistically significant. A larger sample size could possibly reveal statistically significant differences. Nevertheless, this has to be further examined with a well-designed randomized clinical trial. It should be mentioned that within the 24-month periods, a total of six teeth treated with Biodentine failed, four of which demonstrated symptoms of irreversible pulpitis during the first month, and the other two lost vitality within 6–12 months after treatment. In this study, a significant association was found between pulp vitality and symptom intensity before treatment, **i.e., more failures were noticed in teeth presenting with more severe symptoms**. Moreover, in this chapter the integrity of the coronal restoration was evaluated, and it was found that resin composite restorations performed well, without differences between the two materials during the 24 months [28].

In another study conducted on children 6–14 years old, the use of CH, Biodentine, and Er,Cr:YSGG laser (Waterlase iPlus, BioLase) in IPC was comparatively evaluated [36]. Thirty vital, carious teeth without signs/symptoms of irreversible pulpitis were included and were followed up for 9 months. Two out of ten teeth treated with Biodentine failed; one presented with abscess, and the other exhibited signs of root resorption at the end of 9 months. Similarly, within this period, two teeth lost vitality in the laser group and one in the CH group. The success rate for Biodentine was 80%, showing no significant difference in relation to the other materials studied [36]. In another clinical trial, vital pulp therapy (IPC/DPC) was evaluated on 12 carious teeth treated with Biodentine [37]. The patients' age ranged between 15 and 40 years, and the overall success rate after 12 months was 83.4%. The two cases that failed, one of which had undergone IPC and the other DPC procedure, presented with spontaneous pain within 3 months after treatment and required root canal treatment, most probably due to wrong estimation of the underlying pulpal pathology [37].

9.4   Studies Evaluating DPC with Biodentine

Results from RCTs evaluating Biodentine as a DPC material in children's permanent teeth showed high success rates after 12 months. In molars with carious pulp exposures of diameter less than 2 mm and normal pulp or reversible pulpitis symptoms, success with Biodentine reached 100% [33, 38]. When Biodentine was used in teeth with symptoms of irreversible pulpitis, early periapical involvement, and pulp exposure up to 2.5 mm, the success rate was 96.4% at a mean follow-up of 18.9 ±12.9 months [39]. In the studies mentioned above, Biodentine showed similar [33] or higher [38, 39] success rates compared with MTA, though, in most cases, failing to reach statistical significance. It is worth mentioning that after 12 months, teeth treated with Biodentine presented dentin bridge formation at a higher rate compared to gray MTA Angelus™ (95.24% and 85.71%, respectively), but still not reaching statistical significance [33]. As opposed to DPC with Biodentine, gray discoloration was observed only in teeth treated with ProRoot™ MTA [39]. This could be a factor to be considered in vital pulp therapy of anterior teeth receiving high-translucency all-ceramic restorations.

In a recent RCT, comparing MTA to Biodentine in vital pulp therapy (DPC and partial pulpotomy), no statistical differences between the two materials were noted [29]. The overall success rate for Biodentine was 91.7% and for MTA Angelus™ 96.0% after 3 years, without statistically significant difference. These results favor the use of both tricalcium silicate materials in DPC and partial pulpotomy in mature permanent teeth. All reported late failures were linked with recurrent caries and fractured fillings, especially in premolars. The five failing cases in the Biodentine group occurred in teeth with prolonged pulp bleeding, where deeper pulp amputation was attempted, possibly because of erroneous evaluation of the clinical pulpal diagnosis and incomplete removal of inflamed pulpal tissue [29]. All these results are promising on the reliability of calcium silicate-based cements, including Biodentine, in vital pulp treatment, which is an important point to be taken into consideration for their potential application in vital pulp treatment of prosthetic abutment teeth.

In an RCT in adult patients evaluating the efficacy of different calcium silicate materials as pulp-capping agents, it was shown that at the end of the 36-month follow-up, the clinical and radiographic success of both MTA+™ (86%, 85%) and Biodentine (79%, 80%) was significantly higher than CH (Dycal: 69%, 70%/light-cured LC Calcihyd: 61%, 61%), as well as light-cured calcium silicate (TheraCal LC: 72%, 73%) [30]. Only in the light-cured groups (TheraCal LC and LC Calcihyd) pulpal exposure size (diameter groups of either ≤0.5 or 0.6–1 mm) affected the success of the materials. MTA+™ and Biodentine™ presented better results when compared with TheraCal LC in larger pulpal exposures of 0.6–1 mm in diameter. The formation and quality of dentin bridge were assessed radiographically, and its importance was emphasized, as it was present in 98% of all successful cases. Dentin bridge formation was observed in all groups after a 6-month follow-up period, without significant difference between the materials analyzed. However, it was shown that the calcium silicate materials induced significantly higher rates of complete dentin bridge formation (>1 mm thickness), as compared to the CH materials after 3 years. In particular, complete dentin bridge formation was observed in 86.7% of MTA+™ group, 85.7% of Biodentine group, and 85.0% of TheraCal LC group. The authors conclude that tricalcium silicate materials (MTA+™ and Biodentine) are the most appropriate materials in vital pulp treatments [30].

Factors affecting the outcomes of DPC using Biodentine were studied using 86 teeth with signs/symptoms of reversible pulpitis [31]. The overall success rate was 82.6% at 12–16 months. In total, 15 teeth failed by showing evidence of pulp necrosis, requiring root canal treatment or extraction. Among the different factors evaluated (age, sex, initial/secondary caries treatment, occlusal or cervical/proximal caries, delayed placement of a permanent filling, tooth position, and arch type), only age had a significant effect on the preservation of pulp vitality. More specifically, the success rate was 90.9% in patients younger than 40 years and 73.8% in patients 40 years or older. The latter raises significant concerns on the reliability of vital pulp treatment with DPC in patients over 40 years that, however, represent the main target group receiving permanent prosthetic restoration and this warrants further investigation with longer term studies including higher sample sizes. As far as the timing of the permanent restoration is concerned, no significant difference was noticed between the cases where Biodentine was used as a temporary material for 2–3 months and cases that were permanently restored immediately after treatment. This can be explained by the good physical properties and sealing ability of Biodentine [31].

The success of DPC using either white ProRoot™ MTA or Biodentine was evaluated in 24 carious, asymptomatic teeth in adults, during a 6-month follow-up [32]. The success rate is in favor of ProRoot™ MTA (91.7%), as compared to Biodentine (83.3%), although the differences did not reach statistical significance. It is worth mentioning that all failures (two teeth treated with Biodentine and one with MTA) developed symptoms of irreversible pulpitis, requiring root canal treatment within the first 3 weeks [32]. This provides some evidence that if vital pulp therapy by means of silicate-based cements is decided for a tooth that will be used as a future abutment of a prosthetic restoration, it would be safer to re-evaluate pulp status at least 1 month or more after DPC, before proceeding to the fabrication of the definitive restoration.

A retrospective study comparatively evaluated ProRoot™ MTA and Biodentine, during a follow-up of 18 months [34]. Young patients (15–30 years old) with molars affected by caries only at the occlusal surface were included. The overall success rate of DPC with Biodentine (92.3%) was higher than that of ProRoot™ MTA (84.6%), although not statistically significant. Coronal discoloration appeared solely in 69.2% of MTA-treated cases. Radiographically, dentin bridge formation was evident without a significant difference between the two materials [34]. In agreement with Hegde et al. [32], all failures occurred within the first 2 weeks after treatment [34], further supporting the notion that the first few weeks after DPC with calcium silicate-based materials are critical for evaluating the treatment outcome.

In a recently published study, the use of Biodentine was evaluated in a series of 15 cases as a pulp capping material in carious molars with class I cavities in young patients, with ages ranging between 15 and 30 years. All 15 teeth remained asymptomatic during the follow-up periods, which ranged from 12 to 24 months, indicating successful treatment [40].

In conclusion, studies provide evidence on the safety and efficacy of application of silicate-based cements, including Biodentine, in IPC and DPC of vital permanent teeth receiving direct restorations, although the observation times do not exceed 3 years and the sample sizes, especially in older patient groups, are relatively small. Based on the above analysis of clinical studies showing a good biological response, in conjunction with the ideal mechanical properties of Biodentine as dentin substitute [22], it is safe to conclude that it could be considered as a promising candidate material for the core buildup of prosthetic abutment teeth bearing deep carious lesions. Further studies are, however, required to support that Biodentine or any other similar material enhances the structural integrity of abutment teeth and provides better retention and resistance form to the preparation.

Surprisingly, as of today, there are no clinical studies of any type, neither RCTs nor retrospective, comparative, or longitudinal, to support these assumptions. The latter, therefore, highlights the urgent unmet clinical need for implementation of such studies to provide a secure vital pulp therapy modality of prosthetic abutment teeth with a safe long-term prognosis.

9.5   Case Series

The presented series of clinical cases were conducted at a private dental practice (Dr. Athina Bakopoulou) limited to prosthodontics and restorative dentistry, between January 2012 and December 2018. All participants signed a consent form.

9.5.1   Clinical Case 1

A 38-year-old female patient, with a free medical history, presented complaining about tooth sensitivity at her maxillary right side, when consuming cold and hot beverages. Clinical diagnostic assessment and radiographical examination revealed secondary carious lesions below existing amalgam restorations in maxillary right first bicuspid (distally) and maxillary right second bicuspid (interproximally) (Fig. 9.1Aa). Both teeth were tested positive on CO_2 snow sensitivity and negative on percussion. The patient was informed about the need of having the carious lesions treated and the amalgam fillings replaced.

After patient's consent, local anesthesia was performed (Articaine HCL 4% with 1:200,000 adrenaline, Ubistesin, 3M ESPE), the amalgam restorations were removed, and the carious dentin was completely excavated (Fig. 9.1Ab). At the proximal cavity area of tooth maxillary right second bicuspid a very thin pulp-facing layer of remaining dentin could be observed (Fig. 9.1Ac). Biodentine was applied as a provisional filling material of the entire cavity of both teeth (Fig. 9.1Ad, e), according to the manufacturer's instructions, and left in place for 6 weeks [31, 41]. The patient reported that she remained symptom-free during the 6-week period, whereas both teeth were positive on CO_2 snow sensitivity and negative on percussion. Biodentine was then partially removed to serve as a base/dentin substitute (Fig. 9.1Af) and both teeth were restored with indirect composite inlays (SR Adoro,

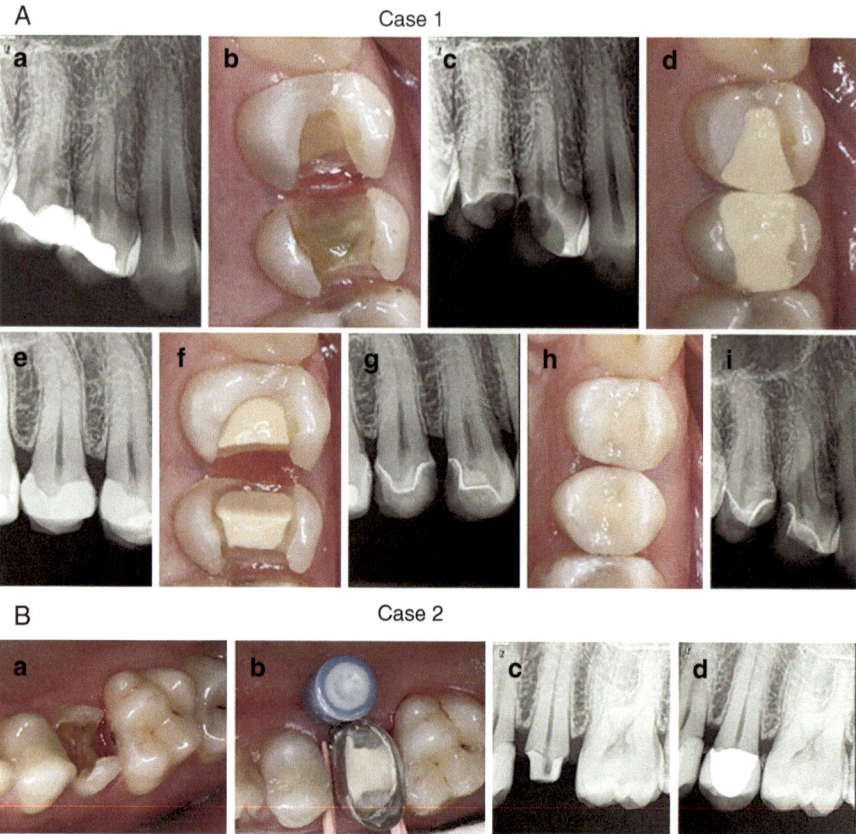

Fig. 9.1 (**A**) a: Preoperative radiograph showing recurrent caries below existing amalgam restorations in maxillary right first and second bicuspids. b: Clinical picture after caries removal. c: Radiograph taken after caries removal, showing close proximity of the cavity walls to the pulp, especially for maxillary right second bicuspid. d: Biodentine was placed as a provisional material to restore both cavities and left in place for 6 weeks. The material has a smooth surface after setting. e: Radiograph after Biodentine placement. f: Biodentine was partially removed to serve as a dentin substitute. g: Radiograph 6 months posttreatment. h: Definitive inlay restorations in place cemented with a dual-cure resin cement. i: Radiograph 1 year posttreatment (Case republished with permission from *Bakopoulou A, About I. Biodentine: a promising bioactive material for the preservation of pulp vitality in restorative dentistry. Septodont Case studies Collection No. 5-June 2013, pages 4–11*). (**B**) a: Clinical picture after deep caries removal. b: Biodentine was placed as a provisional material to restore both cavities and left in place for 6 weeks. The material has a smooth surface after setting. c: Radiograph after Biodentine placement. Definitive inlay restorations in place cemented with a dual-cure resin cement. d: Definitive metal ceramic crown placed after 8 weeks and cemented with conventional glass-ionomer cement (Fuji I, GC)

Ivoclar Vivadent) that were cemented with a dual-cure resin cement (Variolink II, Ivoclar Vivadent) (Fig. 9.1Ag, h). At the follow-up visits of 6 months and 1 year after treatment, both teeth were free from any symptoms and again tested positive for sensitivity and negative for percussion. Radiographical examination showed no signs of periapical pathology (Fig. 9.1Ai).

9.5.2   Clinical Case 2

A 22-year-old male patient, with a free medical history, presented a fracture of the left maxillary second bicuspid, without any symptoms. The tooth had a previous class 2 amalgam restoration and was tested positive on CO_2 snow sensitivity and negative on percussion. The patient was informed about the need of having the carious lesions treated and the amalgam restorations replaced.

After patient's consent, local anesthesia was performed (Articaine HCL 4% with 1:200,000 adrenaline, Ubistesin, 3M ESPE), the amalgam restoration was removed, and the carious dentin was completely excavated (Fig. 9.1Ba). At the proximal cavity area pulp exposure of approximately 2 mm occurred during caries removal (Fig. 9.1Ba). Biodentine was applied as a provisional filling material of the entire cavity of both teeth (Fig. 9.1Bb) and left in place for 6 weeks [31, 41]. The patient reported that he remained symptom-free during the 6-week period, while the tooth remained positive on CO_2 snow sensitivity and negative on percussion. The tooth was then prepared for a full-coverage metal-ceramic crown, due to the significant loss of dental hard tissues after the caries control. The tooth was prepared without removing Biodentine, which served as an abutment core buildup material (Fig. 9.1Bc). The definitive metal-ceramic crown was cemented with a conventional GIC (Fuji I, GC) (Fig. 9.1). At the follow-up visit after 6 months the tooth was symptom-free and negative for percussion, while a radiographic examination showed no signs of periapical pathology (Fig. 9.1Bd).

9.5.3   Clinical Case 3

A 28-year-old female patient, with a free medical history, presented after fracture of her first maxillary left molar during chewing (Fig. 9.2Aa). Clinical and radiographic examination revealed deep caries at high proximity to the pulp in both first and second right maxillary molars (Fig. 9.2Ab). Clinical examination showed that both teeth were positive on CO_2 snow sensitivity and negative on percussion. The patient did not mention any previous symptomatology associated with these teeth in the past. The patient was informed about the need of having the carious lesions treated and the possibility that an endodontic treatment would be required after caries removal.

After patient's consent, local anesthesia was performed (Articaine HCL 4% with 1:200,000 adrenaline, Ubistesin, 3M ESPE) and a rubber dam was placed. After excavation of the carious dentin, the pulp was exposed iatrogenically in the first right maxillary molar, whereas a very thin pulp-facing layer of dentin could be observed in the distal area of this tooth, and in the proximal area of the second right maxillary molar, both requiring IDC (Fig. 9.2Ac, d). Clinically the pulp of the first right maxillary molar at the exposure site was vital without any major bleeding, so the maintenance of tooth vitality by DPC was decided. Cavity disinfection and control of the hemorrhage were performed with sodium hypochlorite. Biodentine was applied as provisional filling material of the entire cavity of both teeth (Fig. 9.2Ae)

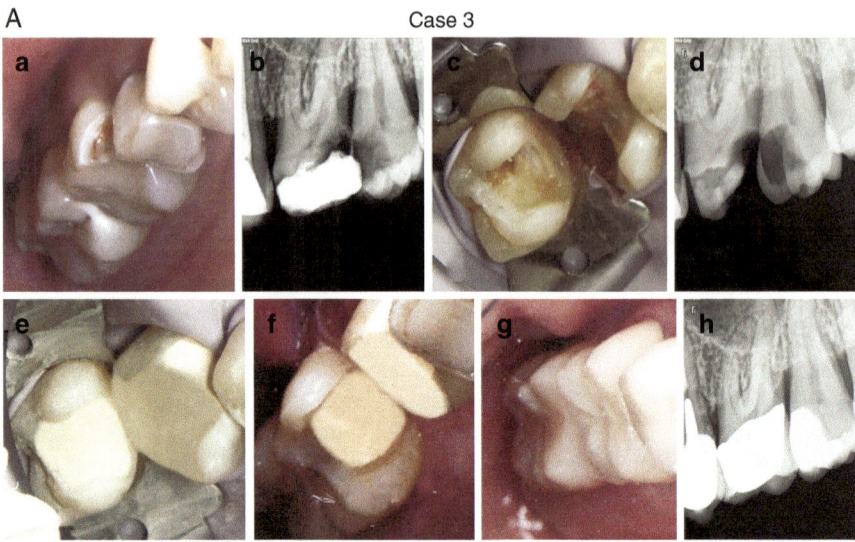

Fig. 9.2 (**A**) a: Preoperative clinical picture showing fracture of maxillary left first molar. b: Preoperative radiograph showing deep caries in both maxillary left first and second molars in close proximity to the pulp. c: After caries removal the pulp was exposed iatrogenically in maxillary left first molar, whereas a very thin pulp-facing layer of dentin could be observed in the distal area of this tooth, as well as the proximal area of maxillary left second molar. d: Radiograph after caries removal. e: Biodentine was placed as a provisional material to restore both cavities and left in place for 6 weeks. A rubber dam was used to avoid bacterial contamination after pulp exposure. f: In maxillary left second molar Biodentine was then partially removed and kept as a base/dentin substitute that was capped by a direct composite resin filling (Tetric EvoCeram, Ivoclar Vivadent). Maxillary left first molar was prepared for a full-coverage restoration and Biodentine remained as an abutment buildup material. g: Postoperative clinical picture with a direct resin composite filling in maxillary left second molar and a metal ceramic crown in maxillary left first molar. h: Radiograph 6 months posttreatment. No signs of periapical pathology could be observed (Case republished with permission from *Bakopoulou A, About I. Biodentine: a promising bioactive material for the preservation of pulp vitality in restorative dentistry. Septodont Case studies Collection No. 5-June 2013, pages 4–11*). (**B**) a: Preoperative clinical photograph of existing crown on maxillary right first molar. b: Preoperative radiograph showing recurrent caries at the distal margin of existing crown on maxillary right first molar. c: Clinical status after crown removal and caries excavation. d: Radiograph taken immediately after caries removal, showing close proximity of the cavity walls to the pulp, especially at the distal abutment wall. e: Biodentine was left in place for 6 weeks. During this period the tooth remained symptom-free, whereas its integrity was maintained. f: Radiographic examination at 6 weeks revealed reparative dentin formation and lack of any periapical pathology. g: Final metal-ceramic crown placed after 8 weeks and cemented with conventional glass-ionomer cement (Fuji I, GC). h: Radiographic examination 1 year posttreatment. The tooth remained free from any periapical pathology. (Case republished with permission from *Bakopoulou A, About I. Biodentine: a promising bioactive material for the long-term preservation of pulp vitality in prosthetic abutments. Septodont Case studies Collection No. 8-May 2014, pages 4–10*)

B   Case 4

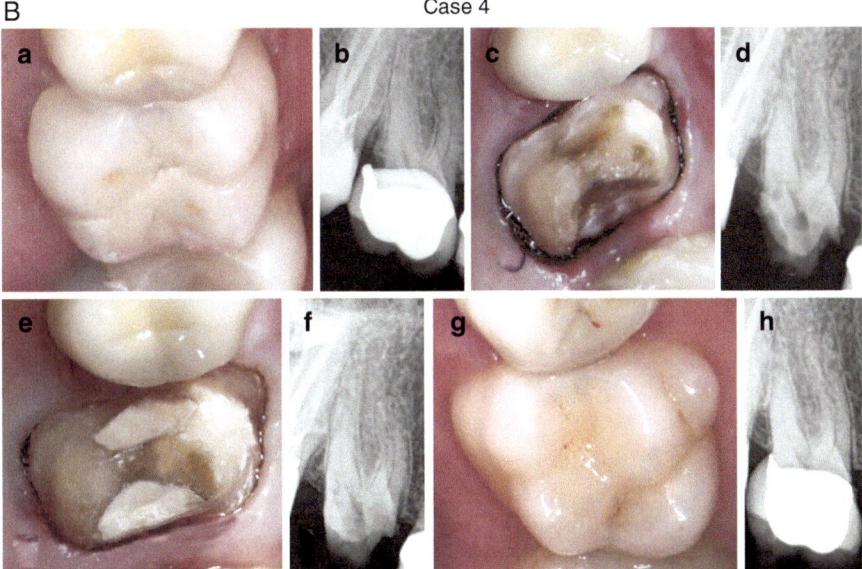

Fig. 9.2   (continued)

and left in place for 6 weeks [31, 41]. During this period the patient was symptom-free, and both teeth remained positive on CO_2 snow sensitivity and negative on percussion. Biodentine was then partially removed in tooth # 27 and kept as a base/dentin substitute that was capped by a direct composite resin filling (Tetric EvoCeram, Ivoclar Vivadent), following normal procedures (acid etching of the cavity with phosphoric acid and application of single-step adhesive of the same manufacturer) (Fig. 9.2Af). The first right maxillary molar was prepared for a full-coverage metal-ceramic restoration due to the significant loss of dental hard tissues. The tooth was prepared without removing Biodentine that remained as an abutment core buildup material. The final metal-ceramic restoration was cemented with a conventional GIC (Fuji I, GC) (Fig. 9.2Ag). At the follow-up visit after 6 months both teeth were symptom-free and again tested positive for sensitivity and negative for percussion. Radiographic examination revealed no signs of periapical pathology (Fig. 9.2Ah).

9.5.4   Clinical Case 4

A 36-year-old female patient, with a medical history of systemic rheumatoid arthritis, presented for her regular scheduled 6-month oral evaluation. The patient had a history of frequent recurrent caries underneath existing restorations that remained symptom-free until the lesion reached the pulp cavity. Radiographic examination revealed a secondary carious lesion at the distal margin of an existing full-coverage restoration in the maxillary right first molar (Fig. 9.2Ba, b). The patient was informed about the need of having the crown removed in order to treat the existing caries and for the possibility that an endodontic treatment might be required before a new restoration could be placed.

After patient's consent, local anesthesia was performed (Articaine HCL 4% with 1:200,000 adrenaline, Ubistesin, 3M ESPE), the crown was removed, and the carious dentin was completely excavated. At the distal area of the prepared maxillary right first molar a very thin pulp-facing layer of remaining dentin could be observed, whereas a shallower cavity was observed at the proximal part of the abutment (Fig. 9.2Bc, d). Biodentine was chosen as a core buildup material to fill both cavities (Fig. 9.2Be) and left in place for 6 weeks [31, 41] in order to ensure preservation of pulp vitality. After the 6-week period, the patient reported that she remained symptom-free and the tooth was positive on CO_2 snow sensitivity and negative on percussion. The patient did not show any signs of periapical pathology (Fig. 9.2Bf). Conventional restorative procedures followed for the placement of a new metal-ceramic extracoronal restoration (Fig. 9.2Bg) with Biodentine remaining as a permanent core buildup material. The crown was cemented with conventional glass-ionomer cement (Fuji I, GC). At the follow-up visit 6 months and 1 year after treatment the tooth remained free from any symptoms. Radiographic examination revealed no signs of periapical pathology or recurrent caries (Fig. 9.2Bh).

9.5.5 Clinical Case 5

A 42-year-old female patient, with free medical history, presented complaining about a spontaneous tooth pain at the left maxillary side. The pain was also present when the patient was consuming cold and hot beverages. Diagnostic assessment and radiographic examination revealed recurrent carious lesions below existing amalgam restorations distally of the left maxillary first molar and mesially of the left maxillary second molar (Fig. 9.3a, b). Both teeth were positive on pulp sensitivity tests at a higher threshold compared to adjacent teeth but negative on percussion. The patient was informed about the need of having the carious lesions treated and restored.

After patient's consent, local anesthesia was performed (Articaine HCL 4% with 1:200,000 adrenaline, Ubistesin, 3M ESPE), the amalgam restorations were removed, and the carious dentin was completely excavated leaving extensive deep cavities (Fig. 9.3c, d). Biodentine was chosen as a provisional filling material of the entire cavities of both teeth (Fig. 9.3e) and left in place for 6 weeks to ensure that pulp sensitivity disappears, while preserving pulp vitality [31, 41]. The patient remained symptom-free during the 6-week period, whereas both teeth were positive

Case 5

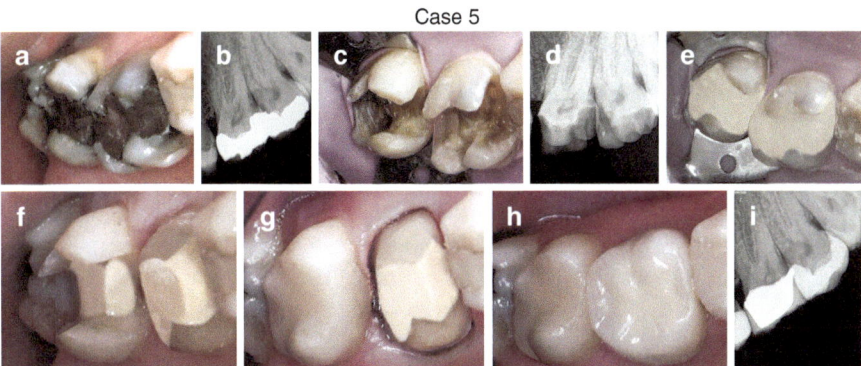

Fig. 9.3 (**a**) Preoperative clinical picture showing existing amalgam restorations on maxillary left first and second molars accompanied with pulp symptomatology. (**b**) Preoperative radiograph showing deep recurrent caries in both maxillary left first and second molars in close proximity to the pulp. (**c**) After caries removal deep cavities in close proximity to the pulp were the case for both teeth. (**d**) Radiographic examination after caries removal confirming the close proximity of the cavity walls to the pulp chamber. (**e**) Biodentine was placed as a provisional material to restore both cavities and left in place for 6 weeks. A rubber dam was used to avoid further bacterial contamination of the symptomatic pulps. (**f**) Biodentine restorations 6 weeks after placement. Marginal integrity of both restorations was fully preserved and no fractures were observed. In maxillary left second molar Biodentine was partially removed and kept as a base/dentin substitute for subsequent filling with a direct composite. Maxillary left first molar was prepared for full coverage and Biodentine remained as an abutment buildup material. (**g**) Maxillary left second molar was capped by a direct composite resin filling (Tetric EvoCeram Bulk Fill, Ivoclar Vivadent) and maxillary left first molar was prepared for a full crown. (**h**) Postoperative clinical picture with a direct resin composite filling in maxillary left second molar and a metal-ceramic crown in maxillary left first molar. (**i**) Radiographic examination 1 year posttreatment. The tooth remained free from any periapical pathology. (Case republished with permission from *Bakopoulou A, About I. Biodentine: a promising bioactive material for the long-term preservation of pulp vitality in prosthetic abutments. Septodont Case studies Collection No. 8-May 2014, pages 4–10*)

on pulp sensitivity tests and negative on percussion. Biodentine was then partially removed from the left maxillary second molar to serve as a base/dentin substitute, whereas the left maxillary first molar was prepared to receive a full crown with Biodentine serving as a dentin substitute for the abutment buildup (Fig. 9.3f). Following conventional restorative procedures, i.e., acid etching of the cavity with phosphoric acid and application of single-step adhesive, Excite F, Ivoclar Vivadent, the left maxillary second molar was filled with a direct composite resin filling (Tetric EvoCeram Bulk, Ivoclar Vivadent) (Fig. 9.3g) and the left maxillary first molar was restored with a full-coverage restoration that was cemented with a conventional GIC (Fuji I, GC) (Fig. 9.3h). At the follow-up visit at 6 months and 1 year after treatment both teeth were free of any symptomatology with no radiographic signs of periapical pathology (Fig. 9.3i).

9.6   Discussion

Maintaining pulp vitality of abutment teeth with deep caries or spontaneous pulp exposure during full-coverage preparation procedures is one of the major dilemmas in clinical prosthodontics. Indeed, on the one hand, maintaining pulp vitality helps to avoid additional restorative challenges and failures related to endodontically treated abutment teeth, including root fractures. On the other hand, vital pulp removal and prophylactic endodontic treatment may be needed to avoid pulp necrosis, infection, and induction of apical periodontitis. The latter is related to more severe consequences, as the definitive restoration might need to be replaced a short time after placement, mainly due to the mechanical failures related to the endodontic treatment access hole through the crown. Another important factor is endodontically treated teeth which serve as abutments for extracoronal restorations that present a success rate of 59.4% after 15–20 years, whereas vital teeth which support full-coverage restorations present a success rate of 81.9% in the same time period [2]. Treatment procedures targeting maintenance of prosthodontic abutment teeth vitality, i.e., ICP or DPC, have not been favored by most clinicians until recently. This was due to the unreliability that these procedures have shown, by the suboptimal results derived from follow-up studies. New techniques employing bioactive materials, including Biodentine, offer new perspectives. However, their promising results need to be validated by well-designed RCTs. Unfortunately, most of the current knowledge is derived from studies supported by definitive direct composite restorations made on single tooth, which allow a safe and predictable reentry in case of failure. Nevertheless, this is not the case for abutment teeth of definitive fixed and removable partial dentures, which complicates the endodontic therapy and the success rates.

9.6.1   Studies of the Preservation of Pulp Vitality After IPC with Biodentine

There is a small number of studies evaluating the use of Biodentine for the IPC of permanent teeth [28, 35–37]. In most studies, except the one by Hashem et al. [28], the follow-up period does not exceed 1 year. This fact and the limited recall intervals do not allow drawing safe conclusions regarding the success of Biodentine. In the latter study, it was concluded that the failed IPC cases were mostly related to the initial presence of severe symptoms of reversible pulpitis (increased pain in the presence of hot/cold stimuli demanding the use of painkillers) rather than the extent of the cavity (1–3 surfaces) [28]. This is an essential factor in decision-making regarding IPC treatment of abutment teeth for definitive prosthetic restorations.

   Another drawback is that in only a few studies, the exact caries excavation procedure, i.e., depth of mechanical excavation, use of chemical agents, and amount of caries left, was presented to allow standardization among the treated teeth [28, 35]. Another critical point of consideration is that in all these studies direct composite resin restorations were used. These restorations were placed either immediately [36,

37] or 1 month after treatment [28, 35]. In this respect, there is no published data regarding the long-term behavior of Biodentine used on teeth which served as abutments of definitive prosthetic restorations.

9.6.2   Studies of the Preservation of Pulp Vitality After DPC with Biodentine

The longest follow-up period for clinical cases (507 in total) of vital pulp therapy by means of DPC (mostly CH based) was 30 years, providing a 73.2% success rate [42]. In a recent systematic review and meta-analysis [43] of randomized and non-randomized comparative studies, the pooled success rates for DPC at 6 months were 91% and 96% for MTA and Biodentine, respectively. The success rates for both materials at 12 months dropped at 86%, while at 2–3 years the success rate for MTA slightly dropped to 84% and for Biodentine remained stable (86%) [39]. Among RCTs, the study by Peskersoy et al. [30] reported an 80% success rate at 36 months, while Awawdeh et al. [29] and Linu et al. [31] reported success rates of 91.7% after 36 months and 92.3% after 18 months, respectively. Similar results were recorded when the definitive restorations (in most cases, direct composite resins) were placed immediately [30], 2 weeks [34], or 3 weeks [32] after treatment. Lipski et al. [31] compared immediate and delayed (2–3 months after treatment) placement, observing no statistically significant differences (85.7% and 78.4% success, respectively). However, according to results from earlier studies, an increased risk of failure after DPC with MTA or CH was noticed when the permanent restoration was performed with a delay of 2 or more days (irrespectively of the type of material applied). This finding highlights the immediate need for a definitive restoration that protects the tooth structures more effectively from microleakage, compared to a provisional filling [44]. On the other hand, the favorable outcomes observed with Biodentine in recent studies demonstrate the improved physical properties and sealing ability of this dentin substitute material, which can restore the treated tooth and endure occlusal forces for up to 6 months [24].

The patients' age appeared to be an essential factor influencing the treatment prognosis, as patients older than 40 years presented lower success rates [31, 45]. However, the evidence in the literature is not clear regarding the influence of age on the success or failure of pulp-capped teeth in adult patients [44, 46]. Besides, RCTs which reported on patients younger than 16 years old showed even more favorable results for Biodentine application in DPC regarding success rates and dentin bridge formation [33, 38, 39]. These studies also included teeth with open apex, which partially explains the very high success rates, as the pulp of immature teeth is highly cellular and has a rich vascular supply, providing a better healing potential [47].

Selection of cases and decision-making in prosthodontics should be based on specific indications and scientific criteria. Ricucci et al. [42] provided guidelines for DPC based on histopathological, histobacteriological, and clinical findings. Based on these, indications in favor of DPC of mature teeth with closed apices include the presence of red, homogeneous, and blood-filled tissue at the exposure site surrounded by sound dentine. The size of the pulp exposure plays an important role, with exposures up to 0.5 mm showing higher success rates than those with a diameter of 0.6–1 mm [30]. Finally, caries location seems to play a role, as well. In the study of Linu et al. [34], only teeth with occlusal caries were included, and the study reported higher success rates for Biodentine after 18 months, compared to other studies evaluating teeth with class II cavities [30] or teeth with either occlusal or proximal defects [31, 32]. In contrast, Lipski et al. [31] concluded that caries location did not play a role in the success of DPC with Biodentine.

Most studies support that DPC should be performed under strict asepsis. Therefore rubber dam isolation is highly recommended. According to the guidelines proposed by Ricucci et al. (2019), hemostasis should be achieved within 2–3 min after rinsing with a mild disinfectant, such as chlorhexidine or 1% sodium hypochlorite, followed by the application of a sterile cotton pellet on the surgical wound [42]. Lastly, the pulp wound should be covered by a biocompatible and bioactive restorative material, extended to the dentin surrounding the exposure. Based on the current evidence provided by clinical studies (Table 9.1), a period of at least 3–6 months with an evaluation of pulp vitality is essential before proceeding to the definitive restoration. According to Koubi et al. [24], Biodentine can be used to restore posterior teeth for up to 6 months due to its favorable physical properties. According to recent studies, when failures with Biodentine occur, these seem to happen 2–3 weeks after its use for direct pulp capping in carious teeth [32, 34]. Therefore, a time period of 2–3 months of waiting and re-evaluation is recommended before proceeding to the definitive restoration [31]. A key evaluation factor with high prognostic value on the final healing and long-term success of DPC is the formation of a dentin bridge protecting the pulp from further bacterial attack [47]. Dentin bridge formation was positively correlated with pulp vitality [27, 29] and was observed in 86% of Biodentine cases, 36 months after treatment, without any significant differences when compared to MTA cases [30]. Case selection and adherence to the clinical guidelines are very important, as this will enhance the treatment outcome and provide favorable long-term prognosis.

9.7   Conclusions

Overall, factors in favor of application of Biodentine in vital pulp therapy of abutment teeth in prosthetic dentistry include its enhanced mechanical properties, which are very similar to those of dentin, good sealing ability, and development of a firm bond with the underlying dentin substrate, which is highly required to ensure the preservation of the abutment integrity and lower the risk for crown detachment. The material can exert its bioactive action within a period of 6 weeks, allowing then for the placement of the permanent restoration. However, in cases of a questionable pulp status, the material can be kept in situ as a provisional filling material for up to 6 months, preserving acceptable surface properties regarding anatomic form, marginal adaptation, and interproximal contact. This is of high importance for the re-evaluation of vital strategic abutment teeth that will be used underneath long-span prosthetic restorations. Another significant advantage is the handling properties of Biodentine, which are superior to other silicate-based materials, such as MTA. Its optical properties are also advantageous, as it causes no discoloration like MTA, and can, therefore, be considered for the restoration of anterior abutment teeth receiving high-translucency all-ceramic restorations. Moreover, its mechanical properties are not affected by restorative procedures, such as acid etching, so that the material can be used in combination with resin-based luting cements. Biodentine is primarily highly indicated for core buildup of teeth of younger patients without severe symptoms of reversible pulpitis following strict IPC or DPC aseptic protocols. It can also be proposed for the vital pulp therapy and core buildup of abutment teeth of older (>40) patients receiving longer span prosthetic restorations. However, a careful case selection is needed. It is important to avoid using Biodentine on teeth with symptoms of reversible pulpitis, adhering to the clinical guidelines for IPC or DPC and re-evaluating the teeth after a substantial time of at least 6 weeks. It is also essential to confirm the successful formation of reparative dentin before the tooth is covered by the definitive extracoronal restoration. Despite promising perspectives, more evidence is required with well-designed RCTs including larger samples, standardized treatment procedures, and longer observation periods, to establish vital pulp therapy of abutment teeth with Biodentine as the treatment modality of choice.

References

1. Pjetursson BE, Sailer I, Makarov NA, Zwahlen M, Thoma DS. All-ceramic or metal-ceramic tooth-supported fixed dental prostheses (FDPs)? A systematic review of the survival and complication rates. Part II: multiple-unit FDPs. Dent Mater. 2015;31(6):624–39. https://doi.org/10.1016/j.dental.2015.02.013.
2. De Backer H, Van Maele G, De Moor N, Van den Berghe L. Long-term results of short-span versus long-span fixed dental prostheses: an up to 20-year retrospective study. Int J Prosthodont. 2008;21(1):75–85.
3. Fransson H. On the repair of the dentine barrier. Swed Dent J Suppl. 2012;226:9–84.
4. Stober T, Rammelsberg P. The failure rate of adhesively retained composite core build-ups in comparison with metal-added glass ionomer core build-ups. J Dent. 2005;33(1):27–32. https://doi.org/10.1016/j.jdent.2004.07.006.
5. Theodosopoulou JN, Chochlidakis KM. A systematic review of dowel (post) and core materials and systems. J Prosthodont. 2009;18(6):464–72. https://doi.org/10.1111/j.1532-849X.2009.00472.x.
6. Tsiagali V, Kirmanidou Y, Pissiotis A, Michalakis K. In vitro assessment of retention and resistance failure loads of teeth restored with a complete coverage restoration and different core materials. J Prosthodont. 2019;28(1):e229–36. https://doi.org/10.1111/jopr.12668.
7. Hilton TJ. Keys to clinical success with pulp capping: a review of the literature. Oper Dent. 2009;34(5):615–25. https://doi.org/10.2341/09-132-0.
8. Dammaschke T, Leidinger J, Schäfer E. Long-term evaluation of direct pulp capping—treatment outcomes over an average period of 6.1 years. Clin Oral Investig. 2010;14(5):559–67. https://doi.org/10.1007/s00784-009-0326-9.
9. Al-Hiyasat AS, Barrieshi-Nusair KM, Al-Omari MA. The radiographic outcomes of direct pulp-capping procedures performed by dental students: a retrospective study. J Am Dent Assoc. 2006;137(12):1699–705. https://doi.org/10.14219/jada.archive.2006.0116.

10. Mohammadi Z, Dummer PM. Properties and applications of calcium hydroxide in endodontics and dental traumatology. Int Endod J. 2011;44(8):697–730. https://doi.org/10.1111/j.1365-25 91.2011.01886.x.

11. Weiner RS, Weiner LK, Kugel G. Teaching the use of bases and liners: a survey of North American dental schools. J Am Dent Assoc. 1996;127(11):1640–5. https://doi.org/10.14219/jada.archive.1996.0100.

12. Kumar G, Shivrayan A. Comparative study of mechanical properties of direct core build-up materials. Contemp Clin Dent. 2015;6(1):16–20. https://doi.org/10.4103/0976-237X.149285.

13. de Souza Costa CA, Teixeira HM, Lopes do Nascimento AB, Hebling J. Biocompatibility of resin-based dental materials applied as liners in deep cavities prepared in human teeth. J Biomed Mater Res B Appl Biomater. 2007;81(1):175–84. https://doi.org/10.1002/jbm.b.30651.

14. Perdigão J. Current perspectives on dental adhesion: (1) dentin adhesion—not there yet. Jpn Dent Sci Rev. 2020;56(1):190–207. https://doi.org/10.1016/j.jdsr.2020.08.004.

15. Isolan CP, Sarkis-Onofre R, Lima GS, Moraes RR. Bonding to sound and caries-affected dentin: a systematic review and meta-analysis. J Adhes Dent. 2018;20(1):7–18. https://doi.org/10.3290/j.jad.a39775.

16. Watts DC, Kisumbi BK, Toworfe GK. Dimensional changes of resin/ionomer restoratives in aqueous and neutral media. Dent Mater. 2000;16(2):89–96. https://doi.org/10.1016/s0109-5641(99)00098-6.

17. Paula AB, Laranjo M, Marto CM, Paulo S, Abrantes AM, Casalta-Lopes J, et al. Direct pulp capping: what is the most effective therapy?—systematic review and meta-analysis. J Evid Based Dent Pract. 2018;18(4):298–314. https://doi.org/10.1016/j.jebdp.2018.02.002.

18. Polydorou O, Hammad M, König A, Hellwig E, Kümmerer K. Release of monomers from different core build-up materials. Dent Mater. 2009;25(9):1090–5. https://doi.org/10.1016/j.dental.2009.02.014.

19. Li Z, Cao L, Fan M, Xu Q. Direct pulp capping with calcium hydroxide or mineral trioxide aggregate: a meta-analysis. J Endod. 2015;41(9):1412–7. https://doi.org/10.1016/j.joen.2015.04.012.

20. Cox CF, Sübay RK, Ostro E, Suzuki S, Suzuki SH. Tunnel defects in dentin bridges: their formation following direct pulp capping. Oper Dent. 1996;21(1):4–11.

21. Barczak K, Palczewska-Komsa M, Sikora M, Buczkowska-Radlińska J. Biodentine™—use in dentistry. Literature review. Pomeranian J Life Sci. 2020;66(2):39–45. https://doi.org/10.21164/pomjlifesci.666.

22. Grech L, Mallia B, Camilleri J. Investigation of the physical properties of tricalcium silicate cement-based root-end filling materials. Dent Mater. 2013;29(2):e20–8. https://doi.org/10.1016/j.dental.2012.11.007.

23. Tran XV, Gorin C, Willig C, Baroukh B, Pellat B, Decup F, et al. Effect of a calcium-silicate-based restorative cement on pulp repair. J Dent Res. 2012;91(12):1166–71. https://doi.org/10.1177/0022034512460833.

24. Koubi G, Colon P, Franquin JC, Hartmann A, Richard G, Faure MO, et al. Clinical evaluation of the performance and safety of a new dentine substitute, Biodentine, in the restoration of posterior teeth—a prospective study. Clin Oral Investig. 2013;17(1):243–9. https://doi.org/10.1007/s00784-012-0701-9.

25. Kayahan MB, Nekoofar MH, McCann A, Sunay H, Kaptan RF, Meraji N, et al. Effect of acid etching procedures on the compressive strength of 4 calcium silicate-based endodontic cements. J Endod. 2013;39(12):1646–8. https://doi.org/10.1016/j.joen.2013.09.008.

26. Odabaş ME, Bani M, Tirali RE. Shear bond strengths of different adhesive systems to Biodentine. ScientificWorldJournal. 2013;2013:626103. https://doi.org/10.1155/2013/626103.

27. Bachoo IK, Seymour D, Brunton P. A biocompatible and bioactive replacement for dentine: is this a reality? The properties and uses of a novel calcium-based cement. Br Dent J. 2013;214(2):E5. https://doi.org/10.1038/sj.bdj.2013.57.

28. Hashem D, Mannocci F, Patel S, Manoharan A, Watson TF, Banerjee A. Evaluation of the efficacy of calcium silicate vs. glass ionomer cement indirect pulp capping and restoration

assessment criteria: a randomised controlled clinical trial-2-year results. Clin Oral Investig. 2019;23(4):1931–9. https://doi.org/10.1007/s00784-018-2638-0.

29. Awawdeh L, Al-Qudah A, Hamouri H, Chakra RJ. Outcomes of vital pulp therapy using mineral trioxide aggregate or Biodentine: a prospective randomized clinical trial. J Endod. 2018;44(11):1603–9. https://doi.org/10.1016/j.joen.2018.08.004.

30. Peskersoy C, Lukarcanin J, Turkun M. Efficacy of different calcium silicate materials as pulp-capping agents: randomized clinical trial. J Dent Sci. 2020; https://doi.org/10.1016/j.jds.2020.08.016.

31. Lipski M, Nowicka A, Kot K, Postek-Stefańska L, Wysoczańska-Jankowicz I, Borkowski L, et al. Factors affecting the outcomes of direct pulp capping using Biodentine. Clin Oral Investig. 2018;22(5):2021–9. https://doi.org/10.1007/s00784-017-2296-7.

32. Hegde S, Sowmya B, Mathew S, Bhandi SH, Nagaraja S, Dinesh K. Clinical evaluation of mineral trioxide aggregate and Biodentine as direct pulp capping agents in carious teeth. J Conserv Dent. 2017;20(2):91–5. https://doi.org/10.4103/0972-0707.212243.

33. Katge FA, Patil DP. Comparative analysis of 2 calcium silicate-based cements (Biodentine and mineral trioxide aggregate) as direct pulp-capping agent in young permanent molars: a Split mouth study. J Endod. 2017;43(4):507–13. https://doi.org/10.1016/j.joen.2016.11.026.

34. Linu S, Lekshmi MS, Varunkumar VS, Sam Joseph VG. Treatment outcome following direct pulp capping using bioceramic materials in mature permanent teeth with carious exposure: a pilot retrospective study. J Endod. 2017;43(10):1635–9. https://doi.org/10.1016/j.joen.2017.06.017.

35. Hashem D, Mannocci F, Patel S, Manoharan A, Brown JE, Watson TF, et al. Clinical and radiographic assessment of the efficacy of calcium silicate indirect pulp capping: a randomized controlled clinical trial. J Dent Res. 2015;94(4):562–8. https://doi.org/10.1177/0022034515571415.

36. Arshad E, Gyanendra K, Dhillon JK. Comparative evaluation of clinical outcome of indirect pulp treatment with calcium hydroxide, calcium silicate and Er,Cr:YSGG laser in permanent molars. Laser Ther. 2019;28(2):123–30. https://doi.org/10.5978/islsm.28_19-OR-09.

37. Kusumvalli S, Diwan A, Pasha S, Devale MR, Chowdhary CD, Saikia P. Clinical evaluation of Biodentine: its efficacy in the management of deep dental caries. Indian J Dent Res. 2019;30(2):191–5. https://doi.org/10.4103/ijdr.IJDR_333_17.

38. Brizuela C, Ormeño A, Cabrera C, Cabezas R, Silva CI, Ramírez V, et al. Direct pulp capping with calcium hydroxide, mineral trioxide aggregate, and Biodentine in permanent young teeth with caries: a randomized clinical trial. J Endod. 2017;43(11):1776–80. https://doi.org/10.1016/j.joen.2017.06.031.

39. Parinyaprom N, Nirunsittirat A, Chuveera P, Na Lampang S, Srisuwan T, Sastraruji T, et al. Outcomes of direct pulp capping by using either ProRoot mineral trioxide aggregate or Biodentine in permanent teeth with carious pulp exposure in 6- to 18-year-old patients: a randomized controlled trial. J Endod. 2018;44(3):341–8. https://doi.org/10.1016/j.joen.2017.10.012.

40. Dube K, Jain P, Rai A, Paul B. Preventive endodontics by direct pulp capping with restorative dentin substitute-Biodentine: a series of fifteen cases. Indian J Dent Res. 2018;29(3):268–74. https://doi.org/10.4103/ijdr.IJDR_292_15.

41. Hashem DF, Foxton R, Manoharan A, Watson TF, Banerjee A. The physical characteristics of resin composite-calcium silicate interface as part of a layered/laminate adhesive restoration. Dent Mater. 2014;30(3):343–9. https://doi.org/10.1016/j.dental.2013.12.010.

42. Ricucci D, Siqueira JF Jr, Li Y, Tay FR. Vital pulp therapy: histopathology and histobacteriology-based guidelines to treat teeth with deep caries and pulp exposure. J Dent. 2019;86:41–52. https://doi.org/10.1016/j.jdent.2019.05.022.

43. Cushley S, Duncan HF, Lappin MJ, Chua P, Elamin AD, Clarke M, El-Karim IA. Efficacy of direct pulp capping for management of cariously exposed pulps in permanent teeth: a systematic review and meta-analysis. Int Endod J. 2020; https://doi.org/10.1111/iej.13449.

44. Mente J, Hufnagel S, Leo M, Michel A, Gehrig H, Panagidis D, Saure D, Pfefferle T. Treatment outcome of mineral trioxide aggregate or calcium hydroxide direct pulp capping: long-term results. J Endod. 2014;40(11):1746–51. https://doi.org/10.1016/j.joen.2014.07.019.

45. Cho SY, Seo DG, Lee SJ, Lee J, Lee SJ, Jung IY. Prognostic factors for clinical outcomes according to time after direct pulp capping. J Endod. 2013;39(3):327–31. https://doi.org/10.1016/j.joen.2012.11.034.
46. Matsuo T, Nakanishi T, Shimizu H, Ebisu S. A clinical study of direct pulp capping applied to carious-exposed pulps. J Endod. 1996;22(10):551–6. https://doi.org/10.1016/S0099-2399(96)80017-3.
47. Fuks AB, Heling I, Nuni E. Pulp therapy for the young permanent dentition. In: Casamassimo PS, Fields HW, McTigue DJ, Nowak AJ, editors. Pediatric dentistry: infancy through adolescence. 5th ed. St. Louis: Saunders; 2013.

Biodentine™ Applications in Furcation Perforation and Root Resorption

10

Till Dammaschke and Mariusz Lipski

10.1 Furcation Perforations

A furcal perforation is a "piercing" or unintentional opening and thus an injury to the dental hard tissue at the bottom of the pulp chamber towards the periodontium. This mainly happens within the process of locating the root canal entrances while the anatomical conditions were disregarded during trepanation. Sometimes, however, a spontaneous perforation may occur due to carious processes. This results in perforation into the periodontal ligament space, so that a communication between the periodontal tissue and the root canal system occurs [1]. Thus, a furcal perforation is a severe outcome of any cleaning and shaping procedure.

As a result of secondary and tertiary dentine formation, the pulp chamber becomes continuously smaller as the patient ages, so that the coronal pulp may be reduced to a minimal residual size. Especially these teeth are at risk of iatrogenically caused perforations of the pulp chamber floor during the search for the root canal orifices [1].

Usually, furcal perforations can be identified easily. Sudden pain during trepanation, especially in non-vital teeth, or an unusually marked bleeding into the pulp chamber can be signs of a perforation of the furcation. Nevertheless, optical magnification aids should be used in order to avoid perforations or to visualize them when they occur. Some cases even require radiographic diagnosis. Perforations can be

T. Dammaschke (✉)
Department of Periodontology and Operative Dentistry, Westphalian Wilhelms-University, Münster, Germany
e-mail: tillda@uni-muenster.de

M. Lipski
Department of Preclinical Conservative Dentistry and Preclinical Endodontics, Pomeranian Medical University, Szczecin, Poland
e-mail: lipam@pum.edu.pl

© Springer Nature Switzerland AG 2022
I. About (ed.), *Biodentine™*, https://doi.org/10.1007/978-3-030-80932-4_10

visualized radiologically by brightening in the furcation area and/or interruptions of the root contour [1].

Due to the location of the perforation close to the clinical crown, it is very likely that a microleakage from the coronal restoration into the endodontic space will develop or continue. Iatrogenic damage in this region must be avoided as otherwise long-term functional stability of the tooth free from endodontic infections cannot be achieved. Furthermore, it is highly problematic that perforations in the furcation area can cause bone resorptions if infections from the root canal system spread to the periodontium. Vice versa, an infection of the root canal system can result via a perforation if it is in contact with the oral cavity through the furcation. The primary goal of perforation repair is therefore a tight, biocompatible seal between the pulp chamber floor and the periodontal tissue to prevent microleakage [1].

Due to their good accessibility, furcal perforations can be restored quite easily. Nevertheless, every attempt should be made carefully to avoid access-related perforations as the tooth is weakened and more susceptible to fracture even if the repair was successful [2].

An ideal perforation repair material should allow easy manipulation and placement, provide an adequate seal, ensure a long-term three-dimensional sealing of all margins (preferably by a molecular bonding to the dentinal walls), be dimensionally stable, be insoluble, be non-absorbable, not be moisture sensitive, not be affected by blood contamination, not be extruded during condensation, be radiopaque, be biocompatible, be bactericidal and be bioactive (induce hard-tissue healing and formation) [3, 4]. In recent decades, numerous materials have been described to cover perforations (such as gutta-percha, amalgam, calcium sulphate, calcium hydroxide, super EBA, glass-ionomer cement, calcium phosphate cement, composite resins), most of which, however, no longer have any clinical relevance for this indication. Sealing properties of many of these materials were negatively affected by wet conditions during perforation repair. Controlling the placement of the materials was problematic and often the defect was not sealed adequately or the periodontal support tissues were chronically irritated from uncontrollable extrusion of repair material [1, 2].

Since the introduction of hydraulic calcium silicate cements such as mineral trioxide aggregates (MTA) and Biodentine, the results from the literature indicate that these cements are considered to be the material of choice for covering perforations of the furcation. Like all hydraulic calcium silicate cements, Biodentine has the following advantages: insensitive to moisture or blood contamination, dimensionally stable, slight expansion during setting, low solubility and antibacterial properties due to the high pH value during the setting phase [5]. Especially the biocompatibility of endodontic materials is essential as the surrounding bone or the periodontium is exposed to these cements during application and even a longer period of time [4].

In many cases, the prognosis of teeth where the furcal perforation was restored with a calcium silicate cement can be considered good. However, the success of a perforation coverage depends on the time between perforation and closure, size of the perforation, possible connection to the oral cavity, infection of the surrounding tissue and avoidance of microbial infection of the perforation [6]. If a perforation of the pulp chamber floor occurs during the canal search, it should therefore be closed again as soon as possible. After disinfecting the perforation area with sodium hypochlorite (NaOCl, approx. 3%), the defect is filled with Biodentine and the root canal treatment can be continued. Alternatively, in case of a single-visit endodontic treatment and the absence of bleeding from the perforation area, the root canal treatment can be completed first. Afterwards the entire floor of the pulp chamber including the perforation area and root canal filling can be covered with Biodentine. Nevertheless, an immediate reparation of the perforation area and an appropriate avoidance of bacterial contamination lead to better results [2].

Due to periodontal disease, especially in older patients, a perforation of the furcation can often be at the level of the alveolar ridge and thus in an unfavourable area for perforation coverage. If the perforation creates a direct connection to the oral cavity, the success of a perforation coverage decreases [7]. Thus, perforation below the crestal bone should be repaired with hydraulic calcium silicate cements like Biodentine. Perforation coronal to the crestal bone (without contact to bone or any soft tissue) should be repaired with an appropriate restorative material, such as dentine adhesive and composite resin [2].

10.1.1 Repair of Fresh Perforations

Ideally, perforations should be restored as quickly as possible. As a rule, fresh perforations do not lead to pronounced bleeding, as no inflammation has formed yet. Bleeding caused by the mechanical injury to the tissue can usually be stopped with low-percentage NaOCl solution (up to 3%). Other haemostatic agents such as iron sulphate or aluminium chloride should not be used, as these materials can damage the tissue and interfere with wound healing [8].

In the absence of bleeding, Biodentine can be applied directly onto the adjacent tissue, bone or granulation tissue in portions under direct visual control using MTA carrier (e.g. MTA gun, MAP-System, MTA applicator) and carefully compacted with cement pluggers or laterally with John West Repair Instruments. Strong pressure is not required during application. Since Biodentine, like all calcium silicate cements, has thixotropic properties, it can be activated by sound or ultrasound energy so that it flows to the defect area. After removal of the sound or ultrasound activation, Biodentine remains in place [9, 10].

The application of Biodentine must not interfere with further endodontic treatment (instrumentation of the root canals). Thus, paper points, gutta-percha points or root canal instruments should be placed in the canals to prevent blockage of the canals with Biodentine [1, 2].

10.1.2 Repair of Old Perforations

In cases of older perforations that have not been treated so far, an infection of the adjacent tissue in the furcation area must be assumed. This infection can lead to local limited osteolysis. In addition, granulation tissue may have grown into the perforation. In these cases, sufficient disinfection of the area, for example by rinsing with NaOCl (approx. 3%), is crucial for healing of the periodontal tissue.

Any foreign material (filling remnants) should be completely removed before covering with Biodentine. If necessary, ingrown granulation tissue can be removed in a controlled manner by electrosurgery (high-frequency current). Granulation tissue beyond the root contour in the furcation area can remain and forms a scaffold for the Biodentine. If the stability of the granulation tissue is not sufficient for the application of Biodentine, the matrix technique can be used [1] (Fig. 10.1).

10.1.3 Matrix Technique

The aim of a matrix technique is to create a scaffold in the tissue which completes the shape of the root corresponding to its original contour that had been destroyed through perforation. While the matrix is located on the outer surface of the root to seal up the perforation, Biodentine can be applied on top of the scaffold material. It is necessary to use the matrix technique if infected perforations led to osteolysis of the bone or if the granulation tissue beyond the perforation is not sufficiently stable. Resorbable collagen fleece of animal origin is usually described as such a scaffold. After disinfecting the perforation area by rinsing with NaOCl, a piece of resorbable collagen, which is previously cut to size, is pushed through the perforation with a plugger, so that a scaffold is created in the tissue and the outer root contour is restored. Biodentine is then applied against the collagen fleece and covered with composite resin [11, 12]. However, for a successful treatment the necessity of a matrix technique has not been scientifically proven [2].

10.1.4 Push-Out Bond Strength

In order to prevent dislodgement from the dentinal walls, a perforation repair material should have sufficient push-out bond strength. Thus, the push-out bond strength of Biodentine was evaluated in several in vitro studies on simulated furcal perforations. After 10-min, 24-h and 1-week storing of the samples, the push-out bond strength was significantly higher for Biodentine than for ProRoot MTA [3, 13–15]. Also the shear bond strength of Biodentine to a dentine surface is higher than for MTA [16]. The significantly higher push-out bond strength of Biodentine compared to ProRoot MTA may be explained by the fact that the Vickers microhardness for Biodentine is significantly higher compared to MTA and more comparable to dentine [17].

The push-out bond strength of Biodentine increased significantly with increased setting time [3]. In contrast to MTA, blood contamination of the dentine surface had no negative effect on the push-out bond strength of Biodentine [3, 18]. But the push-out bond strengths of Biodentine significantly decreased after exposure to 2.5% NaOCl in the early setting phase (10 min after mixture) [19]. In contrast, Guneser

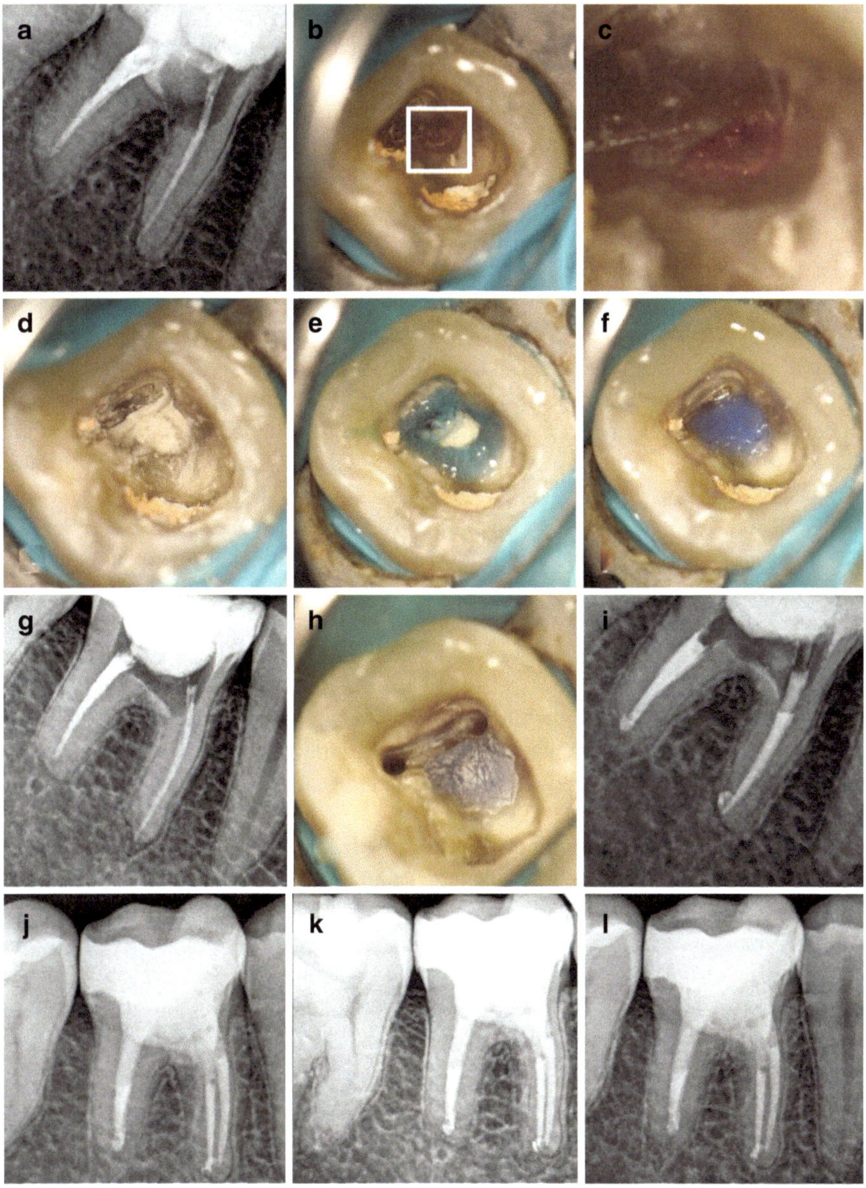

Fig. 10.1 A two-appointment non-surgical retreatment and perforation repair with Biodentine in a mandibular first molar. First appointment: (**a**) A radiograph showing a technically poor root canal treatment and furcal perforation. (**b**) The pulp chamber floor just prior to perforation repair. (**c**) Magnification of perforation site. (**d**) Perforation repaired with Biodentine. Second appointment: (**e**) Pulp chamber floor dentine etching before application of flowable composite resin. (**f**) Biodentine covered with a flowable composite resin (blue). (**g**) A radiograph showing repaired perforation. (**h**) A pulp floor after gutta-percha removal and root canal system preparation. (**i**) A final radiograph showing well-obturated root canals. (**j**) Three-month radiographic follow-up. (**k**) Eighteen-month radiographic follow-up. (**l**) Forty-eight-month radiographic follow-up

et al. [13] reported that exposure of Biodentine to NaOCl (3.5%), CHX (2%) or saline solution (0.9%) 10 min after mixture did not affect the push-out bond strength at all. Rinsing the surface of freshly mixed Biodentine with EDTA 17% or 0.2% chitosan significantly decreases the push-out bond strength [15]. When Biodentine was allowed to set for 1 week, NaOCl (5.25%) irrigation had no influence on the push-out bond strength [14].

10.1.5 Reactions of Cells of the Periodontium to Biodentine

10.1.5.1 Reactions of Cells of the Periodontium In Vitro
Furcal perforation repair materials are in contact with periodontal tissues for an extended period of time. Ideally, these reparative materials should provide a biocompatible and bioactive capacity, especially on periodontal ligament cells (PDL) and osteoblasts. Hence, an in vitro morphological study proved good proliferation and cell attachment of PDL cells and osteoblasts to Biodentine. Biodentine as well as ProRoot MTA leads to an up-regulating of osteoblasts and PDL cell activity after 1–20 days. Thus, Biodentine and MTA resulted in a significantly higher cell density in osteoblasts and PDL cell culture compared to an untreated control group in an ideal cell culture medium. Only in contact with Biodentine the PDL cells matured in a second cell layer crossway to the first one, though from 8th day onward Biodentine even showed a statistically significant higher quantity of PDL cells than ProRoot MTA. Thus, Biodentine has favourable properties regarding biologic response of the cells within the periodontium and may induce periodontal regeneration and/or repair. Hence, Biodentine—besides MTA—can be called a bioactive cement [4].

If Biodentine is plated with PDL cells in vitro, the PDL cells on the surfaces of Biodentine are abundant and well attached, and the fibroblasts appeared to preserve their original morphology and are spindle shaped and clustered. This might show the nontoxicity of Biodentine [20]. Also human gingival fibroblasts exhibited good attachment to the surfaces of Biodentine [21]. Hence, Biodentine had a positive effect on the adhesion, proliferation and biomineralization of human PDL cells [22]. In addition, in an in vitro study on human osteosarcoma cell line Saos-2 is an osteoblastic cell line in which Biodentine had a significantly superior effect on mineralization than MTA [23].

10.1.5.2 Reactions of Cells of the Periodontium in Rats
In vivo studies in animal demonstrated that Biodentine is involved in inflammatory reaction modulations and promotes fibroblast and osteoblast differentiation. It stimulates the formation of collagen bundles of the periodontal ligament and bone matrix of the alveolar process, and therefore consequently favours the periodontal tissues repair in rats [24]. Using Biodentine for sealing artificial furcal perforations in rat molar teeth the tissue reactions were identical to MTA [25].

10.1.5.3   Reactions of Cells of the Periodontium in Dogs

When Biodentine was used for the treatment of experimental furcal perforation in dogs and compared to ProRoot MTA, significantly less inflammation and lower volume of extruded material were observed 4 months after treatment. Teeth repaired with Biodentine showed similar histological morphology and integrity in the furcation area, but larger cementum formation than those treated with ProRoot MTA. In conclusion, Biodentine presented good tissue compatibility and mineralized tissue formation [26]. These results are in contrast with the outcomes of another study which was performed on dogs. Four months after application, MTA induced a significantly thicker formation of mineralized tissue in comparison to Biodentine. Nevertheless, comparable to ProRoot MTA, Biodentine induced the repair of a furcal perforation by formation of mineralized tissue sealing totally or partially in almost all examined cases. New mineralized tissue formed adjacent to Biodentine and MTA. The use of Biodentine and MTA did not cause bone resorption in the furcation region and only few inflammatory cells appeared. In immunofluorescence assay it became obvious that mineralization marker expression like RUNX2, an essential transcription factor for osteoblast differentiation, increased in the periodontal ligament in direct contact to Biodentine and MTA [27]. MTA and Biodentine had satisfactory tissue response, with formation of mineralized tissue and partial reinsertion of fibres, and could be indicated for sealing furcal perforations. But only MTA stimulated the expression of proteins associated with the formation of a cementum-like mineralized tissue [28].

10.1.5.4   Reactions of Cells of the Periodontium in Humans

In a histological study on humans investigating the response of the periodontium to Biodentine it was shown that Biodentine is able to seal the perforation area. PDL fibres were clearly detectable parallel to the material. The inflammatory infiltrate was mild. Few lymphocytes, plasma cells and spindle cells, as well as several small and middle-sized vessels, were observed in the soft tissues surrounding the material. Root resorption, ankylosis or downward epithelial proliferation was not observed. Even though mineralized tissue was observed, Biodentine seems not to induce cementum regeneration. This was in contrast to ProRoot MTA. A new mineralized cementum-like tissue incorporating periodontal fibres was visible in all cases treated with MTA. Thus, Biodentine was less capable of inducing regeneration of cementum compared with MTA [29].

10.1.6 Advantages of Biodentine in the Repair of Furcation Perforations

As known from all other calcium silicate cements Biodentine allows tissue regeneration and healing. An advantage of Biodentine over MTA is that in most cases the use of this cement does not lead to staining of the dentine, especially in the visible clinical crown. The staining is due to heavy metals contained in the MTA, such as bismuth oxide (for radiopacity) [30, 31] or iron [32]. It is mainly caused by the oxidation of these metals after contact with NaOCl or the absorption of blood components [32–34]. Biodentine does not contain heavy metals or bismuth oxide but contains zirconium dioxide as an X-ray contrast medium and therefore is particularly colour stable [35].

Another advantage of Biodentine over MTA is the shorter setting time. Whereas the initial setting time of ProRoot MTA is about 4 h, Biodentine sets in 12 min and its mechanical properties improve with time. Therefore, according to the manufacturer's recommendations, Biodentine should set for at least 12 min before a final restoration can be placed. To overcome this clinical disadvantage and to avoid the long setting time, it was suggested to cover Biodentine with an RMGI (resin-modified glass ionomer cement), compomer or flowable composite resin (in combination with a self-etching dentine adhesive). It should be noted that the overlaying material should completely cover Biodentine and extend into the adjacent dentine. The final restoration is then placed on top so that the cement can set beneath the interlayer [36, 37].

Just 3 min after mixing Biodentine, this cement can be covered with a thin layer of a self-etching, self-adhesive, flowable composite (Vertise Flow), a RMGI or a composite. All these restorative materials achieved shear bond strengths to Biodentine similar to those after 12 min and 2 days. A longer waiting time after mixing did not increase the adhesion of these overlay materials to Biodentine [38]. The time between mixing the cement and application of such an intermediate layer does not influence the setting reaction of the cement. The moisture of calcium silicate cements has no influence on the curing reaction or curing time of these materials or on the structural interface between calcium silicate cements and overlaying material [39, 40]. A definitive permanent restoration or a continuation of the root canal treatment can therefore be performed at the same appointment.

10.2 Root Resorption

Apart from the physiological resorption of the deciduous tooth root by the permanent teeth, there are other, mostly pathological forms of root resorptions. They result from dentinoclastic (odontoclastic) and/or osteoclastic activity and all hard tooth substances can be affected. Thus, root resorption is mediated by osteoclasts and/or odontoclasts, leading to loss of dentine, tooth cementum and bone [41–43]. Different types of root resorptions can be distinguished:

- **Internal resorption**: an inflammatory process initiated within the pulp space with loss of dentine and possible invasion of the cementum.
- **External resorption**: resorption initiated in the periodontium and initially affecting the external surfaces of a tooth (root cement and dentine). An external resorption can also affect the pulp tissue.

- *Replacement resorption*: a pathologic loss of cementum, dentine and periodontal ligament with subsequent replacement of such structures by bone. The replacement resorption results in ankyloses, fusion of bone and tooth.
- *Surface resorption*: a physiologic process causing small superficial defects in the cementum and underlying dentine that undergo repair by deposition of new cementum.
- *Cervical resorption*: a type of external resorption that occurs in the coronal third of the root.
- *Transient resorption*: a response to tooth luxation consisting of radiographic apical bone and root resorption that resolves spontaneously without intervening treatment.
- **Inflammatory resorption**: an internal or external pathologic loss of tooth structure and possibly bone. This resorption occurs as the result of microbial infection and is characterized radiographically by radiolucent areas along the root [41, 44].

10.2.1 Internal Resorptions

The pathogenesis of internal resorptions is based on a long-lasting chronic pulp inflammation [45, 46]. Initially transient internal inflammatory resorptions may change to a progressive stage when the odontoblasts are destroyed to such an extent that new dentine formation and attachment no longer occur and the initially only slight root resorptions cannot be repaired [41–43]. It should be noted that bacteria are always detectable in the pulp or in the dentinal tubules adjacent to the internal resorption [46]. Consequently, resorption is induced by bacterial infection of the pulp with a localized pulp necrosis, which is located coronally to the resorption lacuna [41–43]. This results in the transformation of the pulp tissue into connective tissue similar to periodontal tissue [47]. In case of complete tissue necrosis or removal of the inflamed pulp tissue by endodontic treatment, the resorption is stopped but without subsequent repair [46].

In supragingival position of internal resorption in the area of the crown pulp, a pink-spot discoloration of the tooth crown is impressive in individual cases, caused by the shimmering of the granulation tissue through the hard tooth substance thinned out in the area (= pink spot disease). The subgingival internal resorption is often found as an incidental radiographic finding, since the affected teeth are usually free of symptoms. Radiographs usually show uniformly round or rounded lesions in the middle of the root, which are spatially related to the pulp or root canal lumen. Usually, the sensitivity test is positive, since vital, innervated pulp tissue is still present [41–43]. The process of resorption is able to progress as long as vital pulp tissue is present from apical resorption lacuna, since blood supply is a basic prerequisite for the continued activity of the osteoclasts [46]. Internal resorption can therefore perforate the root surface and thus be connected to the periodontium [41–43].

The most common causes of internal inflammatory resorption are the presence of apical periodontitis and dental trauma. Teeth associated with apical periodontitis should be carefully inspected for the presence of internal resorption. Other predisposing factors for the development of internal resorption can be herpes zoster infections, invaginations, tooth fractures, orthodontic treatment and extensive restorations [41–43].

10.2.2 Management of Internal Resorption

Radiological signs of internal resorption are always an indication for a root canal treatment. After trepanation and coronal canal enlargement, necrotic and vital tissue must be completely removed from the root canal system. As the tissue in the area of an internal resorption is poorly accessible or even inaccessible to instrumentation and root canal preparation, it can be difficult to remove the tissue completely. Therefore, chemical dissolution with NaOCl is necessary. The resorption lacuna is cleaned by excessive irrigation with this tissue-dissolving rinsing fluid. The tissue-dissolving and disinfecting effect of NaOCl can be increased by using higher concentrated solutions, ultrasound or heating. As a rule, endodontic treatment should be carried out over several appointments. Single or multiple root canal medications with calcium hydroxide are recommended in case of pulp inflammation [45, 46], since calcium hydroxide may significantly increase the solubility of pulp tissue remaining in the resorption lacuna in the event of subsequent irrigation with NaOCl. The filling of the resorption lacuna is traditionally done with heated gutta-percha in a thermoplastic obturation method. The liquefaction of the gutta-percha by heat enables an entire obturation of the resorption lacuna, which is difficult when cold obturation methods such as lateral compaction or single-cone technique are being used. However, one should recall that the root is mechanically weakened in the area of inflammatory internal resorption. Gutta-percha is not able to compensate for this weakening. Therefore, root canal obturation and filling of the resorption lacuna should be performed using a calcium silicate cement, as those materials offer clear advantages in terms of stability. In addition, calcium silicate cements alkalize the acidic environment characteristic of resorption. If the internal inflammatory resorption reaches the root surface and has led to a perforation, a conventional root canal filling with gutta-percha and sealer is basically inappropriate. Accordingly, calcium silicate cements such as Biodentine are indicated in this situation [41–43, 48–50] (Figs. 10.2 and 10.3).

10.2.3 External Resorptions

Causes for external resorption can be orthodontic treatment, infection of the endodontium or traumatic luxation injuries [41–43].

It has been shown that orthodontic treatment can cause resorptions or can reinforce existing resorptions, especially when stronger forces are applied [51]. The resorption stops after removal of the orthodontic force application without any need

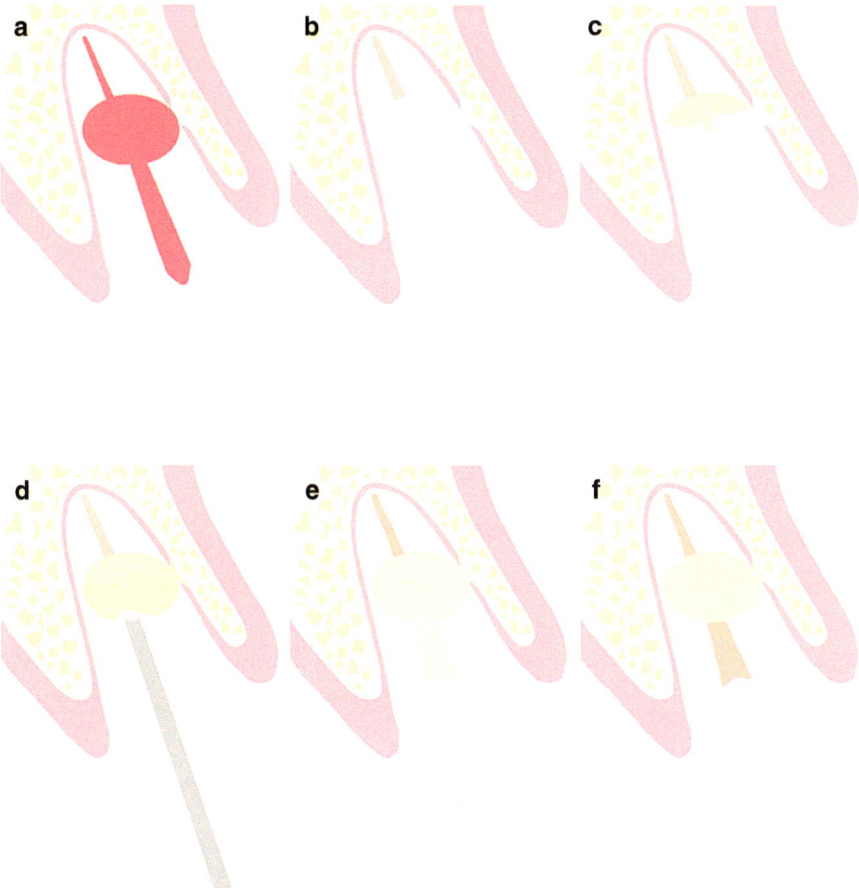

Fig. 10.2 (**a**) Internal inflammatory resorption with perforation localized on the labial surface of the root. (**b**) After trepanation and coronal root canal enlargement, necrotic and vital tissues completely removed from the root canal system. (**c**) The part of the root up to the resorption filled by gutta-percha and sealer, and the resorption lacuna with Biodentine placed with an MTA carrier. (**d**) The calcium silicate cement condensed with plugger. (**e**) The coronal part of root canal filled with Biodentine or (**f**) with gutta-percha and sealer and the crown reconstructed with composite resin material

for a root canal treatment. If the sensibility test is positive, a root canal treatment is not necessary [41–43].

An apical periodontitis is always accompanied by signs of resorptions on the outer root surface. These signs can usually not be diagnosed but can only histologically be detected which is unessential due to their clinical irrelevance. In case of long-term chronic apical periodontitis, resorption-related changes occur in the area of the apical foramen though. The resorption stagnates after a sufficient root canal treatment and disinfection of the root canal system has been performed [41–43].

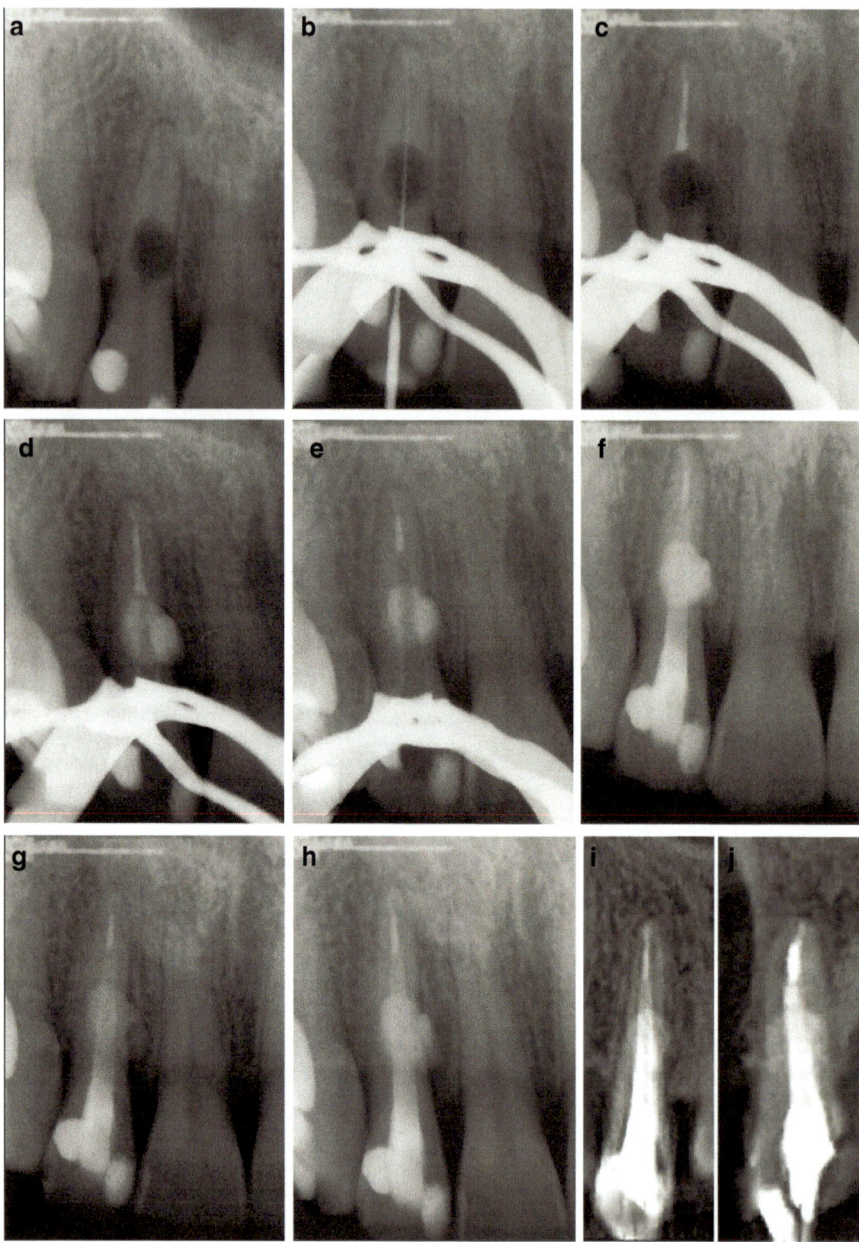

Fig. 10.3 Management of inflammatory internal resorption (IIR) with Biodentine in a maxillary lateral incisor. (**a**) Preoperative radiography showing IIR localized in the middle part of the root with perforation on the mesial surface; (**b**) working length determination using radiography; (**c**) the apical third of the root canal obturation with gutta-percha and sealer; (**d**) the resorption lacuna filling with Biodentine; (**e**) gutta-percha removal and post-space preparation; (**f**) the FRC post-cementation and crown reconstruction with composite resin; (**g**) three-month radiographic follow-up; (**h**) six-month radiographic follow-up; (**i, j**) six-months CBCT follow-up—coronal and sagittal view. (Courtesy of Dr. Wojciech Krajewski)

As a result of the deflection and displacement of the root in the alveolus, damage or destruction of the structures of the root surface and denudation of the root surface may occur. Chemotactic activation of hard tissue-resorbing cells and progressive inflammatory external resorption are the consequences, up to perforation into the pulp chamber. This happens often while clinically undetectable. In many cases, these perforations and other trauma-related damage (e.g. exposed dentine, pulp exposure) lead to pulp infection and even pulp necrosis. This bacterial infection keeps the primarily traumatically imitated resorption going. These resorptions sometimes proceed extremely fast and can lead to complete dissolution of the root. Even though the sensibility test is usually negative, it can also be positive in some cases. The resorptions appear in the radiograph as irregularly shaped lacunae that are often located eccentrically and always apically to the epithelial attachment. The pulp or the root canal lumen is often still visible without any interruption of continuity [41–43].

10.2.3.1 Replacement Resorption

This form of external resorption occurs mainly after traumatic tooth injuries, especially after avulsion with prolonged extraoral dry storage of the teeth or storage in an unsuitable storage medium. This results in damage to the periodontal membrane and necrosis of the periodontal cells. In the area of the denuded root surface there is a direct accumulation of osteoblasts. As a result, hard tooth substance is degraded and replaced by bone.

Basically, two forms of replacement resorption can be distinguished: transient and inflammatory. In the first, the periodontal tissue is only damaged over a very small area and is able to regenerate. In this case, the resorption does not progress any further. On the other hand, the inflammatory replacement resorption is not self-limiting and progresses until the root is dissolved completely. This process can last for months and years. Finally, the root is completely replaced by bone. A reliable therapy has not yet been found [41–43]. Nevertheless, a promising treatment alternative for immature permanent teeth after trauma with necrotic pulp tissue and external inflammatory or replacement resorption was reported recently. The teeth were treated with a regenerative endodontic procedure using plasma-rich fibrin as a scaffold covered by Biodentine as a bioactive cement. In all cases an arresting of the external root resorption was observed [52].

10.2.3.2 Cervical Resorption

Progressive inflammatory cervical resorption is a special form of external resorption, which is often very aggressive and leads to the loss of the affected tooth [53, 54]. Clinically, a single-resorption lacuna is found in the cervical area, directly below the epithelial attachment in the area of the cement [54]. Bacteria and plaque are regularly found in the area of the resorption lacuna. Starting from one, but usually several very small "entry ports" into the dentine, cervical resorption is penetrating and strongly undermining the root dentine. In addition to root dentine, root cement and enamel are also resorbed. The pulp is not involved for a long time, as it is protected by the approximately 70–300 μm thick predentine layer. However, intrapulpal mineralizations (pulp stones, denticles) are often found in the pulp tissue. In the advanced stages, ingrowth of bone-like hard tissue, which is deposited on the dentine, often occurs through the entry ports. This is to be understood as a kind of repair mechanism [55]. Pulp tissue and adjacent alveolar bones are only affected at a very advanced stage. The decisive factor for the mostly rapid progression of the resorption process seems to be a local lack of oxygen. A lack of oxygen in the bone seems to lead to an activation of osteoclasts and an inhibition of osteoblast activity. Cervical invasive resorption may also occur in teeth that have already been root canal treated [56].

Cervical resorption is usually asymptomatic and the aetiology is not fully understood [53, 54]. Predisposing factors that have been proven so far include dental trauma, orthodontic treatment, internal and external bleaching, periodontal treatment, oral surgical treatment, bruxism, extensive coronal restorations, systemic diseases (hyperoxaluria), feline herpesvirus type I (contact with cats) or playing of wind instruments [41–43].

10.2.3.3 Transient Resorptions

Transient resorptions often occur after trauma or orthodontic treatment. In these cases, if there is no long-lasting, continuous stimulation of the resorption cells, the resorption process is not progressive but stagnates. The bowl-shaped resorption lacunae are repaired by cement-like tissue and new Sharpey's fibres. Due to their small size, such resorptions are usually not detected clinically and/or radiologically. They are of only minor clinical relevance and do not require treatment due to their transient character. The transient resorption can change into a progressive form if the root surface becomes colonized by permanently stimulated phagocyting and resorbing cells (macrophages, osteoclasts). Possible stimulants are sharp edges and corners (e.g. after transverse root fractures), increased tissue pressure (e.g. during tooth eruption, cysts, orthodontic treatment), inflammatory reaction due to infection (endodontic or periodontal infections) and systemic diseases (for example Paget's disease). Depending on the starting point of the infection, internal or external resorption occurs [41–43].

10.2.4 Management of External Resorption

In case of traumatic and external resorptions, a multistage root canal treatment is necessary. In addition to mechanical preparation of the root canals, intensive disinfecting irrigation with NaOCl and a medication with an aqueous calcium hydroxide suspension are necessary. The strongly basic pH value of both materials causes death of vital cells in the resection lacuna, as well as destruction of bacteria. It also leads to a neutralization of lactic acid that is secreted by the macrophages and osteoclasts. This should stop the demineralization of the root hard substance [57]. In addition, calcium hydroxide inhibits the genesis of dentinoclasts by neutralizing bacterial lipopolysaccharides [58] and promotes mineralization processes by activating alkaline phosphatase [57]. In order to ensure sufficient dental alkalization, an intracanal calcium hydroxide medication is recommended to remain in place for 2–4 weeks [57].

For progressive resorptions, a water-soluble paste with corticosteroid and tetracycline is recommended as an intracanal medication (Ledermix; Riemser, Greifswald, Germany). Both pharmacologically active ingredients seem to be able to inhibit the activity of osteoclasts. The corticoid also suppresses inflammatory processes and has an antiresorptive effect. Initially, an intracanal medication with, for example, Ledermix should be applied for at least 1 week, which is then replaced by a calcium hydroxide medication for a period of 2–4 weeks [57].

If an apical resorption is accompanied by a very wide open apical foramen, an apical plug with Biodentine or MTA should be performed. Apexification using calcium silicate cements seems preferable in order to achieve an early root canal obturation, to limit the risk of root fracture, and to stop the resorption [59].

10.2.5 Management of External Cervical Resorption

The treatment involves the complete removal of granulation tissue from the tooth and the surrounding periodontium by curettage and closure of the resorption lacuna with restorative materials [41–43]. For complete chemical dissolution of the granulation tissue while preserving the dentine, very careful topical application of trichloroacetic acid (TCA) on a small cotton wool pellet to the lacuna is recommended. Care must be taken when using TCA due to potential irritation of skin and/or oral mucosa caused by inadvertent contact. Alternatively NaOCl (3–5%) may be used [60].

If the pulp is still vital, root canal treatment is not indicated. Rather, the pulp should be indirectly capped before closure of the resorption lacuna. If there is a direct connection between the resorption and the oral cavity, calcium silicate cements can be used for indirect pulp capping, which are coated with composite resin restoration in a second step (sandwich technique). If the restoration does not communicate with the oral cavity, the defect can be completely restored with a calcium silicate cement. This requires the preparation of a mucoperiosteal flap to show the entire defect [61]. However, if the resorption already perforates the root canal system, an additional root canal treatment as described above must be performed [41–43] (Fig. 10.4).

10.2.6 Advantages of Biodentine in the Treatment of Root Resorptions

10.2.6.1 Antiresorptive Effect of Biodentine
Reducing osteoclastic activity is a key factor to inhibit the progression of root resorption. Biodentine showed an inhibitory effect on osteoclast differentiation and activities on osteoclasts originated from murine bone marrow macrophages. Hence, the application of Biodentine (or other calcium silicate cements) is a choice of

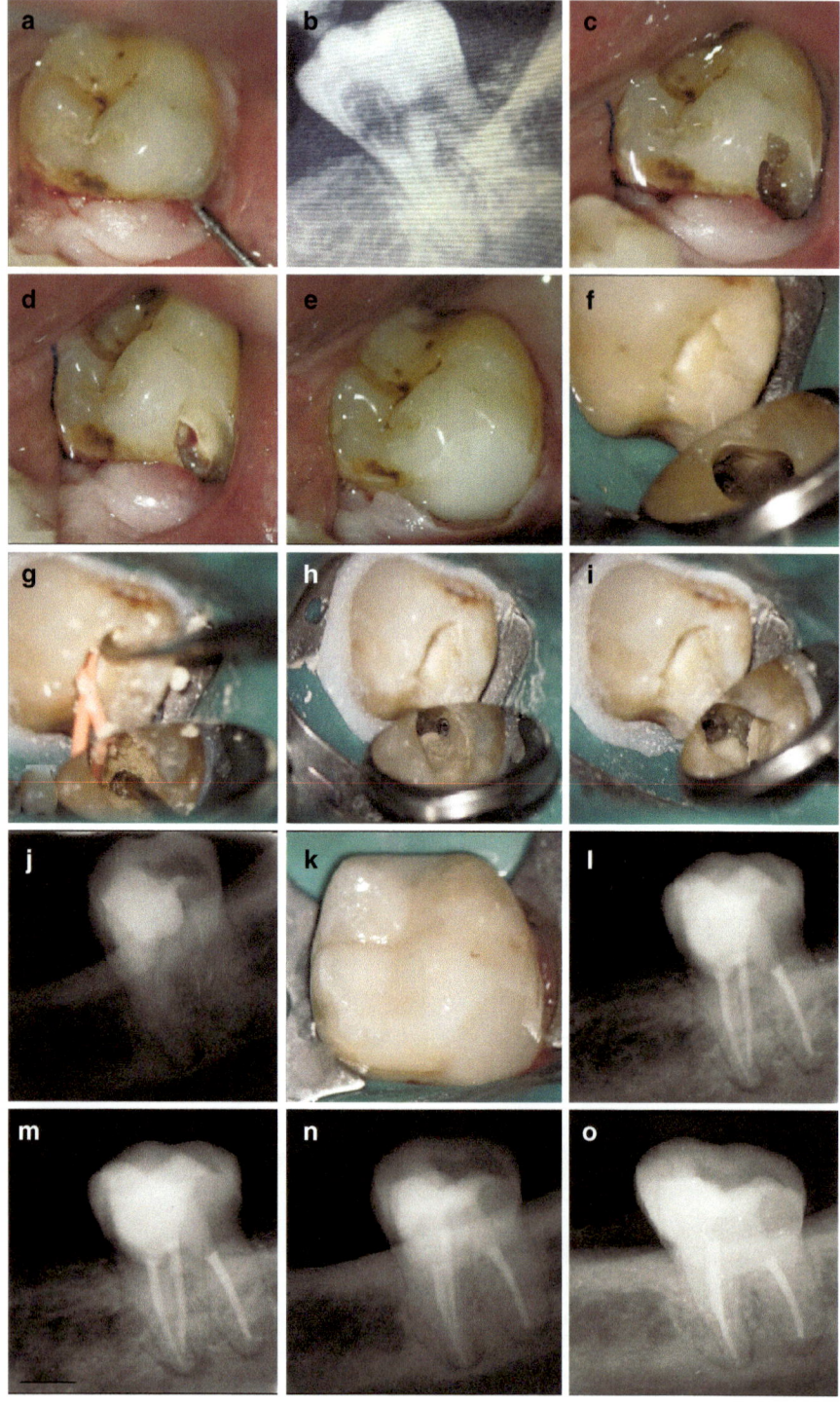

treatment to prevent root resorption [62]. It was suggested that silicate may take part in the inhibitory behaviour of calcium silicate cements on osteoclastogenesis [63, 64]. Biodentine showed significantly higher levels of silicon ion release than MTA [65, 66].

Since Biodentine releases calcium hydroxide as well as silicon ions after setting [67], it has been shown that Biodentine may maintain an alkaline pH of 10–11 and above in the surrounding dentine over a period of 4 weeks [68, 69] and thereby presumably leads to a neutralization of lactic acid and lipopolysaccharides, inhibition of dentinoclasts and activation of alkaline phosphatase [5, 70]. This can stop the resorptive process caused by possible remaining tissue residues, since it is known that a high pH value has a negative effect on osteoclasts [71]. In addition, due to particle size and shape, Biodentine can penetrate and seal dentinal tubules that may harbour microorganisms [9]. The growth of microorganisms may be suppressed in contact with Biodentine [72].

10.2.6.2   Bioactivity and Biocompatibility of Biodentine

When treating external resorptions or internal resorptions that have already perforated the root canal wall to the root surface, direct contact of Biodentine with the surrounding periodontal tissue and bone does not cause severe side effects. Biodentine is cytocompatible with human primary osteoblasts [73] and promotes the growth of human osteoblasts and periodontal ligament cells (PDL cells) [4] and can therefore be used in direct contact to the periodontium. In an animal model Biodentine demonstrated marked osteoinductivity and mineralizing properties [68, 74]. Implanted intramedullary in the tibia of rabbits, Biodentine induced osteoblast differentiation, angiogenesis and finally bone neoformation with a high mineralization degree [74]. The use of calcium silicate cements such as Biodentine seems to be the best choice to restore resorptive cavities for the frequent presence of connection to the periodontium [75]. One reason for the biocompatibility of Biodentine may be the formation of a hydroxyapatite-like surface after contact with calcium- and phosphate-containing (tissue) fluid on the cement [17].

If the external cervical resorption is subgingival and without communication with the oral cavity, Biodentine can be used for the complete restoration of the whole resorption lacuna [60]. PDL cells may attach and proliferate on the Biodentine surface [4]. For example, in a class 3 cervical resorption with a probing depth of up

Fig. 10.4 Management of invasive cervical resorption (ICR) in a second mandibular molar. (**a**) Probing the resorption defect using a periodontal probe; (**b**) preoperative radiograph; (**c**) resorption defect after hard-tissue removal; (**d**) communication with the pulp chamber; (**e**) filling with composite resin; (**f**) damaged floor and buccal wall of pulp chamber seen after access cavity preparation; (**g**) condensation of Biodentine, gutta-percha cones placed in canal orifices to prevent any reparative material dislodging into root canals; (**h**, **i**) resorption lacuna filled with Biodentine; (**j**) radiograph taken after sealing the defect; (**k**) radiograph taken after filling of the root canals; (**l**) crown reconstruction with composite resin; (**m**) radiograph after 3-month follow-up; (**n**) radiograph after 6-month follow-up; (**o**) radiograph after 18-month follow-up. (Courtesy of Dr. Jacek Bilbin)

to 8 mm a treatment of the resorption lacuna with Biodentine resulted in clinical healing of the periodontal tissue and bone regeneration in direct contact with Biodentine, which was still stable after 4 years [76].

To a certain extent Biodentine is resistant to hydrolysis while setting [77]. On the other hand it was shown that Biodentine is significantly more soluble in distilled water and in PBS solution than MTA [17, 68]. Therefore Biodentine cannot be used as a definitive restoration material if the resorption defect is in contact with the oral cavity and therefore in contact with saliva. In case of partly supragingival external cervical resorptions with contact to the oral cavity, this part of the cavity should be restored with a composite resin restoration in direct contact to Biodentine (sandwich technique) [61].

If the resorption lacuna is located in the middle or apical area of the root surface and is not accessible for external therapy or orthograde root canal treatment, it is discussed whether an intentional extraction and replantation after treatment of the resorption with a calcium silicate cement is a possible alternative therapy [60].

In external cervical resorptions with vital and non-inflamed pulp tissue, the tissue should be protected to maintain pulp vitality and an extirpation must be refrained. In these special cases of root resorption an indirect or even direct pulp capping using Biodentine may be indicated. Biodentine is well suitable to be used in pulp capping to maintain pulp vitality and may induce hard-tissue formation in the pulp [78–81].

10.2.6.3   Stabilization of the Tooth Structure Through Biodentine

Reinforcement of teeth with internal root resorption is essential to reduce the risk of root fracture. Thus, another advantage of Biodentine in the treatment of root resorption is its ability to strengthen the tooth structure and increase its stability. Filling the internal resorption cavities with Biodentine provides more strength to the tooth structure in comparison to other calcium silicate-based cements and—more importantly—to injected warm gutta-percha in combination with a sealer [82–84]. Biodentine has a Vickers microhardness that is in the range of dentine, whereas the Vickers microhardness of ProRoot MTA is significantly lower [17]. Furthermore, the shear bond strength of Biodentine on dentine surfaces is significantly higher than that of MTA [16].

An in vitro study examined different obturation techniques on extracted teeth with simulated internal resorption defects. Teeth with defects and root canals filled with Biodentine showed statistically higher resistance to fracture compared to teeth that were conventionally filled with gutta-percha and a sealer or other silicate-based materials [82]. In order to strengthen the roots after internal resorptions, a backfilling with Biodentine (or other calcium silicate cements) may be the preferable method, in comparison to a gutta-percha/sealer combination [83]. However, it is generally advisable to avoid gutta-percha altogether and to obturate the root canals with calcium silicate cement entirely, as they own positive biological effects [85]. The fracture resistance of teeth whose root canals have been filled with Biodentine is higher than in teeth whose root canals have been obturated also with gutta-percha [84]. Thus, the advantage of a root canal obturation with Biodentine is an increased stability of a tooth that had been weakened by resorption and therefore leads to an enhanced prognosis of the tooth. There are concerns about a prolonged contact of calcium silicate cements with dentine as this might have a negative effect on the integrity of the collagen matrix and on the strength and stiffness of the dentine [86, 87]. This fear of an increased fracture susceptibility is not appropriate though. The physical properties of Biodentine and its bond to healthy dentine seem to be clinically adequate to maintain the mechanical strength of the restored teeth [16, 75].

Furthermore, compared to thermoplasticized gutta-percha, MTA and Biodentine showed a statistically significant lower number of voids (especially between resorptive cavity walls and obturation material) when obturating teeth with a simulated internal resorption in vitro. Hence, Biodentine enables a better sealing of internal resorption than warm injected gutta-percha [88, 89].

However, a root canal obturation with Biodentine has some disadvantages: the clinical procedure is technically demanding and difficult, especially in narrow, curved root canals. Since Biodentine can set and achieve dentine strength within approx. 12 min, root canal fillings cannot be repaired and post insertion is hardly possible.

There have been comparatively few scientific studies on the complex of Biodentine and perforation and root resorption. However, there are several case reports in the literature (Tables 10.1 and 10.2). Although case reports are important resources of confirming the material's suitability for clinical usage, it is undeniable that more reliable results can be achieved through randomized long-term clinical trials.

10.3   Conclusion

Biodentine is a biocompatible and bioactive hydraulic calcium silicate cement. The cement is well tolerated by periodontal tissues even in direct contact, exhibits antiresorptive effects and supports healing. In addition, Biodentine adheres to dentine and has similar mechanical properties to those of the natural dentine. This can lead to a stabilization of the Biodentine-treated tooth structure. An advantage of Biodentine as compared to most MTAs is its fast setting time. In addition, Biodentine does not lead to staining of the visible crown. This explains why the cement can be successfully used for the treatment of perforations and of root resorptions.

Table 10.1 Case reports on the treatment of furcal perforations using Biodentine—an overview of the clinical data and treatment procedures

Author (year)	Tooth number	Jaw	Sex	Age	Endodontic treatment	Symptoms	Periodontal defect	Radiolucency adjacent to perforation	Direct contact between perforation and oral cavity	Prior repair	Duration of perforation	Size of perforation	Cause of perforation	Perforation treatment/ barrier	Recall (months)	Success
Heredia et al. (2016) [90]	36	Mandible	M	28	Treatment started	Pain, abscess	Unknown	Unknow	Unknown	No	6 months	1.5 × 2 mm	Iatrogenic	Non-surgical	4	Yes
Indurkar and Maurya (2016) [91]	46	Mandible	F	18	Treatment started	Swelling, pus discharge	Yes	Yes	Yes	No	3 months	Unknown	Iatrogenic	Surgical	6	Yes
Kumar et al. (2016) [92]	36	Mandible	F	35	Treatment started	Mild tenderness to percussion and palpation test	No	Yes	Unknown	No	2 days	2 mm	Iatrogenic	Non-surgical/ gelatin sponge	12	Yes
Mukherjee and Shekhawat (2017) [93]	37	Mandible	M	24	Treatment started	Pain, occasional pus discharge	Unknown	Unknown	Unknown	No	6 months	Unknown	Iatrogenic	Non-surgical	3	Yes
Thakur et al. (2017) [94]	36	Mandible	F	45	Treatment started	Continuous pain aggravated by chewing	Unknown	Yes	Unknown	No	Probably 7 days	Unknown	Iatrogenic	Non-surgical	24	Yes
Kapil et al. (2019) [95]	36	Mandible	M	59	Untreated	No	No	Unknown	Unknown	No	Unknown	<1 mm	Iatrogenic	Non-surgical	12	Yes
Nisar et al. (2020) [96]	46	Mandible	M	14	Treatment started	No	No	No	Unknown	No	Immediately	Unknown	Caries	Non-surgical	–	Yes

F female, M male

Table 10.2 Case reports on the treatment of resorptions using Biodentine—an overview of the clinical data and treatment procedures

Author (year)	Tooth number	Jaw	Localization/root surface	Sex	Age	Clinical symptoms	Type of resorption	Endodontic treatment	Perforation/ treatment	Use of TCA	Recall (months)	Success
Nikhil et al. (2012) [97]	12	Maxilla	Unknown	M	28	No	ICR (class 3)	Yes	Non-surgical	Yes	15	Yes
Borkar and de Noronha de Ataide (2015) [98]	36	Mandible	Coronal and middle thirds of mesial root with multiple perforations (mesial, buccal and furcal)	M	25	Pain	IIR with multiple perforations	Yes	Non-surgical	No	43	Yes
Costa et al. (2015) [99]	13	Maxilla	Palatal	M	28	Crown discoloration	ICR (class 2)	No	Surgical	No	36	Yes
Costa et al. (2015) [99]	13	Maxilla	Palatal	F	38	Sensitive to vertical and lateral percussion	ICR (class 3)	Yes	Non-surgical	No	18	Yes
Jerin et al. (2015) [100]	11	Maxilla	Palatal	F	30	Crown discoloration, bleeding and swelling	ICR (class 4)	Yes	Surgical	Yes	12	Yes
Pruthi et al. (2015) [48]	12	Maxilla	Middle third of the root with perforation (palatal)	M	28	Pain	Resorption with perforation	Yes	Replantation	Yes	18	Yes
Salzano and Tirone (2015) [101]	35	Mandible	Distolingual	F	14	No	ICR (class 4)	Yes	Non-surgical	No	4	Yes

(continued)

Table 10.2 (continued)

Author (year)	Tooth number	Jaw	Localization/root surface	Sex	Age	Clinical symptoms	Type of resorption	Endodontic treatment	Perforation/ treatment	Use of TCA	Recall (months)	Success
Umashetty et al. (2015) [49]	24	Maxilla	Junction of coronal and middle third of the root	F	30	Food lodgement due to caries cavity	IIR without perforation	Yes	Non-surgical	No	10	Yes
Baranwal (2016) [102]	21	Maxilla	Distal	M	23	Crown discoloration, swelling, sinus tract	ICR	Yes	Surgical	No	11	Yes
Baranwal (2016) [102]	11	Maxilla	Distal	M	23	Crown discoloration	ICR	Yes	Surgical	No	11	Yes
Karypidou et al. (2016) [61]	11	Maxilla	Distolabial	F	20	Crown discoloration	ICR	No	Surgical	No	36	Yes
Karypidou et al. (2016) [61]	21	Maxilla	Distolabial	F	20	Crown discoloration, gingival overgrowth	ICR	Yes	Surgical	No	36	Yes
Salzano and Tirone (2016) [103]	27	Maxilla	Distal	F	34		ICR	Yes	Non-surgical	No	3	Yes
Salzano and Tirone (2016) [103]	45	Mandible	Distolingual	M	14		ICR	Yes	Non-surgical	No	11	Yes

Sharma et al. (2016) [104]	22	Maxilla	Labial	F	22	Grade I mobility of tooth, palpation and percussion test-induced pain	ICR (class 3)	Yes	Surgical	No	1/4	Yes
Sharma et al. (2016) [104]	21	Maxilla	Labial	F	22	Grade I mobility of tooth, palpation and percussion test-induced pain	ICR (class 3)	Yes	Surgical	No	1/4	Yes
Ambu et al. (2017) [105]	21	Maxilla	Apical third	M	11	Sinus tract	IAR	Yes	Non-surgical (apical plug)	No	12	Yes
Ambu et al. (2017) [105]	11	Maxilla	Apical third	M	11	No	IAR	Yes	Non-surgical (apical plug)	No	12	Yes
Eftekhar et al. (2017) [106]	33	Mandible	Labial	F	51	Pain	ICR (class 3)	Yes	Surgical	Yes	24	Yes
Mishra et al. (2017) [107]	21	Maxilla	Distal	F	22	Gingival pocket, bleeding	ICR (class 3)	Yes	Surgical	No	6	Yes
Amin et al. (2018) [108]	11	Maxilla	Middle third with perforation (distolabial)	M	21	Sensitive to percussion, mild mobility, swelling	IIR with perforation	Yes	Non-surgical	No	24	Yes
Karunakar et al. (2018) [109]	45	Maxilla	Distopalatal	M	45	Sinus tract	ICR	Yes	Surgical	Yes	6	Yes

(continued)

Table 10.2 (continued)

Author (year)	Tooth number	Jaw	Localization/root surface	Sex	Age	Clinical symptoms	Type of resorption	Endodontic treatment	Perforation/treatment	Use of TCA	Recall (months)	Success
Karunakar et al. (2018) [109]	21	Maxilla	Distopalatal	M	25	Crown discoloration, sinus tract	ICR (class 3)	Yes	Surgical	Yes	6	Yes
Mehra et al. (2018) [76]	23	Maxilla	Labial and palatal	M	43	Pain, periodontal pocket	ICR (class 3)	Yes	Surgical	No	48	Yes
Patni et al. (2018) [110]	12	Maxilla	Labial	M	22	Crown discoloration	ITR	Yes	Non-surgical	No	60	Yes
Baranwal et al. (2019) [111]	21	Maxilla	Distal	M	24	Mobility of bridge	ICR	Early endodontically treated	Surgical	Yes	11	Yes
Baranwal et al. (2019) [111]	13	Maxilla	Labial	F	26	Crown discoloration, percussion to tender, swelling	ICR	Yes	Surgical	No	12	Yes
Nayak et al. (2019) [50]	12	Maxilla	Middle part of the root	F	42	Pain	IIR with perforation	Yes	Non-surgical	No	10	Yes

TCA trichloroacetic acid, *F* female, *M* male, *ICR* invasive cervical resorption, *IIR* inflammatory internal resorption, *IAR* inflammatory apical resorption, Class 2—a well-defined invasive resorptive lesion that has penetrated close to the coronal pulp chamber but shows little or no extension into the radicular dentine, Class 3—a deeper invasion of dentine by resorbing tissue not only involving the coronal dentine but also extending into the coronal third of the root, Class 4—a large invasive resorptive process that has extended beyond the coronal third of the root [112]

References

1. Bargholz C. Perforations. In: Hülsmann M, Schäfer E, editors. Problems in endodontics. Etiology, diagnosis and treatment. Berlin: Quintessence; 2009. p. 385–400.
2. Torabinejad M, Lemon R. Use of MTA as root perforation repair. In: Torabinejad M, editor. Mineral trioxide aggregate. Properties and clinical applications. Ames: Wiley Blackwell; 2014. p. 177–205.
3. Aggarwal V, Singla M, Miglani S, Kohli S. Comparative evaluation of push-out bond strength of ProRoot MTA, Biodentine, and MTA Plus in furcation perforation repair. J Conserv Dent. 2013;16:462–5.
4. Jung S, Mielert J, Kleinheinz J, Dammaschke T. Human oral cells' response to different endodontic restorative materials: an in vitro study. Head Face Med. 2014;10:55. https://doi.org/10.1186/s13005-014-0055-4.
5. Rajasekharan S, Martens LC, Cauwels RG, Verbeeck RM. Biodentine™ material characteristics and clinical applications: a review of the literature. Eur Arch Paediatr Dent. 2014;15:147–58.
6. Torabinejad M, Parirokh M, Dummer PMH. Mineral trioxide aggregate and other bioactive endodontic cements: an updated overview—part II: other clinical applications and complications. Int Endod J. 2018;51:284–317.
7. Krupp C, Bargholz C, Brüsehaber M, Hülsmann M. Treatment outcome after repair of root perforations with mineral trioxide aggregate: a retrospective evaluation of 90 teeth. J Endod. 2013;39:1364–8.
8. Lemon RR, Steele PJ, Jeansonne BG. Ferric sulfate hemostasis: effect on osseous wound healing. Left in situ for maximum exposure. J Endod. 1993;19:170–3.
9. Aksel H, Arslan E, Puralı N, Uyanık Ö, Nagaş E. Effect of ultrasonic activation on dentinal tubule penetration of calcium silicate-based cements. Microsc Res Tech. 2019;82:624–9.
10. Küçükkaya Eren S, Aksel H, Askerbeyli Örs S, Serper A, Koçak Y, Ocak M, et al. Obturation quality of calcium silicate-based cements placed with different techniques in teeth with perforating internal root resorption: a micro-computed tomographic study. Clin Oral Investig. 2019;23:805–11.
11. Kratchman SI. Perforation repair and one-step apexification procedures. Dent Clin N Am. 2004;48:291–307.
12. Bargholz C. Perforation repair with mineral trioxide aggregate: a modified matrix concept. Int Endod J. 2005;38:59–69.
13. Guneser MB, Akbulut MB, Eldeniz AU. Effect of various endodontic irrigants on the push-out bond strength of Biodentine and conventional root perforation repair materials. J Endod. 2013;39:380–4.
14. Nagas E, Kucukkaya S, Eymirli A, Uyanik MO, Cehreli ZC. Effect of laser-activated irrigation on the push-out bond strength of ProRoot mineral trioxide aggregate and Biodentine in furcal perforations. Photomed Laser Surg. 2017;35:231–5.
15. Prasanthi P, Garlapati R, Nagesh B, Sujana V, Naik KMK, Yamini B. Effect of 17% ethylenediaminetetraacetic acid and 0.2% chitosan on pushout bond strength of Biodentine and ProRoot mineral trioxide aggregate: an in vitro study. J Conserv Dent. 2019;22:387–90.
16. Kaup M, Dammann CH, Schäfer E, Dammaschke T. Shear bond strength of Biodentine, ProRoot MTA, glass ionomer cement and composite resin on human dentine ex vivo. Head Face Med. 2015;11:14. https://doi.org/10.1186/s13005-015-0071-z.
17. Kaup M, Schäfer E, Dammaschke T. An in vitro study of different material properties of Biodentine compared to ProRoot MTA. Head Face Med. 2015;11:16. https://doi.org/10.1186/s13005-015-0074-9.
18. Singla M, Verman KG, Goyal V, Jusuja P, Kakkar A, Ahuja L. Comparison of push-out bond strength of furcation perforation repair materials—glass ionomer cement type II, hydroxyapatite, mineral trioxide aggregate, and Biodentine: an in vitro study. Contemp Clin Dent. 2018;9:410–4.

19. Alsubait SA. Effect of sodium hypochlorite on push-out bond strength of four calcium silicate-based endodontic materials when used for repairing perforations on human dentin: an in vitro evaluation. J Contemp Dent Pract. 2017;18:289–94.
20. Akbulut MB, Arpaci PU, Eldeniz AU. Effects of novel root repair materials on attachment and morphological behaviour of periodontal ligament fibroblasts: scanning electron micros-copy observation. Microsc Res Tech. 2016;79:1214–21.
21. Zhou HM, Shen Y, Wang ZJ, Li L, Zheng YF, Häkkinen L, et al. In vitro cytotoxicity evalua-tion of a novel root repair material. J Endod. 2013;39:478–83.
22. Luo T, Liu J, Sun Y, Shen Y, Zou L. Cytocompatibility of Biodentine and iRoot FS with human periodontal ligament cells: an in vitro study. Int Endod J. 2018;51:779–88.
23. Rodrigues EM, Gomes-Cornélio AL, Soares-Costa A, Salles LP, Velayutham M, Rossa-Junior C, et al. An assessment of the overexpression of BMP-2 in transfected human osteoblast cells stimulated by mineral trioxide aggregate and Biodentine. Int Endod J. 2017;50(Suppl 2):e9–18.
24. da Fonseca TS, Silva GF, Guerreiro-Tanomaru JM, Delfino MM, Sasso-Cerri E, Tanomaru-Filho M, et al. Biodentine and MTA modulate immunoinflammatory response favor-ing bone formation in sealing of furcation perforations in rat molars. Clin Oral Investig. 2019;23:1237–52.
25. de Sousa RM, Kochenborger Scarparo R, Steier L, Poli de Figueiredo JA. Periradicular inflammatory response, bone resorption, and cementum repair after sealing of furcation perforation with mineral trioxide aggregate (MTA Angelus™) or Biodentine™. Clin Oral Investig. 2019;23:4019–27.
26. Cardoso M, dos Anjos PM, Correlo V, Reis R, Paulo M, Viegas C. Biodentine for furca-tion perforation repair: an animal study with histological, radiographic and micro-computed tomographic assessment. Iran Endod J. 2018;13:323–30.
27. Silva LAB, Pieroni KAMG, Nelson-Filho P, Silva RAB, Hernandéz-Gatón P, Lucisano MP, et al. Furcation perforation: periradicular tissue response to Biodentine as a repair material by histopathologic and indirect immunofluorescence analyses. J Endod. 2017;43:1137–42.
28. Silva RAB, Borges ATN, Hernandéz-Gatón P, de Queiroz AM, Arzate H, Romualdo PC, et al. Histopathological, histoenzymological, immunohistochemical and immunofluores-cence analysis of tissue response to sealing materials after furcation perforation. Int Endod J. 2019;52:1489–500.
29. Tirone F, Salzano S, Piattelli A, Perrotti V, Iezzi G. Response of periodontium to min-eral trioxide aggregate and Biodentine: a pilot histological study on humans. Aust Dent J. 2018;63:231–41.
30. Berger T, Baratz AZ, Gutmann JL. In vitro investigations into the ethology of mineral trioxide tooth staining. J Conserv Dent. 2014;17:526–30.
31. Dettwiler CA, Walter M, Zaugg LK, Lenherr P, Weiger R, Krastl G. In vitro assessment of the tooth staining potential of endodontic materials in a bovine tooth model. Dent Traumatol. 2016;32:480–7.
32. Shokouhinejad N, Nekoofar MH, Pirmoazen S, Shamshiri AR, Dummer PMH. Evaluation and comparison of occurrence of tooth discoloration after the application of various calcium silicate-based cements: an ex vivo study. J Endod. 2016;42:140–4.
33. Lenherr P, Allgayer N, Weiger R, Filippi A, Attin T, Krastl G. Tooth discoloration induced by endodontic materials: a laboratory study. Int Endod J. 2012;45:942–9.
34. Camilleri J. Color stability of white mineral trioxide aggregate in contact with hypochlorite solution. J Endod. 2014;40:436–40.
35. Możyńska J, Metlerski M, Lipski M, Nowicka A. Tooth discoloration induced by differ-ent calcium silicate-based cements: a systematic review of in vitro studies. J Endod. 2017;43:1593–601.
36. Cao Y, Bogen G, Lim J, Shon WJ, Kang MK. Bioceramic materials and the changing con-cepts in vital pulp therapy. J Calif Dent Assoc. 2016;44:278–90.
37. Bogen G, Dammaschke T, Chandler N. Vital pulp therapy. In: Berman LH, Hargreaves KM, editors. Cohen's pathways of the pulp. 12th ed. St. Louis: Elsevier; 2021. p. 902–38.

38. Schmidt A, Schäfer E, Dammaschke T. Shear bond strength of lining materials to calcium silicate cements at different time intervals. J Adhes Dent. 2017;19:129–35.
39. Ballal S, Venkateshbabu N, Nandini S, Kandaswamy D. An in vitro study to assess the setting and surface crazing of conventional glass ionomer cement when layered over partially set mineral trioxide aggregate. J Endod. 2008;34:478–80.
40. Eid AA, Komabayashi T, Watanabe E, Shiraishi T, Watanabe I. Characterization of the mineral trioxide aggregate-resin modified glass ionomer cement interface in different setting conditions. J Endod. 2012;38:1126–9.
41. Hülsmann M, Schäfer E. Resorption. In: Hülsmann M, Schäfer E, editors. Problems in endodontics. Etiology, diagnosis and treatment. Berlin: Quintessence; 2009. p. 421–34.
42. Andreasen JO, Heithersay GS, Bakland LK. Pathologic tooth resorption. In: Rotstein I, Ingle JI, editors. Ingle's endodontics. 7th ed. Cary: PMPH USA; 2019. p. 421–37.
43. Patel S, Durack C, Ricucci D, Bakhsh AA. Root resorption. In: Berman LH, Hargreaves KM, editors. Cohen's pathways of the pulp. 12th ed. St. Louis: Elsevier; 2021. p. 711–36.
44. Tronstad L. Root resorption—ethology, terminology and clinical manifestations. Endod Dent Traumatol. 1988;4:241–52.
45. Haapasalo M, Endal U. Internal inflammatory root resorption: the unknown resorption of the tooth. Endod Top. 2006;14:60–79.
46. Patel S, Ricucci D, Durak C, Tay FT. Internal root resorption: a review. J Endod. 2010;36:1107–21.
47. Wedenberg C, Zetterqvist L. Internal resorption in human teeth—a histological, scanning electron microscopic, and enzyme histochemical study. J Endod. 1987;13:255–9.
48. Pruthi PJ, Dharmani U, Roongta R, Talwar S. Management of external perforating root resorption by intentional replantation followed by Biodentine restoration. Dent Res J (Isfahan). 2015;12:488–93.
49. Umashetty G, Hoshing U, Patil S, Ajgaonkar N. Management of inflammatory internal root resorption with Biodentine and thermoplasticised gutta-percha. Case Rep Dent. 2015;2015:452609. https://doi.org/10.1155/2015/452609.
50. Nayak N, Priyanka RI, Shenoy V. Conservative management of inflammatory root resorption with perforation—a case report. Indian J Appl Res. 2019;9:24–5.
51. Weltman B, Vig KW, Fields HW, Shanker S, Kaizar EE. Root resorption associated with orthodontic tooth movement: a systematic review. Am J Orthod Dentofac Orthop. 2010;137:462–76.
52. Yoshpe M, Einy S, Ruparel N, Lin S, Kaufman AY. Regenerative endodontics: a potential solution for external root resorption (case series). J Endod. 2020;46:192–9.
53. Heithersay G. Invasive cervical resorption. Endod Top. 2004;7:73–92.
54. Patel S, Mavridou AM, Lambrechts P, Saberi N. External cervical resorption—part 1: histopathology, distribution and presentation. Int Endod J. 2018;51:1205–23.
55. Mavridou AM, Hauben E, Wevers M, Schepers E, Bergmans L, Lambrechts P. Understanding external cervical resorption patterns in vital teeth. Int Endod J. 2016;49:1737–51.
56. Mavridou AM, Hauben E, Wevers M, Schepers E, Bergmans L, Lambrechts P. Understanding external cervical resorption patterns in endodontically treated teeth. Int Endod J. 2017;50:1116–33.
57. Panzarini SR, Trevisan CL, Brandini DA, Poi WR, Sonoda CK, Luvizuto ER, et al. Intracanal dressing and root filling materials in tooth replantation: a literature review. Dent Traumatol. 2012;28:42–8.
58. Jiang J, Zuo J, Chen SH, Holliday LS. Calcium hydroxide reduces lipopolysaccharide-stimulated osteoclast formation. Oral Surg Oral Med Oral Pathol Oral Radiol Endod. 2003;95:348–54.
59. Bonte E, Beslot A, Boukpessi T, Lasfargues JJ. MTA versus Ca(OH)$_2$ in apexification of non-vital immature permanent teeth: a randomized clinical trial comparison. Clin Oral Investig. 2015;19:1381–8.
60. Patel S, Foschi F, Condon R, Pimentel T, Bhuva B. External cervical resorption: part 2—management. Int Endod J. 2018;51:1224–38.

61. Karypidou A, Chatzinikolaou I-D, Kouros P, Koulaouzidou E, Economides N. Management of bilateral invasive cervical resorption lesions in maxillary incisors using a novel calcium silicate-based cement: a case report. Quintessence Int. 2016;47:637–42.

62. Kim M, Kim S, Ko H, Song M. Effect of ProRoot MTA® and Biodentine® on osteoclastic differentiation and activity of mouse bone marrow macrophages. J Appl Oral Sci. 2019;27:e201801501. https://doi.org/10.1590/1678-7757-2018-0150.

63. Hashiguchi D, Fukushima H, Yasuda H, Masuda W, Tomikawa M, Morikawa K, et al. Mineral trioxide aggregate inhibits osteoclastic bone resorption. J Dent Res. 2011;90:912–7.

64. Cheng X, Zhu L, Zhang J, Yu J, Liu S, Lv F, et al. Antiosteoclastogenesis of mineral trioxide aggregate through inhibition of the autophagic pathway. J Endod. 2017;43:766–73.

65. Han L, Okiji T. Uptake of calcium and silicon released from calcium silicate-based endodontic materials into root canal dentine. Int Endod J. 2011;44:1081–7.

66. Han L, Okiji T. Bioactivity evaluation of three calcium silicate-based endodontic materials. Int Endod J. 2013;46:808–14.

67. Natale LC, Rodrigues MC, Xavier TA, Simões A, de Souza DN, Braga RR. Ion release and mechanical properties of calcium silicate and calcium hydroxide materials used for pulp capping. Int Endod J. 2015;48:89–94.

68. Quintana RM, Jardine AP, Grechi TR, Grazziotin-Soares R, Ardenghi DM, Scarparo RK, et al. Bone tissue reaction, setting time, solubility, and pH of root repair materials. Clin Oral Investig. 2019;23:1359–66.

69. Mahmoud O, Al-Meeri WA, Farook MS, Al-Afifi NA. Calcium silicate-based cements as root canal medicament. Clin Cosmet Investig Dent. 2020;12:49–60.

70. Rathinam E, Rajasekharan S, Chitturi RT, Martens L, De Coster P. Gene expression profiling and molecular signaling of dental pulp cells in response to tricalcium silicate cements: a systematic review. J Endod. 2015;41:1805–17.

71. Arnett TR. Extracellular pH regulates bone cell function. J Nutr. 2008;138:415S–8S.

72. Poggio C, Beltrami R, Colombo M, Ceci M, Dagna A, Chiesa M. In vitro antibacterial activity of different pulp capping materials. J Clin Exp Dent. 2015;7:e584–8.

73. Scelza MZ, Nascimento JC, da Silva LE, Gameiro VS, De Deus G, Alves G. Biodentine™ is cytocompatible with human primary osteoblasts. Braz Oral Res. 2017;31:e81. https://doi.org/10.1590/1807-3107BOR-2017.vol31.0081.

74. Gandolfi MG, Iezzi G, Piattelli A, Prati C, Scarano A. Osteoinductive potential and bone-bonding ability of ProRoot MTA, MTA Plus and Biodentine in rabbit intramedullary model: microchemical characterization and histological analysis. Dent Mater. 2017;33:e221–38.

75. Malkondu Ö, Kazandağ MK, Kazazoğlu E. A review on Biodentine, a contemporary dentine replacement and repair material. Biomed Res Int. 2014;2014:160951. https://doi.org/10.1155/2014/160951.

76. Mehra N, Yadav M, Kaushik M, Roshni R. Clinical management of root resorption: a report of three cases. Cureus. 2018;10:e3215. https://doi.org/10.7759/cureus.3215.

77. Koubi G, Colon P, Franquin JC, Hartmann A, Richard G, Faure M-O, et al. Clinical evaluation of the performance and safety of a new dentine substitute, Biodentine, in the restoration of posterior teeth—a prospective study. Clin Oral Investig. 2013;17:243–9.

78. Nowicka A, Lipski M, Parafiniuk M, Sporniak-Tutak K, Lichota D, Kosierkiewicz A, et al. Response of human dental pulp capped with Biodentine and mineral trioxide aggregate. J Endod. 2013;39:743–7.

79. Nowicka A, Wilk G, Lipski M, Kołecki J, Buczkowska-Radlińska J. Tomographic evaluation of reparative dentin formation after direct pulp capping with $Ca(OH)_2$, MTA, Biodentine, and dentin bonding system in human teeth. J Endod. 2015;41:1234–40.

80. Lipski M, Nowicka A, Kot K, Postek-Stefańska L, Wysoczańska-Jankowicz I, Borkowski L, et al. Factors affecting the outcomes of direct pulp capping using Biodentine. Clin Oral Investig. 2018;22:2021–9.

81. Harms CS, Schäfer E, Dammaschke T. Clinical evaluation of direct pulp capping using a calcium silicate cement-treatment outcomes over an average period of 2.3 years. Clin Oral Investig. 2019;23:3491–9.

82. Ulusoy Öİ, Paltun YN. Fracture resistance of roots with simulated internal resorption defects and obturated using different hybrid techniques. J Dent Sci. 2017;12:121–5.
83. Türker SA, Uzunoğlu E, Sungur DD, Tek V. Fracture resistance of teeth with simulated perforating internal resorption cavities repaired with different calcium silicate-based cements and backfilling materials. J Endod. 2018;44:860–3.
84. Sarraf P, Nekoofar MH, Sheykhrezae MS, Dummer PMH. Fracture resistance of immature incisors following root filling with various bioactive endodontic cements using an experimental bovine tooth model. Eur J Dent. 2019;13:156–60.
85. Aggarwal V, Singla M. Management of inflammatory root resorption using MTA obturation—a four year follow up. Br Dent J. 2010;208:287–9.
86. Leiendecker AP, Qi Y-P, Sawyer AN, Niu L-N, Agee KA, Loushine RJ, et al. Effects of calcium silicate-based materials on collagen matrix integrity of mineralized dentin. J Endod. 2012;38:829–33.
87. Sawyer AN, Nikonov SY, Pancio AK, Niu LN, Agee KA, Loushine RJ, et al. Effects of calcium silicate-based materials on the flexural properties of dentin. J Endod. 2012;38:680–3.
88. Patel MH, Yagnik KN, Patel NK, Bhavsar BA. Obturating the pink tooth: an in vitro comparative evaluation of different materials. Endodontology. 2018;30:119–24.
89. Tek V, Türker SA. A micro-computed tomography evaluation of voids using calcium silicate-based materials in teeth with simulated internal root resorption. Restor Dent Endod. 2020;45:e5. https://doi.org/10.5395/rde.2020.45.e5.
90. Heredia AL, Bhagwat SA, Mandke LP. Biodentine as material of choice for furcal perforation repair—a case report. Ann Prosthodont Restor Dent. 2016;2:54–7.
91. Indurkar MS, Maurya AS. Effective seal completes the deal: periodontal management of an iatrogenic endodontic perforation. J Interdisc Dent. 2016;6:87–90.
92. Kumar P, Noronha de Ataide I, Fernandes M, Lambor R. Furcal perforation repair with Biodentine: one year follow up of a case. Int J Curr Res. 2016;8:34221–3.
93. Mukherjee M, Shekhawat K. Perforation repair using Biodentine: a nobel approach. Int J Med Dent Sci. 2017;6:1558–60.
94. Thakur S, Damanpreet, Rani A, Garg N. Management of iatrogenic furcation perforation in mandibular first molar with Biodentine—two years follow up. Dent J Adv Stud. 2017;5:47–50.
95. Kapil S, Verma S, Goel M, Singh M. Repair of iatrogenic furcal perforation using Biodentine. Paripex Indian J Res. 2019;8:125–6.
96. Nisar R, Tiwari P, Kumar V, Mahajan S, Baruah S. Management of pulpal floor perforation by using Biodentine: a clinical report. Eur J Pharm Med Res. 2020;7:512–5.
97. Nikhil V, Arora V, Jha P, Verma M. Non-surgical management of trauma induced external root resorption at two different sites in a single tooth with Biodentine: a case report. Endodontology. 2012;24:150–5.
98. Borkar S, de Noronha de Ataide I. Management of a massive resorptive lesion with multiple perforations in a molar: case report. J Endod. 2015;41:753–8.
99. Costa SV, Oliveira JJ, Pinheiro SL, Bueno CEB, Ferrari PHP. Use of a tricalcium silicate cement in invasive cervical resorption. Endo (Lond, Engl). 2015;9:193–200.
100. Jerin J, Shoba K, Tomy Nithya T, Sheena P, Shibu A. Management of invasive cervical resorption with Biodentine: a case report. J Res Dent. 2015;2:660–6.
101. Salzano S, Tirone F. Conservative nonsurgical treatment of class 4 invasive cervical resorption: a case report. J Endod. 2015;41:1907–12.
102. Baranwal AK. Management of external invasive cervical resorption of tooth with Biodentine: a case report. J Conserv Dent. 2016;19:296–9.
103. Salzano S, Tirone F. Mini-invasive nonsurgical treatment of class 4 invasive cervical resorption: a case series. G Ital Endod. 2016;30:52–63.
104. Sharma A, Maria R, Mishra P, Pethiya A. Sealing the cervical defect with Biodentine. J Curr Res Sci Med. 2016;2:125–8.

105. Ambu E, Fimiani M, Vigna M, Grandini S. Use of bioactive materials and limited FOV CBCT in the treatment of a replanted permanent tooth affected by inflammatory external root resorption: a case report. Eur J Paediatr Dent. 2017;18:51–5.
106. Eftekhar L, Ashraf H, Jabbari S. Management of invasive cervical root resorption in a mandibular canine using Biodentine as a restorative material: a case report. Iran Endod J. 2017;12:386–9.
107. Mishra T, Arora S, Sridevi N, Mishra V. Clinical applications of Biodentine: a case series. Int J Contemp Med Surg Radiol. 2017;2:10–4.
108. Amin S, Jamsheed ET, Babu B, Amin V. Endodontic management of internal resorptive defect in maxillary central incisor using Biodentine; with 3 years and 8 months evident follow-up. Res J Pharm Biol Chem Sci. 2018;9:1688–95.
109. Karunakar P, Soloman RV, Anusha B, Nagarjun M. Endodontic management of invasive cervical resorption: report of two cases. J Conserv Dent. 2018;21:578–81.
110. Patni PM, Jain P, Jain S, Hiremath H, Agarwal R, Patni MJ. Internal tunneling resorption associated with invasive cervical resorption. J Conserv Dent. 2018;21:105–8.
111. Baranwal HC, Sami A, Singh N. Management of different challenging causes of invasive cervical root resorption. Ann Prosthodont Restor Dent. 2019;5:42–5.
112. Heithersay GS. Invasive cervical resorption: an analysis of potential predisposing factors. Quintessence Int. 1999;30:83–95.

Clinical Application of Biodentine™ in Regenerative Endodontics/ Revitalization

11

Kerstin M. Galler and Tatiana M. Botero

11.1 Indication of Revitalization Procedures

The information on revitalization, which is also termed revascularization or regenerative endodontics in the literature, as described in this chapter follows the recommendations of the European Society of Endodontology (ESE), who published a Position Statement on revitalization in 2016 [1]. This document provides background information; describes the indication, clinical assessment and details of the procedure; and comments on follow-up and expected outcome. Similar recommendations exist from the American Association of Endodontists (AAE), which were published in 2013 and updated in 2018 and are accessible via the AAE website as "Clinical Considerations for Regenerative Procedures". Both societies comment on the evolving nature of this field and that updates will be necessary, as new clinical and research findings are generated and will add to the body of knowledge, which might be reflected by adjusting the clinical protocol.

Revitalization procedures are indicated in immature teeth with pulp necrosis, also in cases with periapical lesions due to bacterial infection of the root canal. Thus, it is an alternative treatment method to an apexification or apical plug with mineral trioxide aggregate (MTA) or other hydraulic calcium silicate cements. Whereas revitalization has been suggested as the preferred option particularly in cases of early stages of root development [2], general recommendations cannot be given and the selection of cases has to be made on an individual basis. Revitalization

K. M. Galler (✉)
Department of Conservative Dentistry and Periodontology, University Hospital Regensburg, Regensburg, Germany
e-mail: Kerstin.Galler@klinik.uni-regensburg.de

T. M. Botero
Cariology, Restorative Sciences and Endodontics, University of Michigan, School of Dentistry, Ann Arbor, MI, USA
e-mail: tbotero@umich.edu

© Springer Nature Switzerland AG 2022
I. About (ed.), *Biodentine™*, https://doi.org/10.1007/978-3-030-80932-4_11

is technically less challenging compared to the apical plug, but the provocation of bleeding may be unsuccessful or cause pain; thus the patients have to be very cooperative. Given that most patients for this particular treatment are children, compliance is an issue and needs to be evaluated and will co-determine the choice for one treatment or the other.

The cause for pulp necrosis in immature teeth is mostly dental trauma, less frequently caries lesions or pulpal infections due to developmental anomalies, which account for penetration of bacteria into the pulp chamber and pulp necrosis soon after eruption. Therefore, revitalization is commonly performed in maxillary incisors, which are most frequently affected by dental trauma within the dentition, or in premolars that are affected by *dens evaginatus*.

Comprehensive information should be provided to the patients and parents in relation to the problem, treatment options, procedural details, follow-up and potential outcomes. Patients who are medically compromised, in particular with deficient blood clotting, or are known to have allergies to the materials to be used during the procedure should not be treated with revitalization [1]. Further contraindications include inability of field isolation, teeth which require restoration with a post or avulsed teeth with wide-open apex shortly after replantation, where tissue ingrowth may spontaneously occur without any further interventions.

Revitalization is less invasive than the apical plug technique, as it aims at a "biological filling" of the root canal and tissue ingrowth rather than the application of a synthetic material in direct contact with the periapical tissues. However, the clinician's knowledge and understanding of cellular responses and processes of healing may be more important than technical details for this biology-based treatment approach.

11.2 Clinical Procedure

The clinical diagnostics prior to treatment should include the identification of chief complaints, a cold (thermal) or electric pulp test, tenderness to percussion and percussion tone, evaluation of tooth mobility, pain on palpation, swelling, sinus tract, tooth discolouration and probing depths. Radiographic analysis should focus on the identification of a periapical lesion as well as the size of the apical foramen.

11.2.1 First Visit: Disinfection

During the first visit, anaesthesia is optional, but recommended. The access cavity is prepared after field isolation, followed by thorough irrigation and disinfection of the root canal with 1.5–3% sodium hypochlorite (NaOCl). The thickness of the root walls has to be taken into consideration; generally, there is a recommendation to not or only minimally instrument the canal walls in order to avoid further weakening of the root, which might increase the risk of fracture. Antibiotic pastes (triple or double, ciprofloxacin, metronidazole and/or minocycline, replaced by cephalosporine, amoxicillin or clindamycin) have been used and discussed as intracanal medicaments in the past. The recommendation today is to place a non-discolouring calcium hydroxide as dressing, followed by a temporary seal.

11.2.2 Second Visit: Intracanal Blood Clot Induction

A thorough clinical assessment should be performed during the next visit, where signs and symptoms of inflammation should have receded. Prior to the actual treatment, the tooth should be anaesthetized, possibly without vasoconstrictor, as this additive might impair sufficient bleeding into the canal [3]. After field isolation and access, the canal is thoroughly rinsed with 17% EDTA and the excess liquid is removed with paper points. Subsequently, bleeding is induced by mechanical irritation of the periapical tissues, for example with a hand file, until blood starts to flow and rise up to 2–3 mm below the cemento-enamel junction. The induction of the blood clot may require repeated instrumentation and cause discomfort to the patient, despite anaesthesia. In this situation, intraligamentary anaesthesia helps to reduce the discomfort and maintain patient's cooperation throughout the procedure. Once the clot is generated, a collagenous material can be placed on top to facilitate the subsequent placement of a hydraulic calcium silicate cement. Whereas the collagen matrix does not have a therapeutic effect, it may prevent dislocation of the successively applied material towards the middle or apical third of the canal [3, 4]. As soon as the hydraulic calcium silicate is in place as a thin and homogenous layer of about 2–3 mm which ends below the cemento-enamel junction, it can promptly be covered by a layer of a self-adhesive flowable or a light-curable glass-ionomer. The walls of the access cavity can be refreshed with a bur or grit-blasted with aluminium oxide, and an adhesive restoration needs to be placed as a coronal seal.

In the literature, regenerative endodontic procedures are mostly reported as a two-visit approach. Whereas successful revitalization is possible after a single-visit treatment [5–7], it may be speculated that, even though sufficient disinfection may be achieved in one visit, provocation of bleeding in the presence of periapical inflammation will transport inflammatory mediators into the canal, which may impair healing and repair (Fig. 11.1).

11.3 Outcome

Current evidence regarding regenerative endodontics includes not only case reports, case series, and laboratory and animal studies, but also randomized controlled clinical studies [7–10] and even systematic reviews [11–14] and meta-analyses [12, 13]. However, these procedures are still lacking strong clinical evidence. Early and impressive case reports showed mainly premolars with the anatomic anomaly of a *dens evaginatus*, where the completion of root formation after regenerative endodontics was documented radiographically during the follow-up appointments [3, 15, 16]. A recent clinical trial found a higher success on cases with dental anomalies

First Visit steps

Second Visit steps

Follow-up

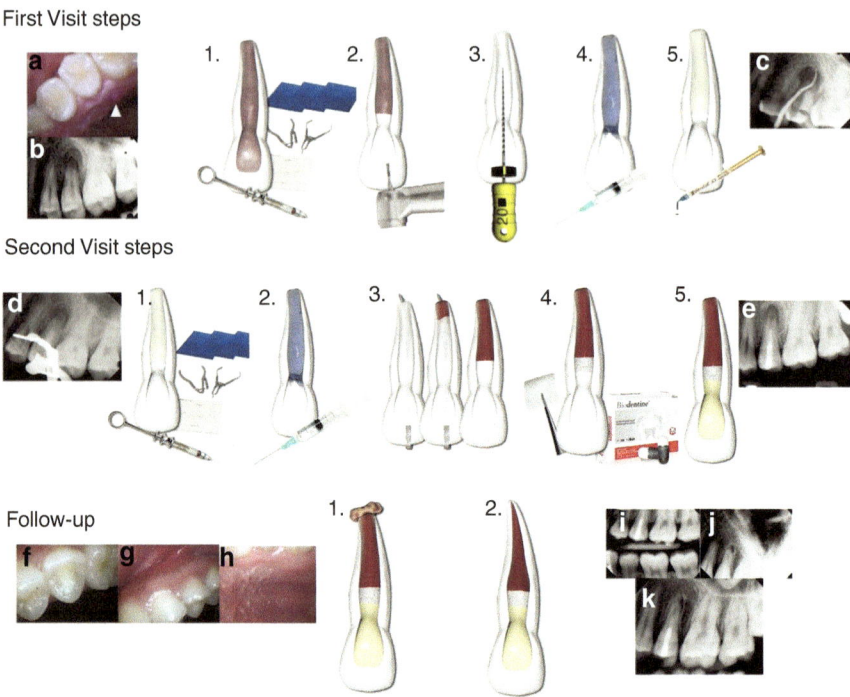

Fig. 11.1 Procedural details of revitalization. *First visit, disinfection, steps*: (1) Local anaesthesia and rubber dam isolation; (2) access opening to confirm pulpal necrosis; (3) minimal instrumentation, root canal length confirmation with apex locator and periapical radiograph; (4) irrigation with 1.5–3% NaOCl; (5) intracanal medication with Ca(OH)$_2$. *Second visit, intracanal blood clot induction, steps*: (1) Local anaesthesia and rubber dam isolation; (2) irrigation with 17% EDTA to remove intracanal medication; (3) induction of bleeding at the periapical level and intracanal blood clot formation; (4) collagen matrix application over the clot and bioceramic (Biodentine) application on top with working time between 10 and 12 min from mix to application; (5) final coronal seal with glass-ionomer and composite. *Follow-up* in (1) 3–6 months with initial periapical healing and (2) 12–24 months reveals root formation (increase in length and thickening of walls) (Drawings by Dr. Diogo Guerriero, Endodontist, private practice, Toronto, Canada). **Clinical case**: 16-year-old female patient referred by her general dentist due to the presence of sinus tract in palatal mucosa of her maxillary left second premolar. The tooth was asymptomatic and diagnosed with pulp necrosis and chronic apical abscess due to *dens evaginatus*. (**a**) Clinical photo of occlusal *dens evaginatus*, (**b**) periapical radiograph showing periapical radiolucency and incomplete root formation. (**c**) *First visit*: after following the steps previously mentioned, periapical radiograph shows intracanal medication and sinus tract traced by the gutta-percha cone. *Second visit*: patient had no symptoms and sinus tract healed. (**d**) Radiograph confirming the level of Biodentine capping material over the formed blood clot and collagen. (**e**) Final radiograph after glass-ionomer and composite occlusal restoration. *Follow-up*: (**f–h**) Clinical photos 12 months post-operative. The treated tooth was asymptomatic with normal periodontal tissues. (**i–k**) Bitewing and periapical radiographs at 12 months showing periapical healing and root formation. (Case by Dr. Tatiana Botero, private practice at Canton Dentist, MI, USA)

than those with trauma. It has been hypothesized that the survival of the apical papilla as well as the damage on the periodontal tissue are key for the success or failure of regenerative endodontics [8]. Therefore, the initial expectation was that new pulp in its original architecture and function would be generated, with the apposition of dentine to thin root walls. However, it became apparent that the new content of the canal consisted mostly of fibrous tissue and mineralized cementum and bone [17–21]. Thus, revitalization results in repair by ectopic tissue formation rather than regeneration [17, 22–26].

Currently, the absence of signs and symptoms of inflammation and healing of periapical lesions after regenerative endodontic procedures are considered the primary goals (AAE, Regenerative Endodontics). These goals can be achieved reliably in 91–94% of cases [12, 13], which implies that true regeneration is not a prerequisite for clinical success. A prospective clinical study of revitalization in traumatized immature teeth showed that a completion of root formation cannot be expected, but healing and apical closure are commonly observed [27]. Systematic reviews and meta-analysis reveal that revitalization and apical plug produce similar results in regard to tooth survival and healing [13, 14]. The apical plug mainly results in apical closure, whereas revitalization shows a higher potential for an increase of root length and thickness [8, 13]. This finding is infrequent and not predictable, though.

Interestingly, a response to thermal or electric pulp testing can be observed in approximately 50% of all cases [28]; thus the ingrowth of nerve fibres into the canal is likely to be independent on the type of new tissue. However, similarly to a cervical pulpotomy, the treatment success cannot be based on sensitivity testing, but has to be evaluated clinically and radiographically. A major adverse effect of revitalization procedures is the risk of discolouration, which may be induced by the various irrigants and materials used during the procedure in contact with dentine or blood. Occurrence of discolouration has been reported in 40% of all studies [12]; the main causes were the use of minocycline [29], but also MTA [30]. Stringent selection of the materials used, e.g. non-discolouring intracanal medicaments and hydraulic calcium silicate cements without bismuth oxide as radiopacifier, can minimize the risk of severe discolouration. It has also been reported that discoloured crowns can be bleached successfully [31].

Recurrent signs and symptoms of infection and inflammation are a possible outcome after revitalization [19, 32, 33], where residual bacteria and insufficient disinfection may be considered as the main causes of failure.

11.4   Material Selection

Several disinfecting agents and dental materials are used during a revitalization treatment. Biological considerations play an important role in this context, as interactions with the surrounding cells and tissues and the blood clot are more critical as for many other applications.

11.4.1 Irrigation and Intracanal Medicament

For revitalization, which ultimately aims at regenerating the dentine-pulp complex, it has to be anticipated that the level of disinfection has to be even higher as for conventional root canal treatment [34]. In a recent study, the microbial profiles of infected immature teeth and primarily infected permanent teeth with closed apices were compared and it was concluded that these are rather similar [35]. Still, during conventional root canal treatment, mechanical preparation and enlargement of the root canal result in the removal of infected dentine and thus the reduction of biofilm. For immature teeth, mechanical instrumentation is not recommended to avoid weakening thin and fragile walls even further. However, instruments can be used to improve the removal of necrotic tissue and the disruption of biofilms. Copious irrigation and an intracanal medicament aid in the removal of necrotic tissue remnants and bacteria. Literature reports of failed cases of revitalization highlight the importance of disinfection [19], and a recent systematic analysis concluded that nearly 80% of failed cases can be attributed to persistent infection [36]. Along these lines, an animal study revealed that persisting bacteria do not necessarily cause periapical lesions but impede mineral deposition and are thus causative for a lack of root lengthening and thickening after revitalization [37].

The treatment should generally be performed after isolation of the affected tooth with rubber dam and be carried out under aseptic conditions. It has to be considered that irrigation solutions and intracanal medicaments have to be most effective regarding disinfection; on the other hand, these agents may compromise the viability of the surrounding cells and tissues, in particular the stem cells from the apical papilla (SCAP) [38, 39]. Whereas sodium hypochlorite (NaOCl) is the irrigant of choice, the recommended concentration ranges between 1% and 3%, as in vitro data clearly show its toxic effects on SCAPs, which increase with increasing concentrations of the agent [38]. However, the use of EDTA can partially reverse toxic effects [38]; furthermore, this agent enables growth factor release from the dentine matrix by surface demineralization [40]. These proteins have bioactive effects: they induce cell migration as well as proliferation and differentiation of stem cells, which are critical for healing and regeneration [41]. Therefore, thorough irrigation with NaOCl in low concentrations (1.5–3%), followed by a rinse with EDTA (17%) during the first visit as well as the sole use of EDTA during the second visit prior to induction of the blood clot, appears beneficial.

As an intracanal medicament, mixtures of antibiotic pastes have been widely used for regenerative endodontic procedures, in particular a triple-antibiotic paste (TAP) of ciprofloxacin, metronidazole and minocycline that goes back to reports by Hoshino, who demonstrated that this combination eliminates bacteria found in carious lesions and in infected root canal dentine [42, 43]. Due to severe discolouration observed after the use of minocycline, variations of the original combination included a modified mTAP, where minocycline was replaced by cefaclor [44], or a double-antibiotic paste (DAP) where minocycline was removed from the mixture [15, 45, 46]. The use of antibiotic pastes in children and adolescents was reconsidered more recently, due to undesirable side effects such as cytotoxicity [39] and risks of sensitization and antibiotic resistance. Therefore, current recommendations advise the use of calcium hydroxide, which is not toxic to SCAP cells in vitro [39] and has been successfully used for regenerative endodontic procedures [45–48].

11.4.2 Hydraulic Calcium Silicate Cement

Due to the fact that hydraulic cements have the specific property to set in the presence of fluids, MTA has been the material of choice for most of the reported cases of regenerative endodontics to cover the blood clot [49]. Its property to set in a moist environment and its biocompatibility along with a lack of suitable alternatives accounted for its use. Although MTA, as other hydraulic calcium silicate cements, can be applied in a moist environment, local conditions and contamination can alter the setting characteristics and affect the mechanical properties. A compromised setting reaction and reduced microhardness have been observed in the presence of tissue fluids [50, 51]. Similarly, blood components can compromise the mechanical properties of the material [52–54].

MTA is a Portland cement-based material, which, in its original formulation, had bismuth oxide added for radiopacity [55–59]. Regardless of its clinical success in multiple clinical cases, MTA has several drawbacks. A contamination of MTA with blood leads to inclusion of blood components into the material's porous structure, which might cause discolouration [60]. Furthermore, the interaction of blood components with bismuth oxide results in dentine staining [58, 61]. Besides the potential of discolouration, other problems include a long setting time of several hours and difficult handling [52]. During revitalization, MTA was often displaced into the canal during its application onto the blood clot. The use of a collagenous matrix has therefore been advocated to keep the material at the desired location, the root canal orifice.

To overcome these disadvantages, synthetic materials produced from laboratory-grade tricalcium silicate have been developed, such as Biodentine. As bismuth oxide has been substituted by zirconium oxide in this material, it exhibits lower radiopacity, but shows a markedly reduced risk of discolouration [62, 63]. As this material has less pores and a more homogenous structure, the risk of discolouration after contact with blood is reduced. Interestingly, formulations without bismuth oxide were also reported to stain dentine after contact with irrigants like NaOCl or chlorhexidine, however, to a much lesser extent [62, 64]. Aesthetic aspects are particularly important for revitalization procedures, as most of the teeth treated with this approach are central and lateral maxillary incisors and therefore are in the most aesthetically critical zone. Compared to other applications such as the apical plug, the material is placed much further coronally where discolouration is much more of an issue.

In regard to the handling properties, the application of Biodentine in regenerative endodontics is suitable. After placement of a collagen matrix, the material can be inserted with ease, due to the coronal location of the site. Subsequent application of a self-adhesive composite or light-curable glass-ionomer is possible without further delay.

As blood is saturated with calcium and phosphate, hydraulic calcium silicate-based materials interact with the clot during revitalization. The bioactivity of these materials, such as hydroxyapatite formation, antibacterial activity and induction of mineralization, has been demonstrated in vitro. However, it is not clear whether these properties are exerted after their use in clinics [61]. Information on the biological behaviour of these materials in contact with blood or resorbable collagen matrices is sparse. One report described a chemical and micromechanical analysis of a Portland-based cement recovered from a patient after failed revitalization [65]. The porous material surface was enriched in calcium carbonate instead of calcium hydroxide or apatite. Therefore, further studies are required to elucidate the properties and behaviour of hydraulic calcium silicate cements after a use in revitalization in a clinical environment (Fig. 11.2).

11.5 Regeneration and Repair

Whereas the process of regeneration restores the physiological structure and function of a tissue, repair might involve the formation of an ectopic tissue; however, both processes result in healing after infections or injuries.

The conventional approach to achieve healing in cases of pulp necrosis with subsequent infections of the root canal and development of periapical lesions is root canal treatment (RCT), where the canal is enlarged, thoroughly disinfected and the void is filled with synthetic materials. Due to the root morphology of immature teeth, the usual root canal filling cannot be placed. Root development is arrested as soon as pulp necrosis occurs, resulting in more or less thin, fragile and fracture-prone roots, depending on the current stage of root development. In particular, a risk of cervical root fracture has been reported [66]. Therefore, it is especially desirable to achieve regeneration in these cases. Initially, expectations were high, as numerous reports showed a completion of root formation in cases of *dens evaginatus*. The

---

Fig. 11.2 Clinical case of a regenerative endodontic procedure/revitalization. Seventeen-year-old male patient was referred for consultation due to inflammation noticed on the buccal aspect of the mandibular second right bicuspid. The tooth was asymptomatic and diagnosed with pulp necrosis and chronic apical abscess associated with *dens evaginatus*. (**a**) Clinical photo and (**b**) periapical radiograph showing sinus tract with a gutta-percha cone. (**c**) *First visit, disinfection*: Periapical radiograph was taken to confirm root length, and periapical lesion was found. (**d**) Calcium hydroxide intracanal medication was placed after minimal instrumentation and irrigation with 2.5% sodium hypochlorite and 17% EDTA. Coronal seal with sterile sponge and glass-ionomer (Fuji II). *Second visit, blood clot induction*: Patient had no symptoms and sinus tract healed. After irrigation as previously described and blood clot induction, collagen was placed and Biodentine was used as capping material over the clot. (**e**) Final periapical radiograph showing Biodentine, glass-ionomer and composite occlusal seal. (**f**) Twelve months post-operative: Clinical photo showing normal periodontal tissues and tooth colour. (**g**) Periapical radiograph showing periapical healing, root apex closure and thickening of dentinal walls. Patient scheduled for yearly follow-up. (Case by Dr. Tatiana Botero and Dr. Mohamad Al-Maaz, Graduate Endodontic Clinic, School of Dentistry, University of Michigan, USA)

hypothesis of pulp regeneration was furthermore supported by reports, which demonstrated that stem cells from the apical papilla (SCAP), which are present in immature teeth until root formation is complete, can be flushed into the canal with the influx of blood [67].

SCAP have been demonstrated to be highly proliferative and to be capable of differentiation into odontoblasts and form dentine [68]. But animal experiments and

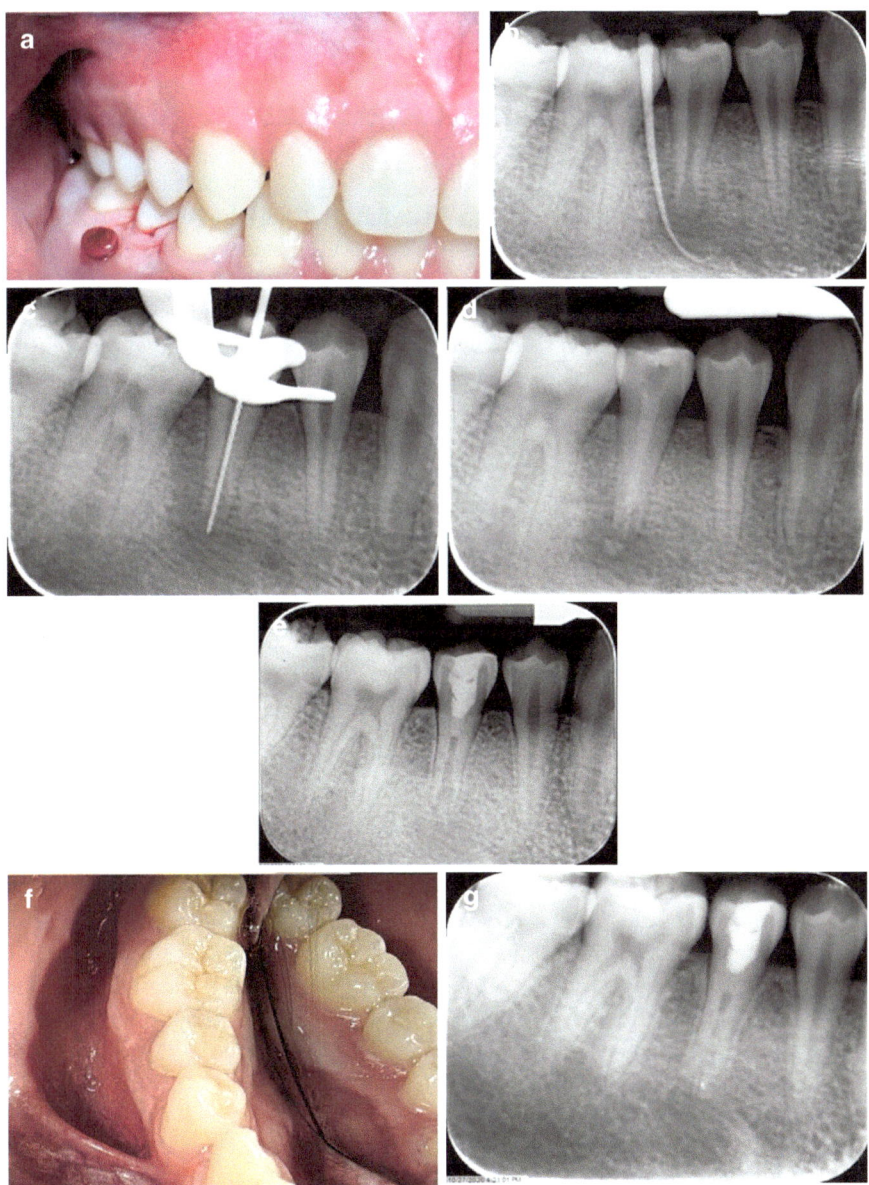

clinical cases after extraction showed the formation of ectopic tissue inside the canal, namely fibrous tissue, cementum and bone [17, 18, 20]. Furthermore, the completion of root formation was absent in numerous trauma cases. It became evident that not regeneration, but mainly repair takes place after revitalization procedures. Since success rates of revitalization are high in terms of tooth survival and healing, this is to date an accepted outcome after this procedure. To date, data support the concept that new pulp tissue formation can only take place if remnants of the original pulp and/or apical papilla remain, as is often the case in the specific situation of a *dens evaginatus*, which was previously demonstrated in the case report by Banchs and Trope [16].

11.6   Future Perspectives

Even though regenerative endodontic procedures are still a fairly new procedure, sound evidence has been gathered to support that the concept is valid and results in high success rates. Initial expectations were high and true regeneration of the dentine-pulp complex with differentiation of odontoblasts from stem cells of the apical papilla and formation of tubular dentine were assumed. The assessment by Diogenes et al. [69] separated patient-based, clinician-based and scientist-based expected outcome and initiated a different way of thinking. Whereas revitalization results in repair, not regeneration, this is considered an acceptable outcome today. The presence of remnant vital pulp tissue as a prerequisite for true regeneration is met in very few cases. With the current realistic assessment of revitalization, more issues arise as we follow patients that were treated with this method. Questions we have to answer include recommendation for orthodontic movement of these teeth, definition of specific success criteria and whether a re-entry is feasible to verify tissue formation inside the canal. The goal is to predict the tooth's long-term prognosis more reliably to facilitate decisions on tooth preservation versus extraction.

To date, revitalization is indicated in immature teeth, but increasing numbers of case series and clinical studies document the outcome after revitalization in mature teeth. After enlargement of the apical foramen, a "biological root canal filling" after provocation of a blood clot inside the canal shows similar outcomes as conventional root canal treatment [9, 70–72]. Thus, an extension of the indication of regenerative endodontics to mature teeth can be anticipated, which leaves the endodontic community to develop more sophisticated concepts for sufficient disinfection.

On a different front, tissue engineering (TE) approaches have been explored to enable regeneration of the dentine-pulp complex. Transplantation of autologous pulp stem cells from deciduous teeth into empty root canals of immature incisors with pulp necrosis after dental trauma may lead to a completion of root formation [73]. Others have implemented successful autotransplantation of dental pulp stem cell [74] and allogenic umbilical cord mesenchymal stem cells in mature teeth [75]. Thus, cell-based approaches hold great promise in the long term, but several hurdles have to be overcome prior to implementation of such concepts in clinical practice. More promising approaches might be based on "cell homing", where carefully selected scaffold materials are laden with growth factors and inserted into the root canal to recruit resident stem cells from remnant pulp or periapical tissues. These cells can migrate, adhere to the matrix, proliferate, degrade the scaffold material and replace it with their own extracellular matrix, and differentiate and form new pulp and dentine [76]. Various promising scaffold materials have been explored for dental pulp TE. Multiple growth factors are present in root dentine [77], where they are embedded and released after dentine demineralization, for example with EDTA [41]. With such approaches, pulp repair or even regeneration might be possible in the future, and regenerative endodontic procedures will be performed more frequently in dental offices.

11.7   Conclusions

During revitalization, hydraulic calcium silicate cements are recommended to cover the blood clot due to their biocompatibility and ability to set in a moist environment. Biodentine appears to be a suitable material due to its handling properties and the low risk of causing discolouration.

References

1. Galler KM, Krastl G, Simon S, Van Gorp G, Meschi N, Vahedi B, Lambrechts P. European Society of Endodontology position statement: revitalization procedures. Int Endod J. 2016;49:717–23.
2. Kim SG, Malek M, Sigurdsson A, Lin LM, Kahler B. Regenerative endodontics: a comprehensive review. Int Endod J. 2018;51:1367–88.
3. Petrino JA, Boda KK, Shambarger S, Bowles WR, McClanahan SB. Challenges in regenerative endodontics: a case series. J Endod. 2010;36:536–41.
4. Jung IY, Lee SJ, Hargreaves KM. Biologically based treatment of immature permanent teeth with pulpal necrosis: a case series. J Endod. 2008;34:876–87.
5. Shin SY, Albert JS, Mortman RE. One step pulp revascularization treatment of an immature permanent tooth with chronic apical abscess: a case report. Int Endod J. 2009;42:1118–26.
6. Topçuoğlu G, Topçuoğlu HS. Regenerative endodontic therapy in a single visit using platelet-rich plasma and Biodentine in necrotic and asymptomatic immature molar teeth: a report of 3 cases. J Endod. 2016;42:1344–6.
7. Botero TM, Tang X, Gardner R, Hu JCC, Boynton JR, Holland GR. Clinical evidence for regenerative endodontic procedures: immediate versus delayed induction? J Endod. 2017;43:S75–81.
8. Lin J, Zeng Q, Wei X, Zhao W, Cui M, Gu J, Lu J, Yang M, Ling J. Regenerative endodontics versus apexification in immature permanent teeth with apical periodontitis: a prospective randomized controlled study. J Endod. 2017;43:1821–7.
9. Arslan H, Ahmed HMA, Şahin Y, Doğanay Yıldız E, Gündoğdu EC, Güven Y, Khalilov R. Regenerative endodontic procedures in necrotic mature teeth with periapical radiolucencies: a preliminary randomized clinical study. J Endod. 2019;45:863–72.
10. Jiang X, Liu H, Peng C. Clinical and radiographic assessment of the efficacy of a collagen membrane in regenerative endodontics: a randomized, controlled clinical trial. J Endod. 2017;43:1465–71.

11. Santos LGPD, Chisini LA, Springmann CG, Souza BDM, Pappen FG, Demarco FF, Felippe MCS, Felippe WT. Alternative to avoid tooth discoloration after regenerative endodontic procedure: a systematic review. Braz Dent J. 2018;29:409–18.
12. Tong HJ, Rajan S, Bhujel N, Kang J, Duggal M, Nazzal H. Regenerative endodontic therapy in the management of nonvital immature permanent teeth: a systematic review-outcome evaluation and meta-analysis. J Endod. 2017;43:1453–64.
13. Torabinejad M, Nosrat A, Verma P, Udochukwu O. Regenerative endodontic treatment or mineral trioxide aggregate apical plug in teeth with necrotic pulps and open apices: a systematic review and meta-analysis. J Endod. 2017;43:1806–20.
14. Duggal M, Tong HJ, Al-Ansary M, Twati W, Day PF, Nazzal H. Interventions for the endodontic management of non-vital traumatised immature permanent anterior teeth in children and adolescents: a systematic review of the evidence and guidelines of the European Academy of Paediatric Dentistry. Eur Arch Paediatr Dent. 2017;18:139–51.
15. Iwaya SI, Ikawa M, Kubota M. Revascularization of an immature permanent tooth with apical periodontitis and sinus tract. Dent Traumatol. 2001;17:185–7.
16. Banchs F, Trope M. Revascularization of immature permanent teeth with apical periodontitis: new treatment protocol? J Endod. 2004;30:196–200.
17. Wang X, Thibodeau B, Trope M, Lin LM, Huang GT. Histologic characterization of regenerated tissues in canal space after the revitalization/revascularization procedure of immature dog teeth with apical periodontitis. J Endod. 2010;36:56–63.
18. da Silva LA, Nelson-Filho P, da Silva RA, Flores DS, Heilborn C, Johnson JD, Cohenca N. Revascularization and periapical repair after endodontic treatment using apical negative pressure irrigation versus conventional irrigation plus triantibiotic intracanal dressing in dogs' teeth with apical periodontitis. Oral Surg Oral Med Oral Pathol Oral Radiol Endod. 2010;109:779–87.
19. Lin LM, Shimizu E, Gibbs JL, Loghin S, Ricucci D. Histologic and histobacteriologic observations of failed revascularization/revitalization therapy: a case report. J Endod. 2014;40:291–5.
20. Nikita B, Ruparel NB, Chrepa V, Gibbs J. Revascularization of immature necrotic teeth. Curr Oral Health Rep. 2017;4(4):319–29.
21. Andreasen JO, Bakland LK. Pulp regeneration after non-infected and infected necrosis, what type of tissue do we want? A review. Dent Traumatol. 2012;28(1):13–8.
22. Torabinejad M, Corr R, Buhrley M, Wright K, Shabahang S. An animal model to study regenerative endodontics. J Endod. 2011;37(2):197–202.
23. Dissanayaka WL, Zhu X, Zhang C, Jin L. Characterization of dental pulp stem cells isolated from canine premolars. J Endod. 2011;37(8):1074–80.
24. Yamauchi N, Nagaoka H, Yamauchi S, Teixeira FB, Miguez P, Yamauchi M. Immunohistological characterization of newly formed tissues after regenerative procedure in immature dog-teeth. J Endod. 2011;37(12):1636–41.
25. Shimizu E, Jong G, Partridge N, Rosenberg PA, Lin LM. Histologic observation of a human immature permanent tooth with irreversible pulpitis after revascularization/regeneration procedure. J Endod. 2012;38(9):1293–7.
26. Martin G, Ricucci D, Gibbs JL, Lin LM. Histological findings of revascularized/revitalized immature permanent molar with apical periodontitis using platelet-rich plasma. J Endod. 2013;39(1):138–44.
27. Nazzal H, Kenny K, Altimimi A, Kang J, Duggal MS. A prospective clinical study of regenerative endodontic treatment of traumatized immature teeth with necrotic pulps using bi-antibiotic paste. Int Endod J. 2018;51:e204–15.
28. Diogenes A, Henry MA, Teixeira FB, Hargreaves KM. An update on clinical regenerative endodontics. Endod Top. 2013;28:2–23.
29. Kim JH, Kim Y, Shin SJ, Park JW, Jung IY. Tooth discoloration of immature permanent incisor associated with triple antibiotic therapy: a case report. J Endod. 2010;36:1086–91.
30. Reynolds K, Johnson JD, Cohenca N. Pulp revascularization of necrotic bilateral bicuspids using a modified novel technique to eliminate potential coronal discolouration: a case report. Int Endod J. 2009;42:84–92.

31. Kirchhoff AL, Raldi DP, Salles AC, Cunha RS, Mello I. Tooth discolouration and internal bleaching after the use of triple antibiotic paste. Int Endod J. 2015;48:1181–7.
32. Shimizu E, Ricucci D, Albert J, Alobaid AS, Gibbs JL, Huang GT, Lin LM. Clinical, radiographic, and histological observation of a human immature permanent tooth with chronic apical abscess after revitalization treatment. J Endod. 2013;39:1078–83.
33. Chaniotis A. Treatment options for failing regenerative endodontic procedures: report of 3 cases. J Endod. 2017;43:1472–8.
34. Fouad AF. The microbial challenge to pulp regeneration. Adv Dent Res. 2011;23:285–9.
35. Nagata JY, Soares AJ, Souza-Filho FJ, Zaia AA, Ferraz CC, Almeida JF, Gomes BP. Microbial evaluation of traumatized teeth treated with triple antibiotic paste or calcium hydroxide with 2% chlorhexidine gel in pulp revascularization. J Endod. 2014;40:778–83.
36. Almutairi W, Yassen GH, Aminoshariae A, Williams KA, Mickel A. Regenerative endodontics: a systematic analysis of the failed cases. J Endod. 2019;45(5):567–77.
37. Verma P, Nosrat A, Kim JR, Price JB, Wang P, Bair E, Xu HH, Fouad AF. Effect of residual bacteria on the outcome of pulp regeneration in vivo. J Dent Res. 2017;96:100–6.
38. Martin DE, De Almeida JF, Henry MA, Khaing ZZ, Schmidt CE, Teixeira FB, Diogenes A. Concentration-dependent effect of sodium hypochlorite on stem cells of apical papilla survival and differentiation. J Endod. 2014;40:51–5.
39. Ruparel NB, Teixeira FB, Ferraz CC, Diogenes A. Direct effect of intracanal medicaments on survival of stem cells of the apical papilla. J Endod. 2012;38:1372–5.
40. Galler KM, Buchalla W, Hiller KA, Federlin M, Eidt A, Schiefersteiner M, Schmalz G. Influence of root canal disinfectants on growth factor release from dentin. J Endod. 2015;41:363–8.
41. Galler KM, Widbiller M, Buchalla W, Eidt A, Hiller KA, Hoffer PC, Schmalz G. EDTA conditioning of dentine promotes adhesion, migration and differentiation of dental pulp stem cells. Int Endod J. 2016;49:581–90.
42. Hoshino E, Kurihara-Ando N, Sato I, Uematsu H, Sato M, Kota K, Iwaku M. In-vitro antibacterial susceptibility of bacteria taken from infected root dentine to a mixture of ciprofloxacin, metronidazole and minocycline. Int Endod J. 1996;29:125–30.
43. Takushige T, Cruz EV, Asgor Moral A, Hoshino E. Endodontic treatment of primary teeth using a combination of antibacterial drugs. Int Endod J. 2004;37:132–8.
44. Thibodeau B, Trope M. Pulp revascularization of a necrotic infected immature permanent tooth: case report and review of the literature. Pediatr Dent. 2007;29:47–50.
45. Cehreli ZC, Isbitiren B, Sara S, Erbas G. Regenerative endodontic treatment (revascularization) of immature necrotic molars medicated with calcium hydroxide: a case series. J Endod. 2011;37:1327–30.
46. Chen MY, Chen KL, Chen CA, Tayebaty F, Rosenberg PA, Lin LM. Responses of immature permanent teeth with infected necrotic pulp tissue and apical periodontitis/abscess to revascularization procedures. Int Endod J. 2012;45:294–305.
47. Chugal N, Mallya SM, Kahler B, Lin LM. Endodontic treatment outcomes. Dent Clin N Am. 2017;61(1):59–80.
48. Cotti E, Mereu M, Lusso D. Regenerative treatment of an immature, traumatized tooth with apical periodontitis: report of a case. J Endod. 2008;34:611–6.
49. Kontakiotis EG, Filippatos CG, Tzanetakis GN, Agrafioti A. Regenerative endodontic therapy: a data analysis of clinical protocols. J Endod. 2015;41(2):146–54.
50. Kim Y, Kim S, Shin YS, Jung I-Y, Lee SJ. Failure of setting of mineral trioxide aggregate in the presence of fetal bovine serum and its prevention. J Endod. 2012;38(4):536–40.
51. Kang JS, Rhim EM, Huh SY, Ahn SJ, Kim DS, Kim SY, et al. The effects of humidity and serum on the surface microhardness and morphology of five retrograde filling material. Scanning. 2012;34(4):207–14.
52. Camilleri J. Mineral trioxide aggregate: present and future developments. Endod Topics. 2015;32(1):31–46.
53. Nekoofar MH, Oloomi K, Sheykhrezae MS, Tabor R, Stone DF, Dummer PMH. An evaluation of the effect of blood and human serum on the surface microhardness and surface microstructure of mineral trioxide aggregate. Int Endod J. 2010;43(10):849–58.

54. Nekoofar MH, Stone DF, Dummer PMH. The effect of blood contamination on the compressive strength and surface microstructure of mineral trioxide aggregate. Int Endod J. 2010;43(9):782–91.
55. Camilleri J. Color stability of white mineral trioxide aggregate in contact with hypochlorite solution. J Endod. 2014;40(3):436–40.
56. Marciano MA, Costa RM, Camilleri J, Mondelli RFL, Guimarães BM, Duarte MAH. Assessment of color stability of white mineral trioxide aggregate angelus and bismuth oxide in contact with tooth structure. J Endod. 2014;40(8):1235–40.
57. Vallés M, Mercadé M, Durán-Sindreu F, Bourdelande JL, Roig M. Color stability of white mineral trioxide aggregate. Clin Oral Investig. 2013;17(4):1155–9.
58. Guimarães BM, Tartari T, Marciano MA, Vivan RR, Mondeli RFL, Camilleri J, et al. Color stability, radiopacity, and chemical characteristics of white mineral trioxide aggregate associated with 2 different vehicles in contact with blood. J Endod. 2015;41(6):947–52.
59. Felman D, Parashos P. Coronal tooth discoloration and white mineral trioxide aggregate. J Endod. 2013;39(4):484–7.
60. Yoldaş SE, Bani M, Atabek D, Bodur H. Comparison of the potential discoloration effect of bioaggregate, Biodentine, and white mineral trioxide aggregate on bovine teeth: in vitro research. J Endod. 2016;42(12):1815–8.
61. Schembri Wismayer P, Lung CYK, Rappa F, Cappello F, Camilleri J. Assessment of the interaction of Portland cement-based materials with blood and tissue fluids using an animal model. Sci Rep. 2016;6(1):34547–9.
62. Keskin C, Demiryurek EO, Ozyurek T. Color stabilities of calcium silicate-based materials in contact with different irrigation solutions. J Endod. 2015;41(3):409–11.
63. Camilleri J. Staining potential of Neo MTA Plus, MTA Plus, and Biodentine used for pulpotomy procedures. J Endod. 2015;41(7):1139–45.
64. Torabinejad M, Parirokh M, Dummer PMH. Mineral trioxide aggregate and other bioactive endodontic cements: an updated overview—part II: other clinical applications and complications. Int Endod J. 2018;51(3):284–317.
65. Meschi N, Li X, Van Gorp G, Camilleri J, Van Meerbeek B, Lambrechts P. Bioactivity potential of Portland cement in regenerative endodontic procedures: from clinic to lab. Dent Mater. 2019;35(9):1342–50.
66. Cvek M. Prognosis of luxated non-vital maxillary incisors treated with calcium hydroxide and filled with gutta-percha. A retrospective clinical study. Endod Dent Traumatol. 1992;8(2):45–55.
67. Lovelace TW, Henry MA, Hargreaves KM, Diogenes A. Evaluation of the delivery of mesenchymal stem cells into the root canal space of necrotic immature teeth after clinical regenerative endodontic procedure. J Endod. 2011;37:133–8.
68. Sonoyama W, Liu Y, Yamaza T, Tuan RS, Wang S, Shi S, Huang GT. Characterization of the apical papilla and its residing stem cells from human immature permanent teeth: a pilot study. J Endod. 2008;34:166–71.
69. Diogenes A, Ruparel NB, Shiloah Y, Hargreaves KM. Regenerative endodontics: a way forward. J Am Dent Assoc. 2016;147:372–80.
70. Nagas E, Uyanik MO, Cehreli ZC. Revitalization of necrotic mature permanent incisors with apical periodontitis: a case report. Restor Dent Endod. 2018;43:e31.
71. Saoud TM, Martin G, Chen YH, Chen KL, Chen CA, Songtrakul K, Malek M, Sigurdsson A, Lin LM. Treatment of mature permanent teeth with necrotic pulps and apical periodontitis using regenerative endodontic procedures: a case series. J Endod. 2016;42:57–65.
72. Paryani K, Kim SG. Regenerative endodontic treatment of permanent teeth after completion of root development: a report of 2 cases. J Endod. 2013;39:929–34.
73. Xuan K, Li B, Guo H, Sun W, Kou X, He X, Zhang Y, Sun J, Liu A, Liao L, Liu S, Liu W, Hu C, Shi S, Jin Y. Deciduous autologous tooth stem cells regenerate dental pulp after implantation into injured teeth. Sci Transl Med. 2018;10:455.

74. Nakashima M, Iohara K, Murakami M, Nakamura H, Sato Y, Ariji Y, Matsushita K. Pulp regeneration by transplantation of dental pulp stem cells in pulpitis: a pilot clinical study. Stem Cell Res Ther. 2017;8(1):61.
75. Brizuela C, Meza G, Urrejola D, Quezada MA, Concha G, Ramírez V, Angelopoulos I, Cadiz MI, Tapia-Limonchi R, Khoury M. Cell-based regenerative endodontics for treatment of peri-apical lesions: a randomized, controlled phase I/II clinical trial. J Dent Res. 2020;99(5):523–9.
76. Galler KM, Widbiller M. Perspectives for cell-homing approaches to engineer dental pulp. J Endod. 2017;43:S40–5.
77. Widbiller M, Schweikl H, Bruckmann A, Rosendahl A, Hochmuth E, Lindner SR, Buchalla W, Galler KM. Shotgun proteomics of human dentin with different prefractionation methods. Sci Rep. 2019;9:4457.